Risk Prediction and New Prophylaxis Strategies for Thromboembolism in Cancer

Risk Prediction and New Prophylaxis Strategies for Thromboembolism in Cancer

Editors

Patrizia Ferroni
Mario Roselli
Fiorella Guadagni

MDPI • Basel • Beijing • Wuhan • Barcelona • Belgrade • Manchester • Tokyo • Cluj • Tianjin

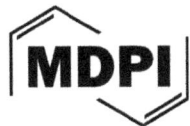

Editors
Patrizia Ferroni
San Raffaele Roma Open
University
Italy

Mario Roselli
University of Rome Tor
Vergata
Italy

Fiorella Guadagni
San Raffaele Roma Open
University
Italy

Editorial Office
MDPI
St. Alban-Anlage 66
4052 Basel, Switzerland

This is a reprint of articles from the Special Issue published online in the open access journal *Cancers* (ISSN 2072-6694) (available at: https://www.mdpi.com/journal/cancers/special_issues/Throm_Cancer).

For citation purposes, cite each article independently as indicated on the article page online and as indicated below:

LastName, A.A.; LastName, B.B.; LastName, C.C. Article Title. *Journal Name* **Year**, *Volume Number*, Page Range.

ISBN 978-3-0365-4707-7 (Hbk)
ISBN 978-3-0365-4708-4 (PDF)

© 2022 by the authors. Articles in this book are Open Access and distributed under the Creative Commons Attribution (CC BY) license, which allows users to download, copy and build upon published articles, as long as the author and publisher are properly credited, which ensures maximum dissemination and a wider impact of our publications.

The book as a whole is distributed by MDPI under the terms and conditions of the Creative Commons license CC BY-NC-ND.

Contents

About the Editors vii

Patrizia Ferroni, Fiorella Guadagni and Mario Roselli
Risk Prediction and New Prophylaxis Strategies for Thromboembolism in Cancer
Reprinted from: *Cancers* 2021, 13, 1556, doi:10.3390/cancers13071556 1

Nicola J. Nasser, Jana Fox and Abed Agbarya
Potential Mechanisms of Cancer-Related Hypercoagulability
Reprinted from: *Cancers* 2020, 12, 566, doi:10.3390/cancers12030566 7

Orly Leiva, Jean M. Connors and Hanny Al-Samkari
Impact of Tumor Genomic Mutations on Thrombotic Risk in Cancer Patients
Reprinted from: *Cancers* 2020, 12, 1958, doi:10.3390/cancers12071958 19

**Laura Pizzuti, Eriseld Krasniqi, Chiara Mandoj, Daniele Marinelli, Domenico Sergi,
Elisabetta Capomolla, Giancarlo Paoletti, Claudio Botti, Ramy Kayal,
Francesca Romana Ferranti, Isabella Sperduti, Letizia Perracchio,
Giuseppe Sanguineti, Paolo Marchetti, Gennaro Ciliberto, Giacomo Barchiesi,
Marco Mazzotta, Maddalena Barba, Laura Conti and Patrizia Vici**
Observational Multicenter Study on the Prognostic Relevance of Coagulation Activation in Risk
Assessment and Stratification in Locally Advanced Breast Cancer. Outline of the ARIAS Trial
Reprinted from: *Cancers* 2020, 12, 849, doi:10.3390/cancers12040849 33

Frits I. Mulder, Floris T. M. Bosch and Nick van Es
Primary Thromboprophylaxis in Ambulatory Cancer Patients: Where Do We Stand?
Reprinted from: *Cancers* 2020, 12, 367, doi:10.3390/cancers12020367 41

**Alice Labianca, Tommaso Bosetti, Alice Indini, Giorgia Negrini and
Roberto Francesco Labianca**
Risk Prediction and New Prophylaxis Strategies for Thromboembolism in Cancer
Reprinted from: *Cancers* 2020, 12, 2070, doi:10.3390/cancers12082070 59

Anne Rossel, Helia Robert-Ebadi and Christophe Marti
Preventing Venous Thromboembolism in Ambulatory Patients with Cancer: A
Narrative Review
Reprinted from: *Cancers* 2020, 12, 612, doi:10.3390/cancers12030612 75

**Marek Z. Wojtukiewicz, Piotr Skalij, Piotr Tokajuk, Barbara Politynska,
Anna M. Wojtukiewicz, Stephanie C. Tucker and Kenneth V. Honn**
Direct Oral Anticoagulants in Cancer Patients. Time for a Change in Paradigm
Reprinted from: *Cancers* 2020, 12, 1144, doi:10.3390/cancers12051144 89

**Dominique Farge, Barbara Bournet, Thierry Conroy, Eric Vicaut, Janusz Rak,
George Zogoulous, Jefferey Barkun, Mehdi Ouaissi, Louis Buscail and Corinne Frere**
Primary Thromboprophylaxis in Pancreatic Cancer Patients: Why Clinical Practice Guidelines
Should Be Implemented
Reprinted from: *Cancers* 2020, 12, 618, doi:10.3390/cancers12030618 105

Despina Fotiou, Maria Gavriatopoulou and Evangelos Terpos
Multiple Myeloma and Thrombosis: Prophylaxis and Risk Prediction Tools
Reprinted from: *Cancers* 2020, 12, 191, doi:10.3390/cancers12010191 129

Stefan Hohaus, Francesca Bartolomei, Annarosa Cuccaro, Elena Maiolo, Eleonora Alma, Francesco D'Alò, Silvia Bellesi, Elena Rossi and Valerio De Stefano
Venous Thromboembolism in Lymphoma: Risk Stratification and Antithrombotic Prophylaxis
Reprinted from: *Cancers* **2020**, *12*, 1291, doi:10.3390/cancers12051291 . . . . **147**

Silvia Riondino, Patrizia Ferroni, Girolamo Del Monte, Vincenzo Formica, Fiorella Guadagni and Mario Roselli
Venous Thromboembolism in Cancer Patients on Simultaneous and Palliative Care
Reprinted from: *Cancers* **2020**, *12*, 1167, doi:10.3390/cancers12051167 . . . . **165**

Ewa Zabrocka and Ewa Sierko
Thromboprophylaxis in the End-of-Life Cancer Care: The Update
Reprinted from: *Cancers* **2020**, *12*, 600, doi:10.3390/cancers12030600 . . . . **183**

About the Editors

Patrizia Ferroni

Patrizia Ferroni is a Full Professor of Clinical Biochemistry and Molecular Biology at the Department of Human Sciences and Quality of Life Promotion of the San Raffaele Roma Open University, Italy. Dr. Ferroni also serves as a senior researcher at the Laboratory of Biomarker Discovery and Advanced Technologies and the InterInstitutional Multidisciplinary Biobank of the IRCCS San Raffaele Rome, a cutting-edge facility for translational research in the medical area. Prof. Ferroni holds an MD Degree from the Sapienza University of Rome (with Honors, 1985), a Residency in Oncology (1988) and a PhD in Experimental Medicine for the development of immunoassays for the detection of cancer biomarkers in tissues, plasma and other body fluids performed as a part of her postdoctoral experience at the Laboratory of Tumor Immunology and Biology, National Cancer Institute, N.I.H., Bethesda, MD, USA. She is currently co-coordinator of the REVERT (taRgeted thErapy for adVanced colorEctal canceR paTients) project GA number 848098 (H2020-SC1- 2019-Two-Stage-RTD—Topic: SC1-BHC-02-2019—Systems approaches for the discovery of combinatorial therapies for complex disorders). Prof. Ferroni has international, long-lasting experience in the field of translational research on the characterization of possible biomarkers to be used in prognostic assessment, or response to treatment and/or drug toxicity. On-going studies in which she is currently involved are focused on translational research and biospecimen sciences. Her major scientific interest is in thrombosis issues both in cardiovascular diseases and in solid cancer, with special reference to new diagnostic/prophylactic strategies for venous thromboembolism and the use and construction of innovative informatics platforms to improve health care organization and efficiency. All these studies have led to the publication of more than 200 articles in international peer-reviewed journals with an H-index of 40.

Mario Roselli

Mario Roselli, Specialist in Oncology (1986) and in Nuclear Medicine (1992), is currently Head of Medical Oncology of the University Hospital Tor Vergata; Full Professor in Medical Oncology at the Department of Systems Medicine, School of Medicine University of Rome "Tor Vergata", Italy; and Head of the Post-graduate School in Medical Oncology of the same University. He is presently member of the Tor Vergata Institutional Review Board (IRB) and participates as Principal Investigator (PI) or co-investigator of several clinical projects, sponsored and granted either by Government Institutions or private companies. Among the funded projects of which Prof. Roselli has been PI, the "MCC—Medical Care Continuity" sponsored by the European Community (2004–2008), in collaboration with the San Raffaele Palliative Care Centers, has been rewarded from 2012 on with the certificate award for "designated centers of integrated oncology and palliative care by the European Society for Medical Oncology" (www.esmo.org). More recently, he is the Clinical Coordinator of European Community-sponsored (Horizon 2020) trial "REVERT – taRgeted thErapy for adVanced colorEctal canceR paTients". As part of an active collaboration with the Laboratory of Tumor Immunology and Biology of the National Cancer Institute, National Institutes of Health, Bethesda, MD, USA, Prof. Roselli has been involved in the investigation of novel strategies for cancer vaccines. Prof. Roselli is member of several national (such as the Italian Society of Immunopharmacology, the Italian Society of Medical Oncology (AIOM), and the Italian Society of Toracic Oncology (AIOT)) and international scientific societies (the European Association for Cancer Research (EACR), the European Society of Medical Oncology (ESMO) and the American Society of Clinical Oncology

(ASCO)). He is also member of the Editorial Boards of several peer-reviewed scientific journals. Prof. Roselli's major scientific interest is focused on translational and clinical research in oncology, which has led to the publication of 235 articles in international peer-reviewed journals with an H-index of 43.

Fiorella Guadagni

Fiorella Guadagni is a Full Professor in Clinical Biochemistry and Molecular Biology at the San Raffaele Roma Open University and the Scientific Coordinator of the InterInstitutional Multidisciplinary Biobank (BioBIM) of the IRCCS San Raffaele Roma, Italy. Prof. Guadagni holds an MD Degree from the University of Perugia (with Honors, 1983), a Residency in Oncology (1988) and in Clinical Pathology (1996) and a PhD in Medical Biotechnologies (2009). In view of her expertise, she is presently a Consultant for the Laboratory of Tumor Immunology and Biology (LTIB), National Cancer Institute (NCI), NIH, Bethesda, MD, USA. As part of this active collaboration, Prof. Guadagni is involved in the investigation of novel strategies for cancer vaccines. She has been an expert evaluator and monitor of the "Fifth Framework Programme—Quality of Life and Management of Living Resources", Key Action 7 (Chronic and degenerative diseases/cancer) and Key Action 2 (Control of infectious diseases). She is also an expert reviewer of several international institutions: the Health Research Board (HRB), Ireland, for the Grant E-Management System (GEMS); the German Federal Ministry of Education and Research (BMBF) for the call 'Methods and Tools for Individualized Medicine' and for the call 'Enabling German Biobank Sites to Connect to BBMRI'; and the NCSTE—National Centre of Science and Technology Evaluation, Ministry of Education and Science, Republic of Kazakhstan. Prof. Guadagni has been the scientific coordinator of several national and international projects funded by governmental funds; in particular, she is the project coordinator of the REVERT (taRgeted thErapy for adVanced colorEctal canceR paTients) GA number 848098 (H2020-SC1- 2019-Two-Stage-RTD—Topic: SC1-BHC-02-2019—Systems approaches for the discovery of combinatorial therapies for complex disorders). Prof. Guadagni's major scientific interest is focused on translational research, which has led to the publication of roughly 250 articles in international peer-reviewed journals with a personal IF greater than 1000 and an H-Index of 42.

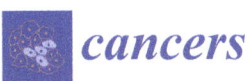

Editorial

Risk Prediction and New Prophylaxis Strategies for Thromboembolism in Cancer

Patrizia Ferroni [1,2,*], Fiorella Guadagni [1,2] and Mario Roselli [3]

1. Department of Human Sciences and Quality of Life Promotion, San Raffaele Roma Open University, 00166 Rome, Italy; fiorella.guadagni@sanraffaele.it
2. InterInstitutional Multidisciplinary Biobank (BioBIM), IRCCS San Raffaele Roma, 00166 Rome, Italy
3. Department of Systems Medicine, Medical Oncology, University of Rome "Tor Vergata", 00133 Rome, Italy; mario.roselli@uniroma2.it
* Correspondence: patrizia.ferroni@sanraffaele.it

Citation: Ferroni, P.; Guadagni, F.; Roselli, M. Risk Prediction and New Prophylaxis Strategies for Thromboembolism in Cancer. *Cancers* **2021**, *13*, 1556. https://doi.org/10.3390/cancers13071556

Received: 24 March 2021
Accepted: 25 March 2021
Published: 29 March 2021

Publisher's Note: MDPI stays neutral with regard to jurisdictional claims in published maps and institutional affiliations.

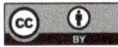

Copyright: © 2021 by the authors. Licensee MDPI, Basel, Switzerland. This article is an open access article distributed under the terms and conditions of the Creative Commons Attribution (CC BY) license (https://creativecommons.org/licenses/by/4.0/).

Venous thromboembolism (VTE) is a compelling challenge across all phases of cancer care as it may result in treatment delays, impaired quality of life (QoL), and increased mortality [1]. This Special Issue of *Cancers* contains a series of articles presented by international leaders, focusing on the current clinical evidence supporting the standard of care and emerging therapeutic/prophylactic options for cancer-associated VTE during both active treatment and simultaneous/palliative care. Tailored approaches based on the use of individualized factors to stratify the thrombotic/bleeding risk in each individual patient are also discussed.

The increased risk of VTE in cancer is typically related to patient [2,3], tumor [2,4], and/or treatment [5–9], which may all cause a disruption of each component of Virchow's triad, altering the haemostatic mechanisms that balance thrombosis and clot lysis and, thus, increasing hypercoagulability. Here, Nasser and colleagues propose an interesting stratification of cancer-related hypercoagulability into two main types: Type I hypercoagulability (resulting from the degradation of endogenous heparin by tumor-secreted heparanase) and Type II hypercoagulability (including all the other etiologies) [10]. Heparanase, indeed, is capable of degrading heparin and low-molecular-weight heparin (LMWH), possibly resulting in neutralization of the anticoagulant properties of these molecules [9]. Interestingly, heparanase was found to be highly expressed in pancreatic, gastric, and lung cancers, which are all correlated with a higher risk of thrombosis compared to other tumor types [10]. Accordingly, Nasser et al. speculate that developing alternative non-invasive methods to deliver heparin—or to mobilize endogenous heparin from its reservoirs (i.e., platelets)—could make this medication more appealing to treat cancer-associated thrombosis [10].

Other tumor-related factors can concur to represent additional triggers of VTE in cancer patients. In this context, the advent of tumor genomic profiling has strongly contributed not only to a deeper comprehension of cancer biology, but also to the discovery of potential VTE risk genomic factors. The subject is addressed in the review by Leiva and colleagues discussing the potential mechanisms by which the tumor mutational status may influence thrombogenesis [11]. Molecular aberrations involving various targetable driver mutations may, in fact, impact thrombotic risk in many tumor types, possibly through a disregulation of tumor tissue factor (TF) expression. This is the case of mutated *KRAS* in colorectal and lung cancer and *IDH1* in brain cancer patients, the former being positively associated with TF upregulation, the latter being associated with hypermethylation of the F3 promoter of the TF gene leading to decreased TF expression and a decreased risk of VTE [11]. Other tumor mutations that have been involved in the prothrombotic state in carcinoma patients include *ALK*, *ROS1*, and *JAK2*, all participating in downstream signaling of inflammatory cytokines [11], while the burden of breast cancer mutational events, using a next-generation sequencing approach, is currently the focus of an ongoing trial [12]. Knowledge that a patient may be at an increased thrombotic risk due to the underlying tumor genotype is another piece of information that the treating clinician can consider when determining VTE risk stratification and may prove to be a significant advancement in the prevention of cancer-associated thrombosis [11].

While many factors contribute to increase the individual thrombotic risk, some co-morbidities and/or chemotherapy-related side effects, such as renal or hepatic insufficiency and thrombocytopenia, can affect the efficacy and safety of anticoagulation, emphasizing the need for a careful evaluation of the risk/benefit assessment of anticoagulant prophylaxis. Hence, the availability of tailored approaches—based on the use of individualized factors to stratify the thrombotic/bleeding risk in each individual patient—undoubtedly represents a significant advance in the prevention of cancer-associated VTE. Several clinical decision models have been developed to guide the oncologist in thromboembolic risk assessment and targeted prophylaxis. The article by Mulder et al. addresses some of the controversies stemming from the translation of the guideline recommendations into clinical practice, discussing the performance of available risk assessment scores, and summarizing the findings of recent trials [13]. From their analysis (performed in light of the most recent prophylactic options), it emerges that the development of an efficient pan-cancer VTE prediction score—as those currently available—is probably not feasible, given the large heterogeneity in tumor biology, cancer treatment, and thromboembolic risk across cancer types [13]. In the authors' opinion, with which we agree, prediction scores should possibly be developed for specific cancer types to help effectively individualize strategies for primary thromboprophylaxis in cancer patients.

The state-of-the-art current guidelines on thromboprophylaxis in cancer patients is addressed in the reviews by Labianca et al. [14] and Rossel et al. [15], summarizing the latest evidence on VTE prophylaxis and treatment in patients with cancer. From their analyses, it emerges that the use of VTE prophylaxis is currently recommended in cancer patients following surgery, or if admitted to hospital for an acute medical condition, but large-scale thromboprophylaxis prescription in ambulatory cancer patients is not advised. Based on the latest recommendations, prophylaxis should always be practiced in high-risk patients with multiple myeloma and in therapy with lenalidomide or thalidomide, unless there are specific clinical contraindications. On the other hand, primary prophylaxis is recommended in outpatients receiving systemic anticancer therapy at an intermediate-to high-risk of VTE—identified by cancer type (i.e., pancreatic) or by a validated risk assessment model (i.e., a Khorana score ≥ 2)—and not at a high risk of bleeding. Thus, patient selection remains the main challenge and improvement of existing VTE risk models, or construction of alternative risk assessment models are needed in order to ameliorate the risk stratification of cancer patients [14,15].

One of the most important novel developments that can be found in the latest recommendations by expert societies is the endorsement of the use of edoxaban and rivaroxaban for VTE treatment/prophylaxis in cancer patients [14,15]. Direct oral anticoagulants (DOACs) represent an interesting option because of their oral administration and lower costs compared to low-molecular-weight heparin (LMWH). Large scale thromboprophylaxis prescription in ambulatory cancer patients is still not advised. However, based on evidence from the AVERT and CASSINI trials, it is now recommended that patients with cancers at very high VTE risk (e.g., pancreas) may be offered thromboprophylaxis with DOACs, whereas caution is needed in patients with GI and genitourinary cancers.

The use of DOACs in VTE treatment and primary prevention in cancer patients is the focus of the review by Wojtukiewicz and coworkers [16]. LMWH has been the recognized standard drug for more than a decade, until recent published results of large randomized clinical trials have confirmed that DOACs may represent a reasonable alternative to LMWH in cancer patients—both in terms of efficacy and safety—and a valuable step forward in the treatment and prevention of cancer-related thrombosis [16]. As stated above, DOACs are an alternative to LMWH in the recommendations of expert societies [14–16] both in the treatment of cancer-associated thrombosis and in VTE primary prevention in high-risk patients [15,16]. Limitations of DOACs are also discussed, including the increased risk of major bleeding, interaction with other drugs, unknown or inappropriate pharmacokinetics in patients with large deviations from normal body weight and in patients with impaired renal function, corroborating the need for careful patient selection [16].

Our digression on the topic of VTE risk stratification and antithrombotic prophylaxis continues with some examples focusing on some high-risk tumor types. The first of these reviews is that by Farge and colleagues [17] who address the issue of clinical practice guidelines on primary thromboprophylaxis in pancreatic cancer (PC) patients [17]. PC is a malignancy with the highest mortality rate of any solid cancer and with the highest rate of VTE. In their article, Farge et al. interestingly point out that despite the fact that Grade 1B evidence has been long since available and thromboprophylaxis is generally recommended in clinical practice guidelines, this remains largely underused in PC patients [17]. Clinical tools could be used to assist clinicians in optimizing treatment in daily clinical practice. However, in the Khorana score, all PC patients have a sum score ≥ 2 and should, therefore, be considered for prophylaxis. Other models, including those reviewed by Mulder et al. [13], have not been externally validated in ambulatory PC patients. The authors conclude that, in the absence of clear evidence to favor either LMWH or DOACs, a "discussion with the patient about the relative benefits and risks, drug cost, duration and tolerance of prophylaxis is warranted before prescribing thromboprophylaxis in PC ambulatory patients" [17].

Fotiou et al. [18] and Hohaus et al. [19] further address the issue of VTE risk stratification and thromboprophylaxis in hematological malignancies. The first article is focused on the need for the development of more accurate risk assessment tools and measures of thrombosis prevention in multiple myeloma (MM) patients [18]. As argued by Fotiou and colleagues, optimum risk stratification and effective thromboprophylaxis can only be achieved through the development of an MM-specific risk score that can successfully capture all aspects of the heterogeneous prothrombotic environment that exists in MM patients to accurately stratify VTE risk and guide thromboprophylaxis [18]. As proposed by the authors, a risk assessment tool including clinical- and treatment-specific risk factors in combination with disease-specific coagulation biomarkers could allow the successful use of the right agent for the right patient and for the sufficient amount of time. An ideal/future algorithm for VTE risk prediction—based on the IMPEDE risk score—using information from current expert society guidelines, data from randomized controlled trials, emerging data on DOACs, retrospective MM VTE risk prediction clinical scores, and clinical experience is also proposed [18]. Similar considerations are raised by Hohaus and co-workers, who review the epidemiology of VTE, its prevalence, and tumor-related factors in lymphoma patients [19]. In agreement with the opinion by Mulder et al. [13], the authors suggest that the pan-cancer Khorana score (developed for patients with solid tumors) is not fitted to capture the disease-specific characteristics associated with VTE risk in lymphoma [19]. Given the absence of a validated risk score, no evidence-based recommendation for VTE prophylaxis in ambulatory patients undergoing anti-neoplastic treatment can be given at present and individual evaluation of the risk–benefit ratio is the current strategy [19].

Finally, Riondino et al. [20] and Zabrocka et al. [21] address the issue of venous thromboembolism in particular settings of cancer care: the transition from active to palliative care, and end-of-life care, respectively. Based on the most recent NICE (National Institute for Health and Care Excellence) guidelines, thromboprophylaxis should be considered for patients receiving palliative care, always taking into account several factors, including risk of bleeding, estimated life expectancy, and the views of the patient and their caregivers. Additionally, VTE prophylaxis should be reviewed daily and should not be offered in the last days of life. Other factors to be considered include the lack of palliative benefits or any unreasonable burden of thromboprophylaxis (e.g., painful injections or frequent monitoring with phlebotomy). Nonetheless, from the analysis by Riondino and colleagues, it emerges that the prevalence of VTE among palliative care unit patients is significant (35 to 50%), and its occurrence is perceived as a physically and emotionally distressing phenomenon that overlaps with the underlying malignancy and strongly decreases QoL [20]. In end-of-life care, where the assurance of the best possible QoL should be the highest priority, VTE prophylaxis may eliminate the symptom burden and psychological distress related to thrombosis [21]. In light of the above, Riondino et al. emphasize that an early integration of VTE preventive strategies in a "simultaneous care program" might help overcoming the problem of deciding in favor or against thromboprophylaxis in the context of palliation [20]. However, specific decision-making tools are needed to avoid under-treatment, and since the continuum of care paradigm is in constant change, a major effort should be made in this area to achieve a broad consensus on how to manage VTE [20].

From the aforementioned data, it emerges that a large series of experimental and clinical data has given a tremendous impulse to disentangle the issue of VTE risk assessment in cancer, tracing new horizons for thromboprophylaxis in selected at-risk patients. A common need for new tools clearly emerges. As a consequence, clinical decision-making is rapidly moving from empiricism to customized healthcare and tailored therapy. Adjunctive clinical risk factors, biomolecular markers, and dynamic risk assessment could all ameliorate VTE prediction, while the introduction of novel computational analyses could help with gaining knowledge from available datasets to obtain accurate and precise personalized risk estimates.

Funding: This work has been partially supported by the European Social Fund, under the Italian Ministry of Economic Development—NET4HEALTH ("HORIZON 2020" PON I&C 2014-2020—F/050383/01-03/X32).

Conflicts of Interest: The authors declare no conflict of interest.

References

1. Leiva, O.; Newcomb, R.; Connors, J.M.; Al-Samkari, H. Cancer and thrombosis: New insights to an old problem. *J. Med. Vasc.* **2020**, *45*, 6S8–6S16. [PubMed]
2. Khorana, A.A.; Dalal, M.; Lin, J.; Connolly, G.C. Incidence and predictors of venous thromboembolism (VTE) among ambulatory high-risk cancer patients undergoing chemotherapy in the United States. *Cancer* **2013**, *119*, 648–655. [CrossRef] [PubMed]
3. Vergati, M.; Della-Morte, D.; Ferroni, P.; Cereda, V.; Tosetto, L.; La Farina, F.; Guadagni, F.; Roselli, M. Increased risk of chemotherapy-associated venous thromboembolism in elderly patients with cancer. *Rejuvenation Res.* **2013**, *16*, 224–231. [CrossRef] [PubMed]
4. Dickmann, B.; Ahlbrecht, J.; Ay, C.; Dunkler, D.; Thaler, J.; Scheithauer, W.; Quehenberger, P.; Zielinski, C.; Pabinger, I. Regional lymph node metastases are a strong risk factor for venous thromboembolism: Results from the Vienna Cancer and Thrombosis Study. *Haematologica* **2013**, *98*, 1309–1314. [CrossRef] [PubMed]
5. Di Nisio, M.; Ferrante, N.; De Tursi, M.; Iacobelli, S.; Cuccurullo, F.; Büller, H.R.; Feragalli, B.; Porreca, E. Incidental venous thromboembolism in ambulatory cancer patients receiving chemotherapy. *Thromb. Haemost.* **2010**, *104*, 1049–1054. [PubMed]
6. Roselli, M.; Ferroni, P.; Riondino, S.; Mariotti, S.; Laudisi, A.; Vergati, M.; Cavaliere, F.; Palmirotta, R.; Guadagni, F. Impact of chemotherapy on activated protein C-dependent thrombin generation—Association with VTE occurrence. *Int. J. Cancer* **2013**, *133*, 1253–1258. [CrossRef] [PubMed]
7. Ferroni, P.; Formica, V.; Roselli, M.; Guadagni, F. Thromboembolic events in patients treated with anti-angiogenic drugs. *Curr. Vasc. Pharmacol.* **2010**, *8*, 102–113. [CrossRef] [PubMed]
8. Bohlius, J.; Wilson, J.; Seidenfeld, J.; Piper, M.; Schwarzer, G.; Sandercock, J.; Trelle, S.; Weingart, O.; Bayliss, S.; Brunskill, S. Erythropoietin or darbepoetin for patients with cancer. *Cochrane Database Syst. Rev.* **2006**, *3*, CD003407.
9. Johannesdottir, S.A.; Horváth-Puhó, E.; Dekkers, O.M.; Cannegieter, S.C.; Jørgensen, J.O.; Ehrenstein, V.; Vandenbroucke, J.P.; Pedersen, L.; Sørensen, H.T. Use of glucocorticoids and risk of venous thromboembolism: A nationwide population-based case-control study. *JAMA Intern. Med.* **2013**, *173*, 743–752. [CrossRef] [PubMed]
10. Nasser, N.; Fox, J.; Agbarya, A. Potential Mechanisms of Cancer-Related Hypercoagulability. *Cancers* **2020**, *12*, 566. [CrossRef]
11. Leiva, O.; Connors, J.; Al-Samkari, H. Impact of Tumor Genomic Mutations on Thrombotic Risk in Cancer Patients. *Cancers* **2020**, *12*, 1958. [CrossRef] [PubMed]
12. Pizzuti, L.; Krasniqi, E.; Mandoj, C.; Marinelli, D.; Sergi, D.; Capomolla, E.; Paoletti, G.; Botti, C.; Kayal, R.; Ferranti, F.; et al. Observational Multicenter Study on the Prognostic Relevance of Coagulation Activation in Risk Assessment and Stratification in Locally Advanced Breast Cancer. Outline of the ARIAS Trial. *Cancers* **2020**, *12*, 849. [CrossRef] [PubMed]
13. Mulder, F.; Bosch, F.; van Es, N. Primary Thromboprophylaxis in Ambulatory Cancer Patients: Where Do We Stand? *Cancers* **2020**, *12*, 367. [CrossRef]
14. Labianca, A.; Bosetti, T.; Indini, A.; Negrini, G.; Labianca, R. Risk Prediction and New Prophylaxis Strategies for Thromboembolism in Cancer. *Cancers* **2020**, *12*, 2070. [CrossRef] [PubMed]

15. Rossel, A.; Robert-Ebadi, H.; Marti, C. Preventing Venous Thromboembolism in Ambulatory Patients with Cancer: A Narrative Review. *Cancers* **2020**, *12*, 612. [CrossRef] [PubMed]
16. Wojtukiewicz, M.; Skalij, P.; Tokajuk, P.; Politynska, B.; Wojtukiewicz, A.; Tucker, S.; Honn, K. Direct Oral Anticoagulants in Cancer Patients. Time for a Change in Paradigm. *Cancers* **2020**, *12*, 1144. [CrossRef]
17. Farge, D.; Bournet, B.; Conroy, T.; Vicaut, E.; Rak, J.; Zogoulous, G.; Barkun, J.; Ouaissi, M.; Buscail, L.; Frere, C. Primary Thromboprophylaxis in Pancreatic Cancer Patients: Why Clinical Practice Guidelines Should Be Implemented. *Cancers* **2020**, *12*, 618. [CrossRef] [PubMed]
18. Fotiou, D.; Gavriatopoulou, M.; Terpos, E. Multiple Myeloma and Thrombosis: Prophylaxis and Risk Prediction Tools. *Cancers* **2020**, *12*, 191. [CrossRef]
19. Hohaus, S.; Bartolomei, F.; Cuccaro, A.; Maiolo, E.; Alma, E.; D'Alò, F.; Bellesi, S.; Rossi, E.; Stefano, V. Venous Thromboembolism in Lymphoma: Risk Stratification and Antithrombotic Prophylaxis. *Cancers* **2020**, *12*, 1291. [CrossRef]
20. Riondino, S.; Ferroni, P.; Del Monte, G.; Formica, V.; Guadagni, F.; Roselli, M. Venous Thromboembolism in Cancer Patients on Simultaneous and Palliative Care. *Cancers* **2020**, *12*, 1167. [CrossRef]
21. Zabrocka, E.; Sierko, E. Thromboprophylaxis in the End-of-Life Cancer Care: The Update. *Cancers* **2020**, *12*, 600. [CrossRef] [PubMed]

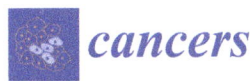

Review

Potential Mechanisms of Cancer-Related Hypercoagulability

Nicola J. Nasser [1,*], Jana Fox [1] and Abed Agbarya [2]

[1] Department of Radiation Oncology, Montefiore Medical Center, Albert Einstein College of Medicine, Bronx, New York, NY 10467, USA; jfox@montefiore.org
[2] Institute of Oncology, Bnai Zion Medical Center, Haifa 31048, Israel; abed.agbarya@b-zion.org.il
* Correspondence: Nicola.Nasser@gmail.com

Received: 3 February 2020; Accepted: 26 February 2020; Published: 29 February 2020

Abstract: The association between cancer and thrombosis has been known for over a century and a half. However, the mechanisms that underlie this correlation are not fully characterized. Hypercoagulability in cancer patients can be classified into two main categories: Type I and Type II. Type I occurs when the balance of endogenous heparin production and degradation is disturbed, with increased degradation of endogenous heparin by tumor-secreted heparanase. Type II hypercoagulability includes all the other etiologies, with factors related to the patient, the tumor, and/or the treatment. Patients with poor performance status are at higher risk of venous thromboembolism (VTE). Tumors can result in VTE through direct pressure on blood vessels, resulting in stasis. Several medications for cancer are correlated with a high risk of thrombosis. These include hormonal therapy (e.g., tamoxifen), chemotherapy (e.g., cisplatin, thalidomide and asparaginase), molecular targeted therapy (e.g., lenvatinib, osimertinib), and anti-angiogenesis monoclonal antibodies (e.g., bevacizumab and ramucirumab).

Keywords: cancer; thrombosis; endogenous heparin; heparanase; heparan sulfate

1. Introduction

Since Trousseau described the correlation between cancer and thrombosis in 1867 [1], there has been no consensus regarding the etiology connecting the two. Virchow's triad of factors that contribute to thrombosis includes hemodynamic changes, endothelial injury/dysfunction, and alterations in the constituents of the blood [2]. Stasis due to pressure of tumor on venous vessels results in alterations in blood flow and endothelial injury. Poor performance status of patients with cancer has been correlated with a higher risk of thrombosis (Figure 1). This may be due to stasis as well as an indication of the aggressive nature of the malignancy in these patients that results in degradation of their functional capabilities. Several systemic therapies of cancer are correlated with thrombosis, including venous thromboembolism (VTE) and arterial thrombosis. Surgical interventions are also known to be associated with an increased risk of VTE.

Procoagulant molecules secreted from tumor cells are the main cause of hypercoagulability in cancer patients. Heparanase is a mammalian endoglycosidase that degrades heparan sulfate (HS) at the cell surface and in the extracellular matrix. Heparanase is physiologically expressed in platelets and the placenta and is pathologically overexpressed in most malignant tumors. We have shown that heparanase is able to degrade heparin and low-molecular-weight heparin (LMWH) [3]. Transgenic mice overexpressing heparanase in all their tissues have shorter activated partial thromboplastin time (APTT) compared to control mice [3]. We found that a substantial proportion of cancer patients suffering from VTE and treated with standard LMWH doses had subtherapeutic anti-Xa activity [4]. Heparanase overexpression and secretion by cancer cells results in degradation of endogenous heparin and hypercoagulability. Heparanase was also found to induce tissue factor expression in vascular endothelial and cancer cells [5] and to induce dissociation of tissue factor pathway inhibitor from the vascular surface [6].

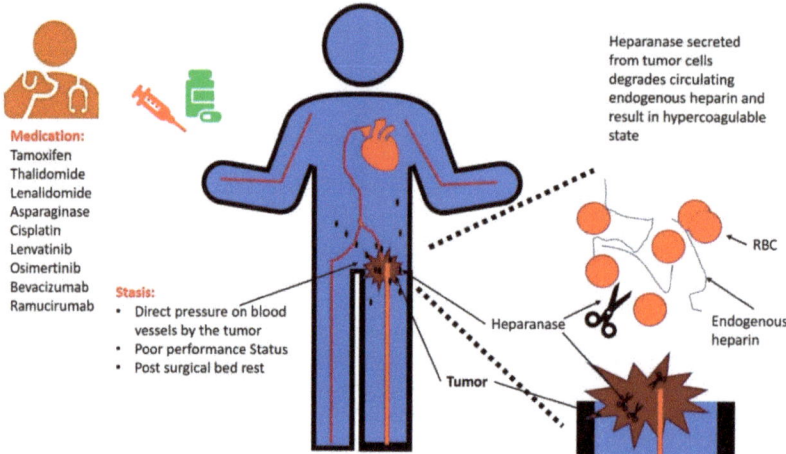

Figure 1. Cancer-associated thrombosis can result from: (1) stasis, i.e., direct pressure on blood vessels by the tumor mass, poor performance status, and bed rest following surgical procedures; (2) iatrogenic, due to treatment with antineoplastic medications; and (3) secretion of heparanase from malignant tumors that results in degradation of endogenous heparin.

We propose stratifying cancer-related hypercoagulability into two main types. Type I hypercoagulability results from the degradation of endogenous heparin by tumor-secreted heparanase. Type II hypercoagulability includes all the other etiologies, with factors related to the patient, the tumor, and/or the treatment. We will initially review the classical mechanism of cancer-associated thrombosis (type II), and then we will focus on the role of degradation of endogenous heparin by tumor-secreted heparanase (type I).

2. Stasis

Direct pressure on blood vessels by a tumor mass can lead to the narrowing of the vessels and subsequent stasis. This results in increased hemodynamic forces on endothelial cells and may induce endothelial dysfunction, thus contributing to the development of vascular pathologies that result in thrombosis [7]. Animal studies on dogs have shown that blood stasis due to an occluded segment of vena cava and/or aorta resulted in blood clot formation within just a few minutes [8,9].

Poor performance status is associated with an increased risk for hypercoagulability. White et al. found that one-third of patients with advanced cancer admitted to specialist palliative care units had a femoral deep vein thrombosis (DVT) [10]. Metcalf et al. [11] studied thrombosis risk in ovarian cancer patients. Patients with thrombosis were found to have a worse performance status, with Eastern Cooperative Oncology Group (ECOG) performance status ≥2 in 29.9% of these patients, compared to 9.5% in patients without thrombosis [11]. A prospective study performed bilateral venous Doppler sonography examination of the lower extremities for 44 nonambulatory cancer patients asymptomatic for lower extremity DVT [12]. Asymptomatic DVT was detected in 34% of the patients. DVT was found in 17.4% of patients with one metastatic site and in 52.3% of patients with two or more sites ($p < 0.01$) [12].

Surgical interventions increase the risk of DVT in general, and in patients with malignancies in particular. A high incidence of 26% DVT was found in the perioperative period of neurosurgical patients, with a preoperative diagnosis of DVT in 11% and postoperatively in 15% of the patients [13]. Chaichana et al. [14] reported the incidence of DVT and pulmonary embolism in adult patients undergoing craniotomy for brain tumors. Poor performance status was associated with thrombosis with an odds ratio of 1.04, p value < 0.0001 [14]. Older age, preoperative motor deficit, high-grade glioma, and hypertension were also independently associated with increased risk of developing perioperative VTE [14]. Osaki et al. studied the risk and incidence of perioperative DVT in patients undergoing gastric cancer surgery. The preoperative and postoperative incidences of DVT were 4.4% and 7.2%, respectively [15].

3. Anti-Neoplastic Medications Associated with Increased Risk of Thrombosis

Multiple cancer therapies are associated with an increased risk of thrombosis. We do not aim to cover all the medications that are associated with increased risk of thrombosis in this report but will highlight some of the more commonly used agents.

3.1. Tamoxifen

The National Surgical Adjuvant Breast and Bowel Project (NSABP), Protocol B-14, was a double-blind, placebo-controlled trial comparing the effectiveness of tamoxifen in patients with breast cancer, histologically negative axillary nodes, and estrogen-receptor positive. Thromboembolism occurred in 0.9% of patients receiving tamoxifen compared to 0.15% of those receiving placebo [16].

Thromboembolic events are more often observed when chemotherapy is given in conjunction with tamoxifen than when tamoxifen is administered alone. The NSABP B-20 study compared chemotherapy plus tamoxifen versus tamoxifen alone in the treatment of patients with axillary lymph node negative, estrogen-receptor-positive breast cancer. VTE was observed in 1.8% of patients treated with tamoxifen alone, compared to 6.5% in patients treated with cyclophosphamide, methotrexate, fluorouracil, and tamoxifen [17]. This increased risk of VTE when tamoxifen is combined with chemotherapy is the main reason that tamoxifen is withheld until chemotherapy treatment is completed.

3.2. Chemotherapy

Multiple studies have shown correlations between chemotherapy and increased incidence of VTE. A retrospective analysis including 17,284 cancer patients found that VTE occurred in 12.6% of the cancer cohort over 12 months after the initiation of chemotherapy, versus 1.4% of controls [18].

(a) Cisplatin. Cisplatin is associated with an increased risk of VTE and arterial thrombosis. A retrospective analysis from the Memorial Sloan Kettering Cancer Center found that 18.1% of cancer patients developed thrombosis during cisplatin treatment. Most of these cases (88%) occurred during the first 100 days from the initiation of cisplatin [19]. A meta-analysis of randomized controlled trials evaluating the incidence and risk of VTE associated with cisplatin-based chemotherapy showed a significantly increased risk of VTE with a relative risk of 1.67 [20]. VTE rates were 1.92% versus 0.79% in patients treated with cisplatin-based and non-cisplatin-based chemotherapy regimens, respectively [20]. A report from the UK National Cancer Research Institute of a randomized trial of patients with advanced gastroesophageal cancer randomized to epirubicin/(fluorouracil or capecitabine) and cisplatin or oxaliplatin found fewer thrombotic events in the oxaliplatin compared with the cisplatin groups, 7.6% vs. 15.1%, respectively; $p = 0.0003$ [21].

(b) Thalidomide. Thalidomide inhibits the production of interleukin (IL)-6, while suppressing proliferation and activating apoptosis of myeloma cells [22]. A study that treated patients with multiple myeloma using thalidomide and dexamethasone in preparation for autologous stem cell transplantation found VTE in 13% and 26% of patients treated with or without low-dose prophylactic warfarin, respectively [23]. A phase III clinical trial of thalidomide plus dexamethasone compared with dexamethasone alone in newly diagnosed multiple myeloma showed that VTE occurred in 19.6% and 2.9% of patients treated with and without thalidomide, respectively [24].

(c) Asparaginase. Asparaginase is an enzyme that degrades L-asparagine, resulting in inhibition of protein synthesis in tumor cells [25]. A retrospective study reported thrombotic complications in adult patients with acute lymphoblastic leukemia receiving L-asparaginase during induction therapy in 4.2% of the patients [26]. A meta-analysis of 1752 patients from 17 prospective trials involving treatment with asparaginase demonstrated a rate of symptomatic thrombosis of 5.2% [27]. The UK ALL 2003 study reported asparaginase-related venous thrombosis in 3.2% of 1824 treated patients [28]. The use of prednisone and asparaginase concomitantly administered in a leukemic patient suffering from a prothrombotic risk factor (such as protein C deficiency, protein S deficiency, antithrombin deficiency, or factor V Leiden) was responsible for the onset of venous thrombosis in the majority of cases [29].

3.3. Molecular Targeted Therapies

(d) Lenvatinib is an oral medication that inhibits multiple receptor tyrosine kinases, including vascular endothelial growth factor receptors, fibroblast growth factor receptors, and platelet-derived growth factor receptor alpha [30]. A phase 2 trial treating patients with advanced, radioiodine-refractory thyroid cancer with lenvatinib, reported pulmonary embolism in 3% of the patients and DVT in 3% of the patients [31].

(e) Osimertinib is an epidermal growth factor receptor inhibitor that is implicated with an enhanced risk of thrombosis. The dose escalation study showed that pulmonary embolism occurred in 2.4% of the treated patients [32]. Osimertinib-induced VTE after initiation of osimertinib treatment was reported recently by Shiroyama et al. [33].

3.4. Anti-angiogenesis Monoclonal Antibodies

(f) Bevacizumab. Bevacizumab is a monoclonal antibody that targets vascular endothelial growth factor (VEGF) in the circulation. The addition of bevacizumab to irinotecan, fluorouracil, and leucovorin resulted in improvement in survival among patients with metastatic colorectal cancer; however, thrombotic events were higher in patients treated with bevacizumab compared to patients treated with chemotherapy alone (19.4% versus 16.2%, respectively, $p = 0.26$) [34]. Analysis of data pooled from five randomized controlled trials found that the combination of bevacizumab and chemotherapy, compared with chemotherapy alone, was associated with an increased risk of arterial thromboembolism with a hazard ratio of 2.0 [35]. A meta-analysis of 20 randomized controlled trials found that the incidence of arterial thrombotic events in patients receiving bevacizumab was 3.3% [36]. This meta-analysis showed the varying risk for arterial thrombotic events with different malignancies treated with bevacizumab, with the highest relative risk of 3.72 for patients with renal cell cancer, and with the relative risk being 1.89 in patients with colorectal cancer treated [36].

(g) Ramucirumab. Ramucirumab is a monoclonal antibody that targets the extracellular domain of VEGF receptor 2, and thus prevents its activation by VEGF [37]. A phase I pharmacologic and biologic study of ramucirumab reported DVT in 5.4% of the patients [37]. A study comparing ramucirumab versus placebo in combination with second-line chemotherapy in patients with metastatic colorectal carcinoma reported a nonsignificant difference in VTE of 8.2% and 6.3% with ramucirumab and placebo, respectively [38].

4. Heparin and Heparan Sulphate

The term 'heparin' was derived from the Greek word 'hepar', or liver, the tissue from which it was first isolated [39]. In 1925, Howell described the role of endogenous heparin for the fluidity of blood [40]. Heparan sulfate is a family of multiple, closely related yet distinct polysaccharide species [41]. Heparin is structurally related to heparan sulfate but has higher N- and O-sulfate contents [41]. Units of N-acetylglucosamine and glucuronic acid form heparan sulphate [42]. Heparan sulfate is ubiquitously expressed on the cell surface and in the extracellular matrix of all mammalian cells [43] and plays multiple roles in cell–cell interactions. Mutations affecting the biosynthesis of heparan sulphate proteoglycans are implicated in multiple diseases including Simpson–Golabi–Behmel syndrome and Ehlers–Danlos syndrome [42].

Most commercial heparin production is derived from pig intestine or bovine lungs [44,45]. Multiple studies have shown that heparin and low-molecular-weight heparin (LMWH) appear to prolong survival in patients with cancer [46–49].

5. Heparanase

Heparanase is produced as a proenzyme and is activated via proteolytic cleavage by cathepsin L [50]. This proteolytic cleavage results in the production of two subunits of heparanase that heterodimerize to form the active enzyme [51]. Heparanase in its enzymatically active form [50,52] degrades heparan sulfate at the cell surface and in the extracellular matrix [53,54]. We and others have shown that heparanase is capable of degrading heparin [3,55] and low-molecular-weight heparin [3]. We showed that heparanase degradation of heparin and low-molecular-weight heparin results in neutralization of the anticoagulant properties of these molecules [3]. Moreover, we showed that transgenic mice overexpressing heparanase in all their tissues have shorter activated partial thromboplastin time compared to control mice [3], which could be due to degradation of endogenous heparin by heparanase.

Under physiologic conditions, heparanase is expressed mainly in the platelets [56–58] and in the placenta [59–63]. Heparanase plays multiple roles in platelets. When an injury occurs, platelets are recruited to the wound region, where they secrete more than 300 active substances from their intracellular granules [64]. One of these molecules is heparanase [55]. The first step in which heparanase is involved is in achieving homeostasis. Heparanase degrades endogenous plasma heparin at the blood–wound microenvironment, facilitating clot formation (Figure 2). The second step is facilitating wound healing. Heparanase degrades the broken heparan sulphate residues at the extracellular matrix of the wounded tissue, clearing the wound area for scar formation and tissue healing. That is followed by the production of a new layer of heparan sulphate covering the healed tissue. Heparanase is expressed at high levels in the placenta [59,61–63] and contributes to the high blood vessel density in this critical organ.

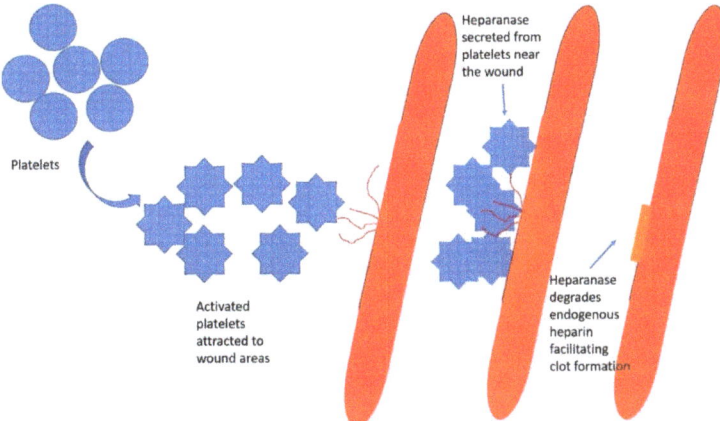

Figure 2. Platelets circulate in the blood. From left to right: Under normal conditions, the platelets are in their nonactive form in the circulation. When an endothelial injury occurs, blood leaks from the injured vessel, and the platelets are recruited to the wound area. The platelets degranulate its content. Heparanase secreted from the platelets degrades endogenous heparin in the blood interface within the wound area to facilitate clot formation. Heparanase also degrades heparan sulphate residues in the injured region as an initial step of wound healing.

We have cloned multiple splice variants of heparanase [54,65–67]; all lack heparanase enzymatic activity. Splice 5 of heparanase, which lacks exon 5, was cloned from human renal cell carcinoma [65]. We cloned heparanase of the subterranean blind mole rat (*Spalax*) and multiple splice variants of it [53,54,66,68] and characterized its heparan sulphate structure [68]. Splice 36 of *Spalax* heparanase functions as a dominant negative to the wild-type enzyme and inhibits heparan sulphate degradation, tumor growth, and metastasis in animal models [54].

6. Type I Cancer-Related Hypercoagulability

Type I cancer-related hypercoagulability is a term that we propose to define thrombotic events in cancer patients that results from lack of sufficient endogenous heparin to maintain the blood in its liquid form. This is mainly due to the degradation of endogenous heparin by tumor-secreted heparanase. Heparanase seems to be the only heparan-sulfate-degrading endoglycosidase [69].

Heparanase was found to be expressed in most malignant tumors. Pancreatic cancers were shown to have heparanase mRNA levels more than 30-fold higher than the levels in normal pancreatic tissues [70]. Kim et al. used in situ hybridization to test for heparanase and found it expressed in 78% of the pancreatic tumors and in none of the normal pancreatic tissues [71]. Heparanase overexpression was associated with angiogenesis and lymphangiogenesis of lung cancer [72]. Cohen et al. showed that heparanase is overexpressed in 75% of lung cancer patients, and its expression correlates inversely with patient survival [73]. A meta-analysis with a total of 27 studies which included 3891 gastric cancer patients showed that higher heparanase expression in gastric cancer is associated with clinicopathologic features of depth of invasion, lymph node metastasis, and TNM stage [74]. All these malignancies are correlated with a high risk of thrombosis, and type I hypercoagulability could be the main reason for that.

Type I hypercoagulability possibly occurs in other situations, such as in pregnancy [75] where degradation of endogenous heparin by placental heparanase could result in thrombosis. The anticoagulant of choice during pregnancy is low-molecular-weight heparin [75], which is a competitive inhibitor of heparanase [3,4,53]. Patients with multiple traumatic injuries could also be at risk of thrombosis [76]. This increased risk of thrombosis could be due to massive secretion of heparanase from activated platelets and degradation of endogenous heparin.

7. Type II Cancer-Related Hypercoagulability

Type II cancer-related hypercoagulability refers to thrombotic events in cancer patients not related to low endogenous heparin levels. This can occur due to a variety of reasons reviewed here. This includes poor performance status, stasis due to pressure on blood vessels by a tumor mass, or drug-associated thrombosis (Figure 1).

8. Thrombosis as Prognostic Factor in Cancer Patients

Cancer diagnosed at the same time as or within one year after an episode of VTE is associated with an advanced stage of cancer and a poor prognosis [77]. Patients with cancer have a greater risk both of VTE and bleeding [78]. Early VTE at the beginning of palliative chemotherapy was shown to be a poor prognostic factor in patients with metastatic pancreatic cancer [79]. Patients with pancreatic cancer with early-onset VTE that occurred within 1.5 months after chemotherapy initiation were found to be negative prognosticators for survival outcomes [80]. In patients with cancer and acute VTE, low-molecular-weight heparin was shown to be more effective than an oral coumarin derivative in reducing the risk of recurrent thromboembolism without increasing the risk of bleeding [47,81]. This could be due to the heparanase-inhibiting function of low-molecular-weight heparin [3].

9. Conclusions and Future Directions

Endogenous heparin is an important component of the balance between blood fluidity and thrombosis. The degradation of endogenous heparin by heparanase seems to play a major role in cancer-associated thrombosis. Developing alternative noninvasive methods to deliver heparin rather than using the subcutaneous or intravenous routes could make this medication more appealing to use in cancer patients, given the introduction of new oral medications [82,83]. Furthermore, developing methods to mobilize endogenous heparin from its reservoirs in the body to the circulation could become the best way to treat cancer-associated thrombosis.

Funding: This research received no external funding.

Conflicts of Interest: The authors declare no conflict of interest.

References

1. Trousseau, A. *Phlegmasia alba dolens in: Lectures on Clinical Medicine, delivered at the Hôtel-Dieu, Paris*; New Sydenham Society: London, UK, 1872; pp. 281–295.
2. Dickson, B.C. Venous thrombosis: On the history of Virchow's triad. *Univ. Tor. Med. J.* **2004**, *81*, 166–171.
3. Nasser, N.J.; Sarig, G.; Brenner, B.; Nevo, E.; Goldshmidt, O.; Zcharia, E.; Li, J.P.; Vlodavsky, I. Heparanase neutralizes the anticoagulation properties of heparin and low-molecular-weight heparin. *J. Thromb. Haemost. JTH* **2006**, *4*, 560–565. [CrossRef]
4. Nasser, N.J.; Na'amad, M.; Weinberg, I.; Gabizon, A.A. Pharmacokinetics of low molecular weight heparin in patients with malignant tumors. *Anti-Cancer Drugs* **2015**, *26*, 106–111. [CrossRef] [PubMed]
5. Nadir, Y.; Brenner, B.; Zetser, A.; Ilan, N.; Shafat, I.; Zcharia, E.; Goldshmidt, O.; Vlodavsky, I. Heparanase induces tissue factor expression in vascular endothelial and cancer cells. *J. Thromb. Haemost.* **2006**, *4*, 2443–2451. [CrossRef] [PubMed]
6. Nadir, Y.; Brenner, B.; Gingis-Velitski, S.; Levy-Adam, F.; Ilan, N.; Zcharia, E.; Nadir, E.; Vlodavsky, I. Heparanase induces tissue factor pathway inhibitor expression and extracellular accumulation in endothelial and tumor cells. *Thromb. Haemost.* **2008**, *99*, 133–141. [CrossRef] [PubMed]
7. Chiu, J.-J.; Chien, S. Effects of disturbed flow on vascular endothelium: Pathophysiological basis and clinical perspectives. *Physiol. Rev.* **2011**, *91*, 327–387. [CrossRef]
8. Sigel, B.; Coelho, J.; Spigos, D.G.; Flanigan, D.P.; Schuler, J.J.; Kasprisin, D.O.; Nyhus, L.M.; Capek, V. Ultrasonography of blood during stasis and coagulation. *Investig. Radiol.* **1981**, *16*, 71–76. [CrossRef]
9. Fareed, J.; Walenga, J.M.; Kumar, A.; Rock, A. A modified stasis thrombosis model to study the antithrombotic actions of heparin and its fractions. *Semin. Thromb. Hemost.* **1985**, *11*, 155–175. [CrossRef]
10. White, C.; Noble, S.I.R.; Watson, M.; Swan, F.; Allgar, V.L.; Napier, E.; Nelson, A.; McAuley, J.; Doherty, J.; Lee, B.; et al. Prevalence, symptom burden, and natural history of deep vein thrombosis in people with advanced cancer in specialist palliative care units (HIDDen): A prospective longitudinal observational study. *Lancet Haematol.* **2019**, *6*, e79–e88. [CrossRef]
11. Metcalf, R.L.; Fry, D.J.; Swindell, R.; McGurk, A.; Clamp, A.R.; Jayson, G.C.; Hasan, J. Thrombosis in ovarian cancer: A case control study. *Br. J. Cancer* **2014**, *110*, 1118–1124. [CrossRef] [PubMed]
12. Beck-Razi, N.; Kuzmin, A.; Koren, D.; Sarig, G.; Brenner, B.; Haim, N.; Gaitini, D. Asymptomatic deep vein thrombosis in advanced cancer patients: The value of venous sonography. *J. Clin. Ultrasound JCU* **2010**, *38*, 232–237. [CrossRef] [PubMed]
13. Natsumeda, M.; Uzuka, T.; Watanabe, J.; Fukuda, M.; Akaiwa, Y.; Hanzawa, K.; Okada, M.; Oishi, M.; Fujii, Y. High Incidence of Deep Vein Thrombosis in the Perioperative Period of Neurosurgical Patients. *World Neurosurg.* **2018**, *112*, e103–e112. [CrossRef] [PubMed]
14. Chaichana, K.L.; Pendleton, C.; Jackson, C.; Martinez-Gutierrez, J.C.; Diaz-Stransky, A.; Aguayo, J.; Olivi, A.; Weingart, J.; Gallia, G.; Lim, M.; et al. Deep venous thrombosis and pulmonary embolisms in adult patients undergoing craniotomy for brain tumors. *Neurol. Res.* **2013**, *35*, 206–211. [CrossRef]
15. Osaki, T.; Saito, H.; Fukumoto, Y.; Kono, Y.; Murakami, Y.; Shishido, Y.; Kuroda, H.; Matsunaga, T.; Sato, K.; Hirooka, Y.; et al. Risk and incidence of perioperative deep vein thrombosis in patients undergoing gastric cancer surgery. *Surg. Today* **2018**, *48*, 525–533. [CrossRef]
16. Fisher, B.; Costantino, J.; Redmond, C.; Poisson, R.; Bowman, D.; Couture, J.; Dimitrov, N.V.; Wolmark, N.; Wickerham, D.L.; Fisher, E.R.; et al. A Randomized Clinical Trial Evaluating Tamoxifen in the Treatment of Patients with Node-Negative Breast Cancer Who Have Estrogen-Receptor–Positive Tumors. *N. Engl. J. Med.* **1989**, *320*, 479–484. [CrossRef]

17. Fisher, B.; Dignam, J.; Wolmark, N.; DeCillis, A.; Emir, B.; Wickerham, D.L.; Bryant, J.; Dimitrov, N.V.; Abramson, N.; Atkins, J.N.; et al. Tamoxifen and chemotherapy for lymph node-negative, estrogen receptor-positive breast cancer. *J. Natl. Cancer Inst.* **1997**, *89*, 1673–1682. [CrossRef]
18. Khorana, A.A.; Dalal, M.; Lin, J.; Connolly, G.C. Incidence and predictors of venous thromboembolism (VTE) among ambulatory high-risk cancer patients undergoing chemotherapy in the United States. *Cancer* **2013**, *119*, 648–655. [CrossRef]
19. Moore, R.A.; Adel, N.; Riedel, E.; Bhutani, M.; Feldman, D.R.; Tabbara, N.E.; Soff, G.; Parameswaran, R.; Hassoun, H. High incidence of thromboembolic events in patients treated with cisplatin-based chemotherapy: A large retrospective analysis. *J. Clin. Oncol.* **2011**, *29*, 3466–3473. [CrossRef]
20. Seng, S.; Liu, Z.; Chiu, S.K.; Proverbs-Singh, T.; Sonpavde, G.; Choueiri, T.K.; Tsao, C.-K.; Yu, M.; Hahn, N.M.; Oh, W.K. Risk of venous thromboembolism in patients with cancer treated with Cisplatin: A systematic review and meta-analysis. *J. Clin. Oncol.* **2012**, *30*, 4416–4426. [CrossRef]
21. Starling, N.; Rao, S.; Cunningham, D.; Iveson, T.; Nicolson, M.; Coxon, F.; Middleton, G.; Daniel, F.; Oates, J.; Norman, A.R. Thromboembolism in patients with advanced gastroesophageal cancer treated with anthracycline, platinum, and fluoropyrimidine combination chemotherapy: A report from the UK National Cancer Research Institute Upper Gastrointestinal Clinical Studies Group. *J. Clin. Oncol.* **2009**, *27*, 3786–3793. [CrossRef] [PubMed]
22. Anderson, K.C. Lenalidomide and thalidomide: Mechanisms of action-similarities and differences. *Semin. Hematol.* **2005**, *42*, S3–S8. [CrossRef] [PubMed]
23. Cavo, M.; Zamagni, E.; Tosi, P.; Cellini, C.; Cangini, D.; Tacchetti, P.; Testoni, N.; Tonelli, M.; de Vivo, A.; Palareti, G. First-line therapy with thalidomide and dexamethasone in preparation for autologous stem cell transplantation for multiple myeloma. *Haematologica* **2004**, *89*, 826–831. [PubMed]
24. Rajkumar, S.V.; Blood, E.; Vesole, D.; Fonseca, R.; Greipp, P.R. Phase III clinical trial of thalidomide plus dexamethasone compared with dexamethasone alone in newly diagnosed multiple myeloma: A clinical trial coordinated by the Eastern Cooperative Oncology Group. *J. Clin. Oncol.* **2006**, *24*, 431–436. [CrossRef]
25. Batool, T.; Makky, E.A.; Jalal, M.; Yusoff, M.M. A comprehensive review on L-asparaginase and its applications. *Appl. Biochem. Biotechnol.* **2016**, *178*, 900–923. [CrossRef]
26. Gugliotta, L.; Mazzucconi, M.G.; Leone, G.; Mattioli-Belmonte, M.; Defazio, D.; Annino, L.; Tura, S.; Mandelli, F.; Group, G. Incidence of thrombotic complications in adult patients with acute lymphoblastic leukaemia receiving L-asparaginase during induction therapy: A retrospective study. *Eur. J. Haematol.* **1992**, *49*, 63–66. [CrossRef]
27. Caruso, V.; Iacoviello, L.; Di Castelnuovo, A.; Storti, S.; Mariani, G.; De Gaetano, G.; Donati, M.B. Thrombotic complications in childhood acute lymphoblastic leukemia: A meta-analysis of 17 prospective studies comprising 1752 pediatric patients. *Blood* **2006**, *108*, 2216–2222. [CrossRef]
28. Qureshi, A.; Mitchell, C.; Richards, S.; Vora, A.; Goulden, N. Asparaginase-related venous thrombosis in UKALL 2003- re-exposure to asparaginase is feasible and safe. *Br. J. Haematol.* **2010**, *149*, 410–413. [CrossRef]
29. Nowak-Göttl, U.; Heinecke, A.; von Kries, R.; Nürnberger, W.; Münchow, N.; Junker, R. Thrombotic events revisited in children with acute lymphoblastic leukemia: Impact of concomitant Escherichia coli asparaginase/prednisone administration. *Thromb. Res.* **2001**, *103*, 165–172. [CrossRef]
30. Nishio, M.; Horai, T.; Horiike, A.; Nokihara, H.; Yamamoto, N.; Takahashi, T.; Murakami, H.; Yamamoto, N.; Koizumi, F.; Nishio, K.; et al. Phase 1 study of lenvatinib combined with carboplatin and paclitaxel in patients with non-small-cell lung cancer. *Br. J. Cancer* **2013**, *109*, 538–544. [CrossRef]
31. Cabanillas, M.E.; Schlumberger, M.; Jarzab, B.; Martins, R.G.; Pacini, F.; Robinson, B.; McCaffrey, J.C.; Shah, M.H.; Bodenner, D.L.; Topliss, D. A phase 2 trial of lenvatinib (E7080) in advanced, progressive, radioiodine-refractory, differentiated thyroid cancer: A clinical outcomes and biomarker assessment. *Cancer* **2015**, *121*, 2749–2756. [CrossRef] [PubMed]
32. Jänne, P.A.; Yang, J.C.-H.; Kim, D.-W.; Planchard, D.; Ohe, Y.; Ramalingam, S.S.; Ahn, M.-J.; Kim, S.-W.; Su, W.-C.; Horn, L.; et al. AZD9291 in EGFR Inhibitor–Resistant Non–Small-Cell Lung Cancer. *N. Engl. J. Med.* **2015**, *372*, 1689–1699. [CrossRef] [PubMed]
33. Shiroyama, T.; Hayama, M.; Satoh, S.; Nasu, S.; Tanaka, A.; Morita, S.; Morishita, N.; Suzuki, H.; Okamoto, N.; Hirashima, T. Successful retreatment with osimertinib after osimertinib-induced acute pulmonary embolism in a patient with lung adenocarcinoma: A case report. *Respir. Med. Case Rep.* **2016**, *20*, 25–27. [CrossRef] [PubMed]

34. Hurwitz, H.; Fehrenbacher, L.; Novotny, W.; Cartwright, T.; Hainsworth, J.; Heim, W.; Berlin, J.; Baron, A.; Griffing, S.; Holmgren, E.; et al. Bevacizumab plus Irinotecan, Fluorouracil, and Leucovorin for Metastatic Colorectal Cancer. *N. Engl. J. Med.* **2004**, *350*, 2335–2342. [CrossRef] [PubMed]
35. Scappaticci, F.A.; Skillings, J.R.; Holden, S.N.; Gerber, H.-P.; Miller, K.; Kabbinavar, F.; Bergsland, E.; Ngai, J.; Holmgren, E.; Wang, J. Arterial thromboembolic events in patients with metastatic carcinoma treated with chemotherapy and bevacizumab. *J. Natl. Cancer Inst.* **2007**, *99*, 1232–1239. [CrossRef]
36. Ranpura, V.; Hapani, S.; Chuang, J.; Wu, S. Risk of cardiac ischemia and arterial thromboembolic events with the angiogenesis inhibitor bevacizumab in cancer patients: A meta-analysis of randomized controlled trials. *Acta Oncol.* **2010**, *49*, 287–297. [CrossRef]
37. Spratlin, J.L.; Mulder, K.E.; Mackey, J.R. Ramucirumab (IMC-1121B): A novel attack on angiogenesis. *Future Oncol.* **2010**, *6*, 1085–1094. [CrossRef]
38. Tabernero, J.; Yoshino, T.; Cohn, A.L.; Obermannova, R.; Bodoky, G.; Garcia-Carbonero, R.; Ciuleanu, T.-E.; Portnoy, D.C.; Van Cutsem, E.; Grothey, A. Ramucirumab versus placebo in combination with second-line FOLFIRI in patients with metastatic colorectal carcinoma that progressed during or after first-line therapy with bevacizumab, oxaliplatin, and a fluoropyrimidine (RAISE): A randomised, double-blind, multicentre, phase 3 study. *Lancet Oncol.* **2015**, *16*, 499–508.
39. Wardrop, D.; Keeling, D. The story of the discovery of heparin and warfarin. *Br. J. Haematol.* **2008**, *141*, 757–763. [CrossRef]
40. Howell, W. The purification of heparin and its presence in blood. *Am. J. Physiol. Leg. Content* **1925**, *71*, 553–562. [CrossRef]
41. Casu, B.; Lindahl, U. Structure and biological interactions of heparin and heparan sulfate. In *Advances in Carbohydrate Chemistry and Biochemistry*; Academic Press: Cambridge, MA, USA, 2001; Volume 57, pp. 159–206.
42. Hacker, U.; Nybakken, K.; Perrimon, N. Heparan sulphate proteoglycans: The sweet side of development. *Nat. Rev. Mol. Cell Biol.* **2005**, *6*, 530–541. [CrossRef] [PubMed]
43. Weiss, R.J.; Esko, J.D.; Tor, Y. Targeting heparin and heparan sulfate protein interactions. *Org. Biomol. Chem.* **2017**, *15*, 5656–5668. [CrossRef] [PubMed]
44. Tremblay, J.F. Making heparin safe. *Chem. Eng. News* **2016**, *94*, 30–34.
45. Kouta, A.; Jeske, W.; Hoppensteadt, D.; Iqbal, O.; Yao, Y.; Fareed, J. Comparative Pharmacological Profiles of Various Bovine, Ovine, and Porcine Heparins. *Clin. Appl. Thromb. Hemost. Off. J. Int. Acad.* **2019**, *25*. [CrossRef] [PubMed]
46. Kakkar, A.K.; Levine, M.N.; Kadziola, Z.; Lemoine, N.R.; Low, V.; Patel, H.K.; Rustin, G.; Thomas, M.; Quigley, M.; Williamson, R.C. Low molecular weight heparin, therapy with dalteparin, and survival in advanced cancer: The fragmin advanced malignancy outcome study (FAMOUS). *J. Clin. Oncol.* **2004**, *22*, 1944–1948. [CrossRef]
47. Lee, A.Y.; Levine, M.N.; Baker, R.I.; Bowden, C.; Kakkar, A.K.; Prins, M.; Rickles, F.R.; Julian, J.A.; Haley, S.; Kovacs, M.J.; et al. Low-molecular-weight heparin versus a coumarin for the prevention of recurrent venous thromboembolism in patients with cancer. *N. Engl. J. Med.* **2003**, *349*, 146–153. [CrossRef]
48. Lebeau, B.; Chastang, C.; Brechot, J.M.; Capron, F.; Dautzenberg, B.; Delaisements, C.; Mornet, M.; Brun, J.; Hurdebourcq, J.P.; Lemarie, E. Subcutaneous heparin treatment increases survival in small cell lung cancer. *Cancer* **1994**, *74*, 38–45. [CrossRef]
49. Lazo-Langner, A.; Goss, G.; Spaans, J.; Rodger, M. The effect of low-molecular-weight heparin on cancer survival. A systematic review and meta-analysis of randomized trials. *J. Thromb. Haemost.* **2007**, *5*, 729–737. [CrossRef]
50. Abboud-Jarrous, G.; Atzmon, R.; Peretz, T.; Palermo, C.; Gadea, B.B.; Joyce, J.A.; Vlodavsky, I. Cathepsin L is responsible for processing and activation of proheparanase through multiple cleavages of a linker segment. *J. Biol. Chem.* **2008**, *283*, 18167–18176. [CrossRef]
51. Levy-Adam, F.; Miao, H.Q.; Heinrikson, R.L.; Vlodavsky, I.; Ilan, N. Heterodimer formation is essential for heparanase enzymatic activity. *Biochem. Biophys. Res. Commun.* **2003**, *308*, 885–891. [CrossRef]
52. Abboud-Jarrous, G.; Rangini-Guetta, Z.; Aingorn, H.; Atzmon, R.; Elgavish, S.; Peretz, T.; Vlodavsky, I. Site-directed mutagenesis, proteolytic cleavage, and activation of human proheparanase. *J. Biol. Chem.* **2005**, *280*, 13568–13575. [CrossRef] [PubMed]
53. Nasser, N.J. Heparanase involvement in physiology and disease. *Cell. Mol. Life Sci. CMLS* **2008**, *65*, 1706–1715. [CrossRef] [PubMed]

54. Nasser, N.J.; Avivi, A.; Shafat, I.; Edovitsky, E.; Zcharia, E.; Ilan, N.; Vlodavsky, I.; Nevo, E. Alternatively spliced Spalax heparanase inhibits extracellular matrix degradation, tumor growth, and metastasis. *Proc. Natl. Acad. Sci. USA* **2009**, *106*, 2253–2258. [CrossRef] [PubMed]
55. Freeman, C.; Parish, R.C. Human platelet heparanase: Purification, characterization and catalytic activity. *Biochem. J.* **1998**, *330*, 1341–1350. [CrossRef]
56. Eldor, A.; Bar-Ner, M.; Yahalom, J.; Fuks, Z.; Vlodavsky, I. Role of heparanase in platelet and tumor cell interactions with the subendothelial extracellular matrix. *Semin. Thromb. Hemost.* **1987**, *13*, 475–488. [CrossRef]
57. Tan, Y.X.; Cui, H.; Wan, L.M.; Gong, F.; Zhang, X.; Vlodavsky, I.; Li, J.P. Overexpression of heparanase in mice promoted megakaryopoiesis. *Glycobiology* **2018**, *28*, 269–275. [CrossRef]
58. Cui, H.; Tan, Y.X.; Osterholm, C.; Zhang, X.; Hedin, U.; Vlodavsky, I.; Li, J.P. Heparanase expression upregulates platelet adhesion activity and thrombogenicity. *Oncotarget* **2016**, *7*, 39486–39496. [CrossRef]
59. Goshen, R.; Hochberg, A.A.; Korner, G.; Levy, E.; Ishai-Michaeli, R.; Elkin, M.; de Groot, N.; Vlodavsky, I. Purification and characterization of placental heparanase and its expression by cultured cytotrophoblasts. *Mol. Hum. Reprod.* **1996**, *2*, 679–684. [CrossRef]
60. Vlodavsky, I.; Friedmann, Y.; Elkin, M.; Aingorn, H.; Atzmon, R.; Ishai-Michaeli, R.; Bitan, M.; Pappo, O.; Peretz, T.; Michal, I.; et al. Mammalian heparanase: Gene cloning, expression and function in tumor progression and metastasis. *Nat. Med.* **1999**, *5*, 793–802. [CrossRef]
61. Haimov-Kochman, R.; Friedmann, Y.; Prus, D.; Goldman-Wohl, D.S.; Greenfield, C.; Anteby, E.Y.; Aviv, A.; Vlodavsky, I.; Yagel, S. Localization of heparanase in normal and pathological human placenta. *Mol. Hum. Reprod.* **2002**, *8*, 566–573. [CrossRef]
62. Eddy, A.C.; Chapman, H.; George, E.M. Heparanase regulation of sFLT-1 release in trophoblasts in vitro. *Placenta* **2019**, *85*, 63–68. [CrossRef] [PubMed]
63. Hambruch, N.; Kumstel, S.; Haeger, J.D.; Pfarrer, C. Bovine placentomal heparanase and syndecan expression is related to placental maturation. *Placenta* **2017**, *57*, 42–51. [CrossRef] [PubMed]
64. Golebiewska, E.M.; Poole, A.W. Platelet secretion: From haemostasis to wound healing and beyond. *Blood Rev.* **2015**, *29*, 153–162. [CrossRef] [PubMed]
65. Nasser, N.J.; Avivi, A.; Shushy, M.; Vlodavsky, I.; Nevo, E. Cloning, expression, and characterization of an alternatively spliced variant of human heparanase. *Biochem. Biophys. Res. Commun.* **2007**, *354*, 33–38. [CrossRef]
66. Nasser, N.J.; Nevo, E.; Shafat, I.; Ilan, N.; Vlodavsky, I.; Avivi, A. Adaptive evolution of heparanase in hypoxia-tolerant Spalax: Gene cloning and identification of a unique splice variant. *Proc. Natl. Acad. Sci. USA* **2005**, *102*, 15161–15166. [CrossRef]
67. Nasser, N.J.; Nevo, E. Heparanase patents: Dim past and bright future. *Recent Pat. Inflamm. Allergy Drug Discov.* **2013**, *7*, 162–167. [CrossRef]
68. Sandwall, E.; Bodevin, S.; Nasser, N.J.; Nevo, E.; Avivi, A.; Vlodavsky, I.; Li, J.P. Molecular structure of heparan sulfate from Spalax. Implications of heparanase and hypoxia. *J. Biol. Chem.* **2009**, *284*, 3814–3822. [CrossRef]
69. Vlodavsky, I.; Gross-Cohen, M.; Weissmann, M.; Ilan, N.; Sanderson, R.D. Opposing Functions of Heparanase-1 and Heparanase-2 in Cancer Progression. *Trends Biochem. Sci.* **2018**, *43*, 18–31. [CrossRef]
70. Koliopanos, A.; Friess, H.; Kleeff, J.; Shi, X.; Liao, Q.; Pecker, I.; Vlodavsky, I.; Zimmermann, A.; Buchler, M.W. Heparanase expression in primary and metastatic pancreatic cancer. *Cancer Res.* **2001**, *61*, 4655–4659.
71. Kim, A.W.; Xu, X.; Hollinger, E.F.; Gattuso, P.; Godellas, C.V.; Prinz, R.A. Human heparanase-1 gene expression in pancreatic adenocarcinoma. *J. Gastrointest. Surg. Off. J. Soc. Surg. Aliment. Tract* **2002**, *6*, 167–172. [CrossRef]
72. Zhang, Q.; Ming, J.; Li, Y.; Zhang, S.; Li, B.; Qiu, X.; Wang, E. Heparanase expression correlates with angiogenesis and lymphangiogenesis in human lung cancer. *Zhongguo Fei Ai Za Zhi Chin. J. Lung Cancer* **2009**, *12*, 864–867. [CrossRef]
73. Cohen, E.; Doweck, I.; Naroditsky, I.; Ben-Izhak, O.; Kremer, R.; Best, L.A.; Vlodavsky, I.; Ilan, N. Heparanase is overexpressed in lung cancer and correlates inversely with patient survival. *Cancer* **2008**, *113*, 1004–1011. [CrossRef] [PubMed]

74. Li, H.L.; Gu, J.; Wu, J.J.; Ma, C.L.; Yang, Y.L.; Wang, H.P.; Wang, J.; Wang, Y.; Chen, C.; Wu, H.Y. Heparanase mRNA and Protein Expression Correlates with Clinicopathologic Features of Gastric Cancer Patients: A Meta-analysis. *Asian Pac. J. Cancer Prev. APJCP* **2015**, *16*, 8653–8658. [CrossRef] [PubMed]
75. Konkle, B.A. Diagnosis and management of thrombosis in pregnancy. *Birth Defects Res. Part. C Embryo Today Rev.* **2015**, *105*, 185–189. [CrossRef] [PubMed]
76. Tomaiuolo, M.; Brass, L.F.; Stalker, T.J. Regulation of Platelet Activation and Coagulation and Its Role in Vascular Injury and Arterial Thrombosis. *Interv. Cardiol. Clin.* **2017**, *6*, 1–12. [CrossRef] [PubMed]
77. Sorensen, H.T.; Mellemkjaer, L.; Olsen, J.H.; Baron, J.A. Prognosis of cancers associated with venous thromboembolism. *N. Engl. J. Med.* **2000**, *343*, 1846–1850. [CrossRef]
78. Iorga, R.A.; Bratu, O.G.; Marcu, R.D.; Constantin, T.; Mischianu, D.L.D.; Socea, B.; Gaman, M.A.; Diaconu, C.C. Venous thromboembolism in cancer patients: Still looking for answers. *Exp. Ther. Med.* **2019**, *18*, 5026–5032. [CrossRef]
79. Kim, J.S.; Kang, E.J.; Kim, D.S.; Choi, Y.J.; Lee, S.Y.; Kim, H.J.; Seo, H.Y.; Kim, J.S. Early venous thromboembolism at the beginning of palliative chemotherapy is a poor prognostic factor in patients with metastatic pancreatic cancer: A retrospective study. *BMC Cancer* **2018**, *18*, 1260. [CrossRef]
80. Chen, J.S.; Hung, C.Y.; Chang, H.; Liu, C.T.; Chen, Y.Y.; Lu, C.H.; Chang, P.H.; Hung, Y.S.; Chou, W.C. Venous Thromboembolism in Asian Patients with Pancreatic Cancer Following Palliative Chemotherapy: Low Incidence but a Negative Prognosticator for Those with Early Onset. *Cancers* **2018**, *10*, 501. [CrossRef]
81. Li, Y.; Shang, Y.; Wang, W.; Ning, S.; Chen, H. Lung Cancer and Pulmonary Embolism: What Is the Relationship? A Review. *J. Cancer* **2018**, *9*, 3046–3057. [CrossRef]
82. Raskob, G.E.; van Es, N.; Verhamme, P.; Carrier, M.; Di Nisio, M.; Garcia, D.; Grosso, M.A.; Kakkar, A.K.; Kovacs, M.J.; Mercuri, M.F.; et al. Edoxaban for the Treatment of Cancer-Associated Venous Thromboembolism. *N. Engl. J. Med.* **2018**, *378*, 615–624. [CrossRef] [PubMed]
83. Dangas, G.D.; Tijssen, J.G.P.; Wöhrle, J.; Søndergaard, L.; Gilard, M.; Möllmann, H.; Makkar, R.R.; Herrmann, H.C.; Giustino, G.; Baldus, S.; et al. A Controlled Trial of Rivaroxaban after Transcatheter Aortic-Valve Replacement. *N. Engl. J. Med.* **2019**, *382*, 120–129. [CrossRef] [PubMed]

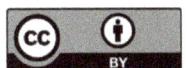

© 2020 by the authors. Licensee MDPI, Basel, Switzerland. This article is an open access article distributed under the terms and conditions of the Creative Commons Attribution (CC BY) license (http://creativecommons.org/licenses/by/4.0/).

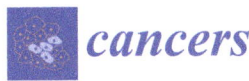

Review

Impact of Tumor Genomic Mutations on Thrombotic Risk in Cancer Patients

Orly Leiva [1,2], Jean M. Connors [2,3] and Hanny Al-Samkari [2,4,*]

1. Department of Medicine, Brigham and Women's Hospital, Boston, MA 02215, USA; oleiva@partners.org
2. Harvard Medical School, Boston, MA 02215, USA; jconnors@bwh.harvard.edu
3. Hematology Division, Brigham and Women's Hospital, Boston, MA 02215, USA
4. Division of Hematology Oncology, Massachusetts General Hospital, Boston, MA 02114, USA
* Correspondence: hal-samkari@mgh.harvard.edu; Tel.: +1-617-643-6214

Received: 3 June 2020; Accepted: 16 July 2020; Published: 19 July 2020

Abstract: Venous thromboembolism (VTE) is common in patients with cancer and is an important contributor to morbidity and mortality in these patients. Early thromboprophylaxis initiated only in those cancer patients at highest risk for VTE would be optimal. Risk stratification scores incorporating tumor location, laboratory values and patient characteristics have attempted to identify those patients most likely to benefit from thromboprophylaxis but even well-validated scores are not able to reliably distinguish the highest-risk patients. Recognizing that tumor genetics affect the biology and behavior of malignancies, recent studies have explored the impact of specific molecular aberrations on the rate of VTE in cancer patients. The presence of certain molecular aberrations in a variety of different cancers, including lung, colon, brain and hematologic tumors, have been associated with an increased risk of VTE and arterial thrombotic events. This review examines the findings of these studies and discusses the implications of these findings on decisions relating to thromboprophylaxis use in the clinical setting. Ultimately, the integration of tumor molecular genomic information into clinical VTE risk stratification scores in cancer patients may prove to be a major advancement in the prevention of cancer-associated thrombosis.

Keywords: molecular subtype; cancer; venous thromboembolism; arterial thrombosis; ALK; ROS1; KRAS

1. Introduction

Thrombotic complications, in particular venous thromboembolism (VTE), are common in patients with cancer where they are a major cause of morbidity and mortality [1]. VTE complicates the clinical course of 5–10% of all cancer patients, with the risk being the greatest during the first year following cancer diagnosis [1,2]. Additionally, cancer patients who have had VTE events have an approximately 4-fold increased risk of death than those without VTE [3].

While thromboprophylaxis would be expected to be of high utility in cancer patients given these statistics, the elevated bleeding risk in this population precludes indiscriminate thromboprophylaxis use [4]. Among those patients receiving anticoagulation, cancer patients have an increased incidence of bleeding compared to non-cancer patients, irrespective of the anticoagulant chosen [5]. Those cancer patients with metastatic disease, gastrointestinal, gynecological or genitourinary malignancies, coagulopathy, thrombocytopenia or a recent major bleeding event have been identified as having the greatest bleeding risk [5]. Primary thromboprophylaxis in cancer patients was initially studied using low molecular weight heparin (LMWH) in the general cancer patient population.

Numerous clinical cancer-associated VTE risk stratification scores have been developed to identify cancer patients with the highest risk of VTE (Table 1). Several of the more well-known scores include the Khorana risk score (the best validated), Vienna Cancer and Thrombosis (CATS), PROTECHT,

CONKO and Tic-ONCO scores [6–10]. These risk scores incorporate patient's histologic tumor type and primary location, prechemotherapy blood counts (hemoglobin, white blood cell and platelets), body mass index (BMI) or performance status, chemotherapy administered and soluble markers (D-dimer and P-selectin). Additionally, the Tic-ONCO score incorporates genetic risk score of germline polymorphisms in the *F5*, *F13* and *SERPINA10* genes [10]. Due to their inability to reliably discriminate between those patients at highest risk for VTE and those with intermediate risk within some cancer types [11,12], the utility of these scores in routine clinical practice is limited.

Table 1. Risk stratification models for venous thromboembolism (VTE) risk in cancer patients. Adapted with permission from Song et al. [13].

Score	Incorporated Risk Factors
Khorana score (KS) [14]	Tumor site of origin: Very high risk: stomach, pancreas High risk: lung, lymphoma, gynecologic, bladder, testicular Prechemotherapy platelet count ≥350 × 10^9/L Hemoglobin level < 10 g/dL or use of erythropoiesis-stimulating agents Prechemotherapy leukocyte count >11 × 10^9/L Body mass index ≥35 kg/m²
Vienna CATS score [7]	KS plus the following: Soluble P-selectin >53.1 ng/L D-dimer ≥1.44 µg/L
PROTECHT score [8]	KS plus the following: Use of platinum-based therapy Use of gemcitabine
CONKO score [9]	Tumor site of origin: Very high risk: stomach, pancreas High risk: lung, lymphoma, gynecologic, bladder, testicular Prechemotherapy platelet count ≥350 × 10^9/L Hemoglobin level < 10 g/dL or use of erythropoiesis-stimulating agents Prechemotherapy leukocyte count >11 × 10^9/L WHO performance status ≥2
Tic-ONCO score [10]	Tumor site of origin: Very high risk: stomach, pancreas High risk: lung, lymphoma, gynecologic, bladder, testicular Genetic risk score (germline polymorphisms in F5, F13 or SERPINA10) Body mass index >25 kg/m² Family history of VTE
ONKOTEV score [15]	KS > 2 Metastatic cancer Personal history of VTE Macroscopic vascular or lymphatic compression
COMPASS-CAT score [16]	Breast, lung, ovarian or colorectal cancer only Cancer-related risk factors: Anthracycline or anti-hormonal therapy in women with breast cancer Time since cancer diagnosis ≤6 months Central venous catheter Advanced cancer stage Predisposing risk factors: Cardiovascular risk factors (≥2 of peripheral artery disease, ischemic stroke, coronary artery disease, hypertension, hyperlipidemia, diabetes, obesity) Recent hospitalization for acute medical illness Personal history of VTE Prechemotherapy platelet count ≥350 × 10^9/L

The advent of routine molecular testing of tumor samples has allowed for the characterization of tumors beyond histological type and location. Given the foundational role of tumor genetics in the behavior and prognosis of tumors, specific mutations or mutational signatures may also play a role in thrombotic risk, and indeed recent studies are beginning to elucidate this link. This review examines the findings of these studies and discusses the implications of these findings on the decisions pertaining to thromboprophylaxis in the clinical setting. Ultimately, the integration of tumor molecular genomic information into clinical VTE risk stratification scores in cancer patients may prove to be a major advancement in the management of cancer-associated thrombosis.

2. Historic and Current Approaches to Patient Selection for Primary Thromboprophylaxis of Cancer-Associated Thrombosis

Several randomized controlled trials have evaluated the use of low molecular weight heparin (LMWH) for primary thromboprophylaxis in patients with cancer. Semuloparin, an ultra-low-molecular weight heparin, was studied for efficacy and safety of thromboprophylaxis in 3212 unselected patients (no risk stratification score was applied to guide selection) with locally advanced or metastatic cancer [17]. After a median follow-up period of 3.5 months, VTE occurred in 1.2% of the semuloparin group and 3.4% of the placebo group with a number needed to treat (NNT) of 45.5 and clinically relevant bleeding occurring in 2.8% of patients receiving semuloparin versus 2.0% receiving placebo [17]. Other studies of LMWH in unselected patients have similarly found NNTs in the 40–50 range [17–21]. When cancer patients at high risk of VTE (Khorana score of three or greater) were selected, LMWH thromboprophylaxis reduced the VTE incidence (12% in LMWH group versus 21% in observation group) but resulted in a seven-fold increase risk of bleeding [21]. Therefore, routine use of LMWH for thromboprophylaxis in cancer patients was not recommended for unselected patients in practice guidelines and is not routinely used in the United States with the possible exception of pancreatic cancer patients undergoing chemotherapy [22].

The advent of direct oral anticoagulant (DOAC) therapy has provided additional options for the treatment and prevention of VTE in cancer patients [13,23] although limitations on reversibility in the case of bleeding remain an ongoing concern. Two large randomized control trials, Apixaban for the Prevention of Venous Thromboembolism in High-Risk Ambulatory Cancer Patients (AVERT) and Rivaroxaban for Thromboprophylaxis in High-Risk Ambulatory Patients with Cancer (CASSINI), investigated the role of thromboprophylaxis in cancer patients deemed to be high risk of VTE (Khorana risk score of ≥ 2) [24,25]. In the AVERT trial, patients with an active malignancy undergoing chemotherapy treatment with a Khorana score of 2 or higher were randomized to apixaban at a dose of 2.5 mg twice a day or placebo for 180 days. In the intention-to-treat analysis, the apixaban group had a reduced incidence of VTE compared to the placebo group (4.2% vs. 10.2%, respectively) at the expense of increased major bleeding (3.5% vs. 1.8%) and clinically relevant non-major bleeding (7.3% vs. 5.5%). There was no difference in overall survival between the two groups, although the trial was not powered to detect a difference. The NNT to prevent VTE (incidental or symptomatic) with apixaban was 17 and the number needed to harm (NNH) for major bleeding was 59 [25]. The CASSINI trial investigated the safety and efficacy of rivaroxaban 10 mg daily in the prevention of cancer associated VTE. In contrast to AVERT, in which patients were not screened for VTE during the trial screening period, participations in CASSINI underwent venous duplex ultrasound screening of VTE in both legs prior to enrollment (and were excluded if an occult VTE was found) and also underwent ultrasound screening every 8 weeks during the study period. Additionally, CASSINI had a higher proportion of pancreatic cancer participants than AVERT (32% vs. 13%, respectively) and AVERT had slightly more patients with Khorana scores of 4 or greater than CASSINI (8.9% vs. 6.6%). In CASSINI, the intention-to-treat analysis found no significant reduction in VTE events in the rivaroxaban group compared to placebo after 180 days and no increased risk of major bleeding [24]. However, in the on-treatment analysis, rivaroxaban did significantly reduce thrombotic events compared to placebo (2.6% vs. 6.4% with a hazard ratio of 0.40). While these trials represent an improvement over the unselected population evaluated in the prior LMWH trials, the overall NNT to prevent one VTE using a Khorana score of 2 or higher and low-dose DOAC therapy was approximately 20–25, with a NNH to cause a major bleed of approximately 75 [26]. These findings suggest that use of the Khorana risk score to guide thromboprophylaxis as was done in AVERT and CASSINI offers a clear tradeoff: prevent three VTE events for every major bleed caused by thromboprophylaxis. Thus, even with the use of the best-validated existing risk-prediction model, optimal patient selection for primary thromboprophylaxis remains challenging.

3. Molecular Aberrations Associated with Increased Thrombotic Risk

The discovery of targetable driver mutations and distinct molecular subtypes in most common cancers has revolutionized clinical oncology. Although decades of data and study have been devoted to targeting driver tumor genomic aberrations with mutation-specific treatments and understanding how different genotypes respond to traditional cancer treatments, our understanding of the contribution of tumor genomics to thrombotic risk is still in its early stages. Nonetheless, several studies have evaluated the contribution of certain molecular aberrations in several tumor types. Specific aberrations of interest are summarized in Table 2 and described in greater detail below.

Table 2. Molecular aberrations associated with increased thromboembolic risk.

Genetic Mutation	Tumor type	Incidence of VTE	Comments	References
ALK rearrangement	Lung	26.9% to 47.1%	2.2-to-5-fold increase compared to no *ALK* rearrangement	[27–32]
ROS1 rearrangement	Lung	34.6% to 41.6%	3-to-5-fold increase compared to no *ROS1* rearrangement	[33,34]
EGFR mutation	Lung	9% to 35%	Data conflicts; also associated with possible reduced risk of VTE	[28,32,35–38]
KRAS mutation	Lung, colon	16.1% to 54%	2.6-fold increase	[28,36,38,39]
JAK2 V617F mutation	Hematopoietic (myeloproliferative neoplasm)	12%	2-fold increase compared to *CALR* or triple negative	[40,41]
IDH1/IDH2 wild type	Brain	18.2% to 25.6%	Mutant *IDH1/IDH2* associated with decreased VTE risk	[42,43]

3.1. Lung Cancer

Lung cancer has been historically associated with an intermediate risk of VTE compared to other malignancies, with a risk of approximately 7–13% [6,44]. A meta-analysis of randomized controlled trials of thromboprophylaxis in lung cancer showed a reduction of thrombosis with prophylactic anticoagulation (NNT of 25) at the expense of increased bleeding risk and no effect on overall survival [45]. Prior studies have demonstrated that the Khorana risk score poorly discriminates between patients with lung cancer at high versus intermediate risk of VTE [11,12]. However, recent evidence has suggested that certain molecular subtypes of lung cancer may have a considerably higher thrombotic risk. Non-small cell lung cancer (NSCLC) patients with rearrangements in the anaplastic lymphoma kinase (*ALK*) and c-ros oncogene1 (*ROS1*) genes have been shown in multiple studies to have an increased risk of VTE events.

The *ALK* rearrangement occurs in 5% of NSCLC patients [46]. Hypercoagulability including recurrent thrombosis despite adequate anticoagulation and disseminated intravascular coagulation have been described in *ALK*-rearranged NSCLC [47–49]. Several initial studies (ranging in size from 17 to 241 patients with the *ALK* rearrangement) suggested an increased risk of VTE in *ALK*-rearranged NSCLC, although findings were not consistent (VTE rates ranged from 8% to 47%, Table 3) [27–32,35,50]. A recently-published large cohort study (807 advanced NSCLC patients, including 422 patients with the *ALK* rearrangement and 385 without the *ALK* rearrangement as a control group) utilizing multivariable time-to-event regression analyses (Cox proportional hazards model) and multivariable time-to-event regression analyses accounting for the competing risk of death (model of Fine and Gray) confirmed an increased VTE rate, finding an approximate four-fold increase in VTE risk for patients with the ALK rearrangement relative to those without (Cox model: hazard ratio (HR) 3.70 (95% CI, 2.51-5.44, $p < 0.001$); competing-risks: subhazard ratio (SHR) 3.91 (95% CI, 2.55–5.99, $p < 0.001$)) [51]. Negative binomial modeling demonstrated higher overall VTE rates in patients with the *ALK* rearrangement, reflective of the much higher rates of single and multiple VTE recurrence in this population (incidence rate ratio 2.47 (95% CI, 1.72–3.55, $p < 0.001$)) and the odds ratio (OR) for recurrent VTE was 4.85 (95% CI 2.60 to 9.52, $p < 0.001$). Additionally, utilizing similar methodology, this study also found an approximate three-fold increase in risk of arterial thrombotic events in patients with the *ALK* rearrangement compared to those without (Cox model: HR 3.15 (95% CI, 1.18–8.37, $p = 0.021$); competing-risks: SHR 2.80 (95% CI, 1.06–7.43, $p = 0.038$)). Strikingly, although patients with the *ALK* rearrangement were nearly two decades younger on average than the non-*ALK* control group, with fewer co-morbidities and lower rates of nearly every arterial and venous thrombotic risk factor, they still had higher venous and arterial thrombotic rates, strongly suggestive of a major role for the *ALK* rearrangement in increasing thrombotic risk.

ROS1 is an oncogene that encodes an orphan receptor tyrosine kinase that is related to *ALK*. The *ROS1* rearrangement occurs in approximately 2% of NSCLC and has also been associated with increased VTE risk that may be comparable to the risk in *ALK*-rearranged lung cancer [34,52]. Patients with *ROS1*- and *ALK*-rearranged NSCLC have similar demographics, including that a majority have never smoked (77.7% and 77.2%, respectively) [34,53,54]. Incidence of thrombotic events among a retrospective cohort study involving 95 *ROS1* and 193 *ALK* rearranged NSCLC patients was 34.7% and 22.3% respectively [34]. A multivariable logistic regression analysis comparing *ROS1* and *ALK* rearranged NSCLC showed no significant difference in the odds of thrombotic events between the two groups. However, in similar analyses, *ROS1* patients had an approximately two-fold increase in odds of thrombotic events compared to patients with *EGFR*- or *KRAS*-mutant NSCLC in the same study [34]. Additionally, a subanalysis of the Crizotinib in the Pretreated Metastatic NSCL With *MET* Amplification or *ROS1* Translocation (METROS) trial including 48 *ROS1*-rearranged patients and 26 *MET*-mutated NSCLC patients demonstrated that *ROS1*-rearranged patients had an increased incidence of VTE compared to *MET*-mutated patients (41.6% vs. 15.3%) [33].

Mutations in *KRAS* and epidermal growth factor receptor (*EGFR*) genes have been studied in the context of VTE risk, with conflicting findings. Compared to patients with *ROS1* and *ALK* rearrangements, patients with *EGFR* and *KRAS* mutations had a lower risk of thrombotic events [34]. In one study of post-operative NSCLC patients, mutations in *EGFR* were associated with increased VTE risk [37]. However, another study in Chinese NSCLC patients showed that wild type *EGFR* NSCLC had a higher VTE risk than mutated *EGFR* [36]. Mutations in the *KRAS* gene have also been associated with increased VTE risk in NSCLC patients in one small trial [38]. However other trials have failed to confirm this increased VTE risk in patients with *KRAS* mutated NSCLC [28,36].

Table 3. *ALK* Rearrangement in Non-Small Cell Lung Cancer (NSCLC) is Associated with Increased Thrombotic Risk.

Study	Study Design	N of Patients with ALK	Median Follow-Up	VTE Rate	Arterial Thrombosis Rate	Hazard Ratio vs. Non-ALK Rearranged	Comments
Zer et al. [27]	Retrospective	55	22 months	42%	Not reported	2.06 (95% CI 1.08–3.55)	Small number of patients, did not employ survival analysis
Verso et al. [28]	Retrospective	17	Not mentioned	47.1%	Not reported	2.45	Stage III and IV patients, only included pulmonary emboli. ALK rearrangement, KRAS and EGFR mutations compared to wild type. Only ALK rearrangement had significant increased risk of PE compared to wild type
Lee et al. [29]	Retrospective	24	45.6 months	Not reported	Not reported	2.47 (95% CI 1.04–5.90)	Small number of patients, only HR reported (VTE rate not reported)
Dou et al. [30]	Prospective	26	7.5 months	26.9%	Not reported	Not reported	Short follow-up, only prospective study, but small number of patients with *ALK* rearrangement. Multivariable time-to-event analyses.
Zugazagoitia et al. [31]	Retrospective	241	30 months	30%	5%	ROS1 vs ALK rearrangement: 1.45 (95% CI 0.79–2.64)	Only included patients with stage III and IV ALK rearrangements and no control group. Studied arterial events.
Ng et al. [34]	Retrospective	193	19.9 months	22.3%	9.8%	Not reported	Compared *ALK* rearranged, *ROS1* rearranged, KRAS and EGFR NSCLC. Multivariable logistic regression analysis.
Gervaso et al. [32]	Retrospective	46	33.1 months	43.5%	Not reported	VTE: 3.70 (95% CI, 2.51–5.44) Arterial: 3.15 (95% CI, 1.18–8.37)	Compared *ALK* rearranged, EGFR and wild type NSCLC patients. urvival analysis
Al-Samkari et al. [51]	Retrospective	422	31 months	42.7%	5%		Non-resectable stage III and IV ALK rearranged and non-ALK-rearranged NSCLC. Employed multivariable time-to-event analyses (Cox proportional hazards, competing risks model of Fine and Gray).

3.2. Colon Cancer

As with lung cancer, colorectal cancer (CRC) is associated with an intermediate risk of VTE [6]. Thromboprophylaxis in CRC may be complicated by the anti-angiogenic therapies commonly used to treat patients with metastatic disease, which can be associated with increased bleeding and thrombotic risk [55,56]. Mutations in the *KRAS* oncogene are found in approximately thirty to fifty percent of CRC [57]. *KRAS* mutations in CRC have been associated with increased risk of VTE compared to wild type *KRAS* [39]. In one study of 172 patients with metastatic CRC (65 *KRAS* mutated and 107 *KRAS* wild type), VTE occurred in 32.3% of patients with *KRAS* mutations compared to 17.8% of patients with wild type *KRAS* (odds ratio of 2.21, 95% confidence internal 1.08–4.53) [39].

3.3. Myeloproliferative Neoplasms

Myeloproliferative neoplasms (MPNs) are clonal stem cell disorders and include essential thrombocythemia (ET), polycythemia vera (PV) and primary myelofibrosis (PMF), among others [58]. Mutations in the Janus kinase 2 (*JAK2*), myeloproliferative leukemia virus (*MPL*) and calreticulin (*CALR*) genes are found in the majority of patients with these three classic MPNs and all lead to hyperactivity of the JAK-STAT signaling pathway normally involved in inflammatory signaling and hematopoietic cell proliferation [59]. Thrombotic and hemorrhagic complications are commonly seen in these patients with approximately 18% of patients developing thrombotic events during a 10 year period [60–62]. In a study of 891 patients with ET, the presence of the *JAK2* V617F mutation, the most common mutation in MPNs, was associated with a two-fold increase in the risk of VTE and arterial thrombosis compared to patients without a *JAK* 2V617F mutation (hazard ratio of 2.04 with 95% confidence interval of 1.19–3.48) [40]. Patients with PMF and *CALR* mutations or triple-negative disease (absence of *JAK2*, *MPL* or *CALR* mutations) disease have been found to have lower rates of cardiovascular events compared to patients with *JAK2* V617F mutations with rates of 0.00%, 0.80%, 0.95% and 2.52% in patients with triple negative, *CALR*-mutant, *MPL*-mutant and *JAK2* V617F-mutant disease, respectively [63]. The risk of thrombotic events is approximately two-fold lower in *CALR*-mutated PMF compared to *JAK2* V617 despite higher platelet counts and a longer overall survival in patients with *CALR* mutated PMF [41]. Though subclonal mutations in *TET2* and *ASXL1* are associated with increased risk of leukemic transformation in certain MPN patients, these mutations have not been associated with increased thrombosis risk [64,65].

3.4. Primary Brain Cancer

Primary brain tumors are associated with a high risk of VTE and a particularly morbid bleeding risk, making decisions about primary thromboprophylaxis more challenging [66,67]. Mutations in isocitrate dehydrogenase 1 or 2 (*IDH1/2*) are commonly found in primary brain tumors (more than 70% in grade II and III astrocytomas and oligodendrogliomas) and are associated with better prognosis [68]. In one retrospective study involving gliomas that were tested for *IDH1/2* mutations, gliomas with wild type *IDH1/2* had a cumulative incidence of VTE of 26% compared to none with mutated *IDH1/2* [42]. Additionally, increased expression of brain tumor podoplanin has been found to be associated with increased risk of VTE in patients with primary brain cancer [69]. A combination of *IDH1/2* mutation status and podoplanin expression may be helpful in identifying those patients with primary brain cancer who are at high risk of VTE with those having wild type *IDH1* and high podoplanin expression having the highest risk and those with mutant *IDH1* tumors and absent podoplanin expression having the lowest (18.2% six month risk of VTE versus 0%, respectively) [43].

4. Potential Mechanisms of Increased Thrombotic Risk

Tumor mutational status may influence thrombogenesis through various potential mechanisms. The tissue factor is an important physiologic trigger of coagulation and its upregulation in certain malignancies likely contributes to the prothrombotic state of malignancy [70,71]. Mutations in *KRAS* have been associated with increased tumor tissue factor expression in CRC and lung cancer [72,73]. Mutations in *IDH1* led to hypermethylation of the F3 promoter of the tissue factor gene leading to decreased expression and may explain the decreased risk of VTE in primary brain cancer patients with mutant *IDH1* [42,74]. Inflammation is known to induce a prothrombotic state and might play a role in cancer associated VTE [75,76]. The mechanisms behind *ALK* rearrangement and increased thrombotic risk in NSCLC are unclear but some studies in lymphomas with *ALK* mutations suggest the *ALK* rearrangement results in increased STAT3 signaling and inflammation [77]. *ALK* fusion proteins activate STAT3, which participates in downstream signaling of inflammatory cytokines. *ALK* has also been shown to be important in the activation of the NLRP3 inflammasome in macrophages [78]. The mechanisms behind increased thrombotic risk in MPNs may also be related to increased JAK-STAT signaling and inflammation [60]. Other potential mechanisms for thrombosis include the upregulation of lysyl oxidase (LOX), an enzyme more commonly known to be involved in collagen cross-linking but may also increase platelet reactivity and thrombosis risk [79–81]. Nasser and colleagues provide a comprehensive review of the mechanisms behind hypercoagulability in cancer patients that is beyond the scope of this review [82].

5. Implications of Tumor Molecular Aberrations on the Use of Primary Thromboprophylaxis

Balancing the scales of bleeding and thrombotic risk in the cancer patient presents unique challenges [83]. Although we have the various cancer-associated VTE risk stratification scores, the present and future bleeding risk must be considered, including risks associated with radiation therapy, chemotherapy-induced thrombocytopenia and other concerns. Although most studies to date have been retrospective and observational, large cohorts have demonstrated significantly increased risk of thrombosis in patients with *ALK* and *ROS1* rearranged NSCLC compared to those without those rearrangements. Therefore, clinicians may contemplate a lower threshold to consider thromboprophylaxis in patients with NSCLC and either *ALK* or *ROS1* rearrangement who otherwise have traditional risk scores in the intermediate risk range. Similarly, in the case of molecular aberrations in other tumors (Table 2), knowledge that a patient may be at increased thrombotic risk due to their underlying tumor genotype is another piece of information that the treating clinician can consider when determining if a patient may be likely to benefit from thromboprophylaxis, along with traditional thrombotic risk factors such as elevated BMI, previous VTE and known hereditary thrombophilia. Further studies on incorporating tumor molecular aberrations into traditional risk scores may enhance the ability of risk scores to identify the patients most likely to benefit from primary thromboprophylaxis.

6. Conclusions

Thrombosis greatly contributes to morbidity and mortality in cancer patients. The use of thromboprophylaxis in clinical practice is based on the balance of benefit and risk of bleeding. Despite recent advances in primary thromboprophylaxis of cancer patients, the current tools available for patient selection are suboptimal given increased bleeding risk that may outweigh any benefit [26]. Available risk stratification scores appear to be inadequate for many groups of patients [11,12]. A reason for this could be the lack of consideration of underlying tumor biology mutational status of the primary tumor. Molecular aberrations involving various driver mutations including *ALK, ROS1, KRAS, IDH1/2* and *JAK2* may impact thrombotic risk in various tumor types. Additional study is needed to understand the precise role that tumor genetics plays in the risk of venous and arterial thrombotic events across the spectrum of malignancies. This could allow for the refinement of clinical risk stratification tools that could improve our ability to select patients for primary thromboprophylaxis.

Author Contributions: O.L. wrote the first draft of the manuscript and contributed to creation of the tables and figures and final approval. J.M.C. contributed to critical revision of the manuscript and final approval. H.A.-S. contributed to concept and design, creation of the tables and figures, critical revision of the manuscript, and final approval. All authors have read and agreed to the published version of the manuscript.

Funding: This research received no external funding

Acknowledgments: H. Al-Samkari is the recipient of the National Hemophilia Foundation-Shire Clinical Fellowship Award, the Harvard Catalyst Medical Research Investigator Training Award, and the American Society of Hematology Scholar Award. O. Leiva is a recipient of the American Society of Hematology Minority Resident Hematology Award Program.

Conflicts of Interest: O.L.: None. J.M.C: Bristol-Myers Squibb (Scientific Advisory Board, Consultant, Personal Fees); Unum Therapeutics (Data Safety Monitoring Board); Portola (Scientific Advisory Boards). H.A: Agios (Consultancy, Research Funding to Institution), Dova (Consultancy, Research Funding to Institution), Amgen (Research Funding to Institution).

References

1. Blom, J.W.; Doggen, C.J.; Osanto, S.; Rosendaal, F.R. Malignancies, prothrombotic mutations, and the risk of venous thrombosis. *JAMA* **2005**, *293*, 715–722. [CrossRef] [PubMed]
2. Timp, J.F.; Braekkan, S.K.; Versteeg, H.H.; Cannegieter, S.C. Epidemiology of cancer-associated venous thrombosis. *Blood* **2013**, *122*, 1712–1723. [CrossRef] [PubMed]
3. Sorensen, H.T.; Mellemkjaer, L.; Olsen, J.H.; Baron, J.A. Prognosis of cancers associated with venous thromboembolism. *N. Engl. J. Med.* **2000**, *343*, 1846–1850. [CrossRef] [PubMed]
4. Lyman, G.H.; Khorana, A.A.; Kuderer, N.M.; Lee, A.Y.; Arcelus, J.I.; Balaban, E.P.; Clarke, J.M.; Flowers, C.R.; Francis, C.W.; Gates, L.E.; et al. Venous thromboembolism prophylaxis and treatment in patients with cancer: American Society of Clinical Oncology clinical practice guideline update. *J. Clin. Oncol.* **2013**, *31*, 2189–2204. [CrossRef] [PubMed]
5. Angelini, D.E.; Radivoyevitch, T.; McCrae, K.R.; Khorana, A.A. Bleeding incidence and risk factors among cancer patients treated with anticoagulation. *Am. J. Hematol.* **2019**, *94*, 780–785. [CrossRef] [PubMed]
6. Khorana, A.A.; Kuderer, N.M.; Culakova, E.; Lyman, G.H.; Francis, C.W. Development and validation of a predictive model for chemotherapy-associated thrombosis. *Blood* **2008**, *111*, 4902–4907. [CrossRef]
7. Ay, C.; Dunkler, D.; Marosi, C.; Chiriac, A.L.; Vormittag, R.; Simanek, R.; Quehenberger, P.; Zielinski, C.; Pabinger, I. Prediction of venous thromboembolism in cancer patients. *Blood* **2010**, *116*, 5377–5382. [CrossRef]
8. Verso, M.; Agnelli, G.; Barni, S.; Gasparini, G.; LaBianca, R. A modified Khorana risk assessment score for venous thromboembolism in cancer patients receiving chemotherapy: The Protecht score. *Intern. Emerg. Med.* **2012**, *7*, 291–292. [CrossRef]
9. Pelzer, U.; Sinn, M.; Stieler, J.; Riess, H. Primary pharmacological prevention of thromboembolic events in ambulatory patients with advanced pancreatic cancer treated with chemotherapy? *Dtsch. Med. Wochenschr.* **2013**, *138*, 2084–2088. [CrossRef]
10. Munoz Martin, A.J.; Ortega, I.; Font, C.; Pachon, V.; Castellon, V.; Martinez-Marin, V.; Salgado, M.; Martinez, E.; Calzas, J.; Ruperez, A.; et al. Multivariable clinical-genetic risk model for predicting venous thromboembolic events in patients with cancer. *Br. J. Cancer* **2018**, *118*, 1056–1061. [CrossRef]
11. Van Es, N.; Di Nisio, M.; Cesarman, G.; Kleinjan, A.; Otten, H.M.; Mahe, I.; Wilts, I.T.; Twint, D.C.; Porreca, E.; Arrieta, O.; et al. Comparison of risk prediction scores for venous thromboembolism in cancer patients: A prospective cohort study. *Haematologica* **2017**, *102*, 1494–1501. [CrossRef] [PubMed]
12. Mansfield, A.S.; Tafur, A.J.; Wang, C.E.; Kourelis, T.V.; Wysokinska, E.M.; Yang, P. Predictors of active cancer thromboembolic outcomes: Validation of the Khorana score among patients with lung cancer. *J. Thromb. Haemost.* **2016**, *14*, 1773–1778. [CrossRef] [PubMed]
13. Song, A.B.; Rosovsky, R.P.; Connors, J.M.; Al-Samkari, H. Direct oral anticoagulants for treatment and prevention of venous thromboembolism in cancer patients. *Vasc. Health Risk Manag.* **2019**, *15*, 175–186. [CrossRef] [PubMed]
14. Khorana, A.A.; Francis, C.W. Risk prediction of cancer-associated thrombosis: Appraising the first decade and developing the future. *Thromb. Res.* **2018**, *164* (Suppl. S1), S70–S76. [CrossRef]
15. Cella, C.A.; Di Minno, G.; Carlomagno, C.; Arcopinto, M.; Cerbone, A.M.; Matano, E.; Tufano, A.; Lordick, F.; De Simone, B.; Muehlberg, K.S.; et al. Preventing Venous Thromboembolism in Ambulatory Cancer Patients: The ONKOTEV Study. *Oncologist* **2017**, *22*, 601–608. [CrossRef] [PubMed]
16. Gerotziafas, G.T.; Taher, A.; Abdel-Razeq, H.; AboElnazar, E.; Spyropoulos, A.C.; El Shemmari, S.; Larsen, A.K.; Elalamy, I.; Group, C.-C.W. A Predictive Score for Thrombosis Associated with Breast, Colorectal, Lung, or Ovarian Cancer: The Prospective COMPASS-Cancer-Associated Thrombosis Study. *Oncologist* **2017**, *22*, 1222–1231. [CrossRef]

17. Agnelli, G.; George, D.J.; Kakkar, A.K.; Fisher, W.; Lassen, M.R.; Mismetti, P.; Mouret, P.; Chaudhari, U.; Lawson, F.; Turpie, A.G.; et al. Semuloparin for thromboprophylaxis in patients receiving chemotherapy for cancer. *N. Engl. J. Med.* **2012**, *366*, 601–609. [CrossRef]
18. Eck, R.J.; Bult, W.; Wetterslev, J.; Gans, R.O.B.; Meijer, K.; Keus, F.; van der Horst, I.C.C. Intermediate Dose Low-Molecular-Weight Heparin for Thrombosis Prophylaxis: Systematic Review with Meta-Analysis and Trial Sequential Analysis. *Semin. Thromb. Hemost.* **2019**, *45*, 810–824. [CrossRef]
19. Eck, R.J.; Bult, W.; Wetterslev, J.; Gans, R.O.B.; Meijer, K.; van der Horst, I.C.C.; Keus, F. Low Dose Low-Molecular-Weight Heparin for Thrombosis Prophylaxis: Systematic Review with Meta-Analysis and Trial Sequential Analysis. *J. Clin. Med.* **2019**, *8*, 2039. [CrossRef]
20. Ben-Aharon, I.; Stemmer, S.M.; Leibovici, L.; Shpilberg, O.; Sulkes, A.; Gafter-Gvili, A. Low molecular weight heparin (LMWH) for primary thrombo-prophylaxis in patients with solid malignancies—Systematic review and meta-analysis. *Acta Oncol.* **2014**, *53*, 1230–1237. [CrossRef]
21. Khorana, A.A.; Francis, C.W.; Kuderer, N.M.; Carrier, M.; Ortel, T.L.; Wun, T.; Rubens, D.; Hobbs, S.; Iyer, R.; Peterson, D.; et al. Dalteparin thromboprophylaxis in cancer patients at high risk for venous thromboembolism: A randomized trial. *Thromb. Res.* **2017**, *151*, 89–95. [CrossRef] [PubMed]
22. Farge, D.; Bournet, B.; Conroy, T.; Vicaut, E.; Rak, J.; Zogoulous, G.; Barkun, J.; Ouaissi, M.; Buscail, L.; Frere, C. Primary Thromboprophylaxis in Pancreatic Cancer Patients: Why Clinical Practice Guidelines Should Be Implemented. *Cancers* **2020**, *12*, 618. [CrossRef] [PubMed]
23. Al-Samkari, H.; Connors, J.M. The Role of Direct Oral Anticoagulants in Treatment of Cancer-Associated Thrombosis. *Cancers* **2018**, *10*, 271. [CrossRef] [PubMed]
24. Khorana, A.A.; Soff, G.A.; Kakkar, A.K.; Vadhan-Raj, S.; Riess, H.; Wun, T.; Streiff, M.B.; Garcia, D.A.; Liebman, H.A.; Belani, C.P.; et al. Rivaroxaban for Thromboprophylaxis in High-Risk Ambulatory Patients with Cancer. *N. Engl. J. Med.* **2019**, *380*, 720–728. [CrossRef]
25. Carrier, M.; Abou-Nassar, K.; Mallick, R.; Tagalakis, V.; Shivakumar, S.; Schattner, A.; Kuruvilla, P.; Hill, D.; Spadafora, S.; Marquis, K.; et al. Apixaban to Prevent Venous Thromboembolism in Patients with Cancer. *N. Engl. J. Med.* **2019**, *380*, 711–719. [CrossRef]
26. Agnelli, G. Direct Oral Anticoagulants for Thromboprophylaxis in Ambulatory Patients with Cancer. *N. Engl. J. Med.* **2019**, *380*, 781–783. [CrossRef]
27. Zer, A.; Moskovitz, M.; Hwang, D.M.; Hershko-Klement, A.; Fridel, L.; Korpanty, G.J.; Dudnik, E.; Peled, N.; Shochat, T.; Leighl, N.B.; et al. ALK-Rearranged Non-Small-Cell Lung Cancer Is Associated With a High Rate of Venous Thromboembolism. *Clin. Lung Cancer* **2017**, *18*, 156–161. [CrossRef]
28. Verso, M.; Chiari, R.; Mosca, S.; Franco, L.; Fischer, M.; Paglialunga, L.; Bennati, C.; Scialpi, M.; Agnelli, G. Incidence of Ct scan-detected pulmonary embolism in patients with oncogene-addicted, advanced lung adenocarcinoma. *Thromb. Res.* **2015**, *136*, 924–927. [CrossRef]
29. Lee, Y.G.; Kim, I.; Lee, E.; Bang, S.M.; Kang, C.H.; Kim, Y.T.; Kim, H.J.; Wu, H.G.; Kim, Y.W.; Kim, T.M.; et al. Risk factors and prognostic impact of venous thromboembolism in Asian patients with non-small cell lung cancer. *Thromb. Haemost.* **2014**, *111*, 1112–1120. [CrossRef]
30. Dou, F.; Zhang, Y.; Yi, J.; Zhu, M.; Zhang, S.; Zhang, D.; Zhang, Y. Association of ALK rearrangement and risk of venous thromboembolism in patients with non-small cell lung cancer: A prospective cohort study. *Thromb. Res.* **2020**, *186*, 36–41. [CrossRef]
31. Zugazagoitia, J.; Biosca, M.; Oliveira, J.; Olmedo, M.E.; Domine, M.; Nadal, E.; Ruffinelli, J.C.; Munoz, N.; Luna, A.M.; Hernandez, B.; et al. Incidence, predictors and prognostic significance of thromboembolic disease in patients with advanced ALK-rearranged non-small cell lung cancer. *Eur. Respir. J.* **2018**, *51*. [CrossRef] [PubMed]
32. Gervaso, L.P.S.; Roopkumar, J.; Reddy, C.; Pennell, N.; Velcheti, V.; McCrae, K.; Khorana, A. Molecular Subtyping to Predict Risk of Venous Thromboembolism in Patients with Advanced Lung Adenocarcinoma: A Cohort Study. *Blood* **2019**, *131*, 3651. [CrossRef]
33. Chiari, R.; Ricciuti, B.; Landi, L.; Morelli, A.M.; Delmonte, A.; Spitaleri, G.; Cortinovis, D.L.; Lamberti, G.; Facchinetti, F.; Pilotto, S.; et al. ROS1-rearranged Non-small-cell Lung Cancer is Associated With a High Rate of Venous Thromboembolism: Analysis From a Phase II, Prospective, Multicenter, Two-arms Trial (METROS). *Clin. Lung Cancer* **2020**, *21*, 15–20. [CrossRef] [PubMed]

34. Ng, T.L.; Smith, D.E.; Mushtaq, R.; Patil, T.; Dimou, A.; Yang, S.; Liu, Q.; Li, X.; Zhou, C.; Jones, R.T.; et al. ROS1 Gene Rearrangements Are Associated With an Elevated Risk of Peridiagnosis Thromboembolic Events. *J. Thorac. Oncol.* **2019**, *14*, 596–605. [CrossRef] [PubMed]

35. Davidsson, E.; Murgia, N.; Ortiz-Villalon, C.; Wiklundh, E.; Skold, M.; Kolbeck, K.G.; Ferrara, G. Mutational status predicts the risk of thromboembolic events in lung adenocarcinoma. *Multidiscip. Respir. Med.* **2017**, *12*, 16. [CrossRef] [PubMed]

36. Dou, F.; Li, H.; Zhu, M.; Liang, L.; Zhang, Y.; Yi, J.; Zhang, Y. Association between oncogenic status and risk of venous thromboembolism in patients with non-small cell lung cancer. *Respir. Res.* **2018**, *19*, 88. [CrossRef]

37. Wang, J.; Hu, B.; Li, T.; Miao, J.; Zhang, W.; Chen, S.; Sun, Y.; Cui, S.; Li, H. The EGFR-rearranged adenocarcinoma is associated with a high rate of venous thromboembolism. *Ann. Transl. Med.* **2019**, *7*, 724. [CrossRef]

38. Corrales-Rodriguez, L.; Soulieres, D.; Weng, X.; Tehfe, M.; Florescu, M.; Blais, N. Mutations in NSCLC and their link with lung cancer-associated thrombosis: A case-control study. *Thromb. Res.* **2014**, *133*, 48–51. [CrossRef]

39. Ades, S.; Kumar, S.; Alam, M.; Goodwin, A.; Weckstein, D.; Dugan, M.; Ashikaga, T.; Evans, M.; Verschraegen, C.; Holmes, C.E. Tumor oncogene (KRAS) status and risk of venous thrombosis in patients with metastatic colorectal cancer. *J. Thromb. Haemost.* **2015**, *13*, 998–1003. [CrossRef]

40. Carobbio, A.; Thiele, J.; Passamonti, F.; Rumi, E.; Ruggeri, M.; Rodeghiero, F.; Randi, M.L.; Bertozzi, I.; Vannucchi, A.M.; Antonioli, E.; et al. Risk factors for arterial and venous thrombosis in WHO-defined essential thrombocythemia: An international study of 891 patients. *Blood* **2011**, *117*, 5857–5859. [CrossRef]

41. Rumi, E.; Pietra, D.; Pascutto, C.; Guglielmelli, P.; Martinez-Trillos, A.; Casetti, I.; Colomer, D.; Pieri, L.; Pratcorona, M.; Rotunno, G.; et al. Clinical effect of driver mutations of JAK2, CALR, or MPL in primary myelofibrosis. *Blood* **2014**, *124*, 1062–1069. [CrossRef] [PubMed]

42. Unruh, D.; Schwarze, S.R.; Khoury, L.; Thomas, C.; Wu, M.; Chen, L.; Chen, R.; Liu, Y.; Schwartz, M.A.; Amidei, C.; et al. Mutant IDH1 and thrombosis in gliomas. *Acta Neuropathol.* **2016**, *132*, 917–930. [CrossRef] [PubMed]

43. Mir Seyed Nazari, P.; Riedl, J.; Preusser, M.; Posch, F.; Thaler, J.; Marosi, C.; Birner, P.; Ricken, G.; Hainfellner, J.A.; Pabinger, I.; et al. Combination of isocitrate dehydrogenase 1 (IDH1) mutation and podoplanin expression in brain tumors identifies patients at high or low risk of venous thromboembolism. *J. Thromb. Haemost.* **2018**, *16*, 1121–1127. [CrossRef]

44. Ay, C.; Unal, U.K. Epidemiology and risk factors for venous thromboembolism in lung cancer. *Curr. Opin. Oncol.* **2016**, *28*, 145–149. [CrossRef] [PubMed]

45. Thein, K.Z.; Yeung, S.J.; Oo, T.H. Primary thromboprophylaxis (PTP) in ambulatory patients with lung cancer receiving chemotherapy: A systematic review and meta-analysis of randomized controlled trials (RCTs). *Asia Pac. J. Clin. Oncol.* **2018**, *14*, 210–216. [CrossRef] [PubMed]

46. Takeuchi, K.; Choi, Y.L.; Soda, M.; Inamura, K.; Togashi, Y.; Hatano, S.; Enomoto, M.; Takada, S.; Yamashita, Y.; Satoh, Y.; et al. Multiplex reverse transcription-PCR screening for EML4-ALK fusion transcripts. *Clin. Cancer Res.* **2008**, *14*, 6618–6624. [CrossRef] [PubMed]

47. Al-Samkari, H.; Connors, J.M. Dual anticoagulation with fondaparinux and dabigatran for treatment of cancer-associated hypercoagulability. *Am. J. Hematol.* **2018**, *93*, E156–E158. [CrossRef]

48. De Giglio, A.; Porreca, R.; Brambilla, M.; Metro, G.; Prosperi, E.; Bellezza, G.; Pirro, M.; Chiari, R.; Ricciuti, B. Fatal acute disseminated intravascular coagulation as presentation of advanced ALK-positive non-small cell lung cancer: Does oncogene addiction matter? *Thromb. Res.* **2018**, *163*, 51–53. [CrossRef]

49. Yoshida, T.; Hida, T.; Yatabe, Y. Rapid and dramatic response to alectinib in an anaplastic lymphoma kinase rearranged non-small-cell lung cancer patient who is critically ill. *Anticancer Drugs* **2016**, *27*, 573–575. [CrossRef]

50. Alexander, M.; Solomon, B.; Burbury, K. Thromboembolism in Anaplastic Lymphoma Kinase-Rearranged Non-Small Cell Lung Cancer. *Clin. Lung Cancer* **2018**, *19*, e71–e72. [CrossRef]

51. Al-Samkari, H.; Leiva, O.; Dagogo-Jack, I.; Shaw, A.T.; Lennerz, J.; Iafrate, A.J.; Bendapudi, P.K.; Connors, J.M. Impact of ALK Rearrangement on Venous and Arterial Thrombotic Risk in Non-Small Cell Lung Cancer. *J. Thorac. Oncol.* **2020**. [CrossRef]

52. Gainor, J.F.; Shaw, A.T. Novel targets in non-small cell lung cancer: ROS1 and RET fusions. *Oncologist* **2013**, *18*, 865–875. [CrossRef] [PubMed]

53. Bergethon, K.; Shaw, A.T.; Ou, S.H.; Katayama, R.; Lovly, C.M.; McDonald, N.T.; Massion, P.P.; Siwak-Tapp, C.; Gonzalez, A.; Fang, R.; et al. ROS1 rearrangements define a unique molecular class of lung cancers. *J. Clin. Oncol.* **2012**, *30*, 863–870. [CrossRef] [PubMed]
54. Shaw, A.T.; Ou, S.H.; Bang, Y.J.; Camidge, D.R.; Solomon, B.J.; Salgia, R.; Riely, G.J.; Varella-Garcia, M.; Shapiro, G.I.; Costa, D.B.; et al. Crizotinib in ROS1-rearranged non-small-cell lung cancer. *N. Engl. J. Med.* **2014**, *371*, 1963–1971. [CrossRef] [PubMed]
55. Nalluri, S.R.; Chu, D.; Keresztes, R.; Zhu, X.; Wu, S. Risk of venous thromboembolism with the angiogenesis inhibitor bevacizumab in cancer patients: A meta-analysis. *JAMA* **2008**, *300*, 2277–2285. [CrossRef]
56. Hurwitz, H.I.; Saltz, L.B.; Van Cutsem, E.; Cassidy, J.; Wiedemann, J.; Sirzen, F.; Lyman, G.H.; Rohr, U.P. Venous thromboembolic events with chemotherapy plus bevacizumab: A pooled analysis of patients in randomized phase II and III studies. *J. Clin. Oncol.* **2011**, *29*, 1757–1764. [CrossRef]
57. Andreyev, H.J.; Norman, A.R.; Cunningham, D.; Oates, J.; Dix, B.R.; Iacopetta, B.J.; Young, J.; Walsh, T.; Ward, R.; Hawkins, N.; et al. Kirsten ras mutations in patients with colorectal cancer: The 'RASCAL II' study. *Br. J. Cancer* **2001**, *85*, 692–696. [CrossRef]
58. Spivak, J.L. Myeloproliferative Neoplasms. *N. Engl. J. Med.* **2017**, *376*, 2168–2181. [CrossRef]
59. Palumbo, G.A.; Stella, S.; Pennisi, M.S.; Pirosa, C.; Fermo, E.; Fabris, S.; Cattaneo, D.; Iurlo, A. The Role of New Technologies in Myeloproliferative Neoplasms. *Front. Oncol.* **2019**, *9*, 321. [CrossRef]
60. Leiva, O.; Bekendam, R.H.; Garcia, B.D.; Thompson, C.; Cantor, A.; Chitalia, V.; Ravid, K. Emerging Factors Implicated in Fibrotic Organ-Associated Thrombosis: The Case of Two Organs. *TH Open* **2019**, *3*, e165–e170. [CrossRef]
61. Hultcrantz, M.; Wilkes, S.R.; Kristinsson, S.Y.; Andersson, T.M.; Derolf, A.R.; Eloranta, S.; Samuelsson, J.; Landgren, O.; Dickman, P.W.; Lambert, P.C.; et al. Risk and Cause of Death in Patients Diagnosed With Myeloproliferative Neoplasms in Sweden Between 1973 and 2005: A Population-Based Study. *J. Clin. Oncol.* **2015**, *33*, 2288–2295. [CrossRef] [PubMed]
62. Rumi, E.; Boveri, E.; Bellini, M.; Pietra, D.; Ferretti, V.V.; Sant'Antonio, E.; Cavalloni, C.; Casetti, I.C.; Roncoroni, E.; Ciboddo, M.; et al. Clinical course and outcome of essential thrombocythemia and prefibrotic myelofibrosis according to the revised WHO 2016 diagnostic criteria. *Oncotarget* **2017**, *8*, 101735–101744. [CrossRef] [PubMed]
63. Finazzi, M.C.; Carobbio, A.; Cervantes, F.; Isola, I.M.; Vannucchi, A.M.; Guglielmelli, P.; Rambaldi, A.; Finazzi, G.; Barosi, G.; Barbui, T. CALR mutation, MPL mutation and triple negativity identify patients with the lowest vascular risk in primary myelofibrosis. *Leukemia* **2015**, *29*, 1209–1210. [CrossRef] [PubMed]
64. Cerquozzi, S.; Barraco, D.; Lasho, T.; Finke, C.; Hanson, C.A.; Ketterling, R.P.; Pardanani, A.; Gangat, N.; Tefferi, A. Risk factors for arterial versus venous thrombosis in polycythemia vera: A single center experience in 587 patients. *Blood Cancer J.* **2017**, *7*, 662. [CrossRef]
65. Andreasson, B.; Pettersson, H.; Wasslavik, C.; Johansson, P.; Palmqvist, L.; Asp, J. ASXL1 mutations, previous vascular complications and age at diagnosis predict survival in 85 WHO-defined polycythaemia vera patients. *Br. J. Haematol.* **2020**. [CrossRef]
66. Horsted, F.; West, J.; Grainge, M.J. Risk of venous thromboembolism in patients with cancer: A systematic review and meta-analysis. *PLoS Med.* **2012**, *9*, e1001275. [CrossRef]
67. Perry, J.R.; Julian, J.A.; Laperriere, N.J.; Geerts, W.; Agnelli, G.; Rogers, L.R.; Malkin, M.G.; Sawaya, R.; Baker, R.; Falanga, A.; et al. PRODIGE: A randomized placebo-controlled trial of dalteparin low-molecular-weight heparin thromboprophylaxis in patients with newly diagnosed malignant glioma. *J. Thromb. Haemost.* **2010**, *8*, 1959–1965. [CrossRef]
68. Yan, H.; Parsons, D.W.; Jin, G.; McLendon, R.; Rasheed, B.A.; Yuan, W.; Kos, I.; Batinic-Haberle, I.; Jones, S.; Riggins, G.J.; et al. IDH1 and IDH2 mutations in gliomas. *N. Engl. J. Med.* **2009**, *360*, 765–773. [CrossRef]
69. Riedl, J.; Preusser, M.; Nazari, P.M.; Posch, F.; Panzer, S.; Marosi, C.; Birner, P.; Thaler, J.; Brostjan, C.; Lotsch, D.; et al. Podoplanin expression in primary brain tumors induces platelet aggregation and increases risk of venous thromboembolism. *Blood* **2017**, *129*, 1831–1839. [CrossRef]
70. Monroe, D.M.; Key, N.S. The tissue factor-factor VIIa complex: Procoagulant activity, regulation, and multitasking. *J. Thromb. Haemost.* **2007**, *5*, 1097–1105. [CrossRef]
71. Rak, J.; Milsom, C.; Yu, J. Tissue factor in cancer. *Curr. Opin. Hematol.* **2008**, *15*, 522–528. [CrossRef] [PubMed]

72. Regina, S.; Rollin, J.; Blechet, C.; Iochmann, S.; Reverdiau, P.; Gruel, Y. Tissue factor expression in non-small cell lung cancer: Relationship with vascular endothelial growth factor expression, microvascular density, and K-ras mutation. *J. Thorac. Oncol.* **2008**, *3*, 689–697. [CrossRef] [PubMed]
73. Yu, J.L.; May, L.; Lhotak, V.; Shahrzad, S.; Shirasawa, S.; Weitz, J.I.; Coomber, B.L.; Mackman, N.; Rak, J.W. Oncogenic events regulate tissue factor expression in colorectal cancer cells: Implications for tumor progression and angiogenesis. *Blood* **2005**, *105*, 1734–1741. [CrossRef] [PubMed]
74. Unruh, D.; Mirkov, S.; Wray, B.; Drumm, M.; Lamano, J.; Li, Y.D.; Haider, Q.F.; Javier, R.; McCortney, K.; Saratsis, A.; et al. Methylation-dependent Tissue Factor Suppression Contributes to the Reduced Malignancy of IDH1-mutant Gliomas. *Clin. Cancer Res.* **2019**, *25*, 747–759. [CrossRef]
75. Saghazadeh, A.; Rezaei, N. Inflammation as a cause of venous thromboembolism. *Crit. Rev. Oncol. Hematol.* **2016**, *99*, 272–285. [CrossRef]
76. Date, K.; Ettelaie, C.; Maraveyas, A. Tissue factor-bearing microparticles and inflammation: A potential mechanism for the development of venous thromboembolism in cancer. *J. Thromb. Haemost.* **2017**, *15*, 2289–2299. [CrossRef]
77. Crescenzo, R.; Abate, F.; Lasorsa, E.; Tabbo, F.; Gaudiano, M.; Chiesa, N.; Di Giacomo, F.; Spaccarotella, E.; Barbarossa, L.; Ercole, E.; et al. Convergent mutations and kinase fusions lead to oncogenic STAT3 activation in anaplastic large cell lymphoma. *Cancer Cell* **2015**, *27*, 516–532. [CrossRef]
78. Zhang, B.; Wei, W.; Qiu, J. ALK is required for NLRP3 inflammasome activation in macrophages. *Biochem. Biophys. Res. Commun.* **2018**, *501*, 246–252. [CrossRef]
79. Leiva, O.; Ng, S.K.; Matsuura, S.; Chitalia, V.; Lucero, H.; Findlay, A.; Turner, C.; Jarolimek, W.; Ravid, K. Novel lysyl oxidase inhibitors attenuate hallmarks of primary myelofibrosis in mice. *Int. J. Hematol.* **2019**, *110*, 699–708. [CrossRef]
80. Abbonante, V.; Chitalia, V.; Rosti, V.; Leiva, O.; Matsuura, S.; Balduini, A.; Ravid, K. Upregulation of lysyl oxidase and adhesion to collagen of human megakaryocytes and platelets in primary myelofibrosis. *Blood* **2017**, *130*, 829–831. [CrossRef]
81. Matsuura, S.; Mi, R.; Koupenova, M.; Eliades, A.; Patterson, S.; Toselli, P.; Thon, J.; Italiano, J.E., Jr.; Trackman, P.C.; Papadantonakis, N.; et al. Lysyl oxidase is associated with increased thrombosis and platelet reactivity. *Blood* **2016**, *127*, 1493–1501. [CrossRef] [PubMed]
82. Nasser, N.J.; Fox, J.; Agbarya, A. Potential Mechanisms of Cancer-Related Hypercoagulability. *Cancers* **2020**, *12*, 566. [CrossRef] [PubMed]
83. Al-Samkari, H.; Connors, J.M. Managing the competing risks of thrombosis, bleeding, and anticoagulation in patients with malignancy. *Blood Adv.* **2019**, *3*, 3770–3779. [CrossRef] [PubMed]

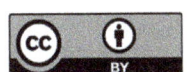

© 2020 by the authors. Licensee MDPI, Basel, Switzerland. This article is an open access article distributed under the terms and conditions of the Creative Commons Attribution (CC BY) license (http://creativecommons.org/licenses/by/4.0/).

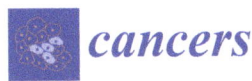

Brief Report

Observational Multicenter Study on the Prognostic Relevance of Coagulation Activation in Risk Assessment and Stratification in Locally Advanced Breast Cancer. Outline of the ARIAS Trial

Laura Pizzuti [1,†], Eriseld Krasniqi [1,†], Chiara Mandoj [2], Daniele Marinelli [3], Domenico Sergi [1], Elisabetta Capomolla [1], Giancarlo Paoletti [1], Claudio Botti [4], Ramy Kayal [5], Francesca Romana Ferranti [5], Isabella Sperduti [6], Letizia Perracchio [7], Giuseppe Sanguineti [8], Paolo Marchetti [3], Gennaro Ciliberto [9], Giacomo Barchiesi [10], Marco Mazzotta [1,*], Maddalena Barba [1,*], Laura Conti [2,‡] and Patrizia Vici [1,‡]

1. Division of Medical Oncology 2, IRCCS Regina Elena National Cancer Institute, Via Elio Chianesi, 00144 Rome, Italy; laura.pizzuti@ifo.gov.it (L.P.); krasniqier@gmail.com (E.K.); domenico.sergi@ifo.gov.it (D.S.); elisabetta.capomolla@ifo.gov.it (E.C.); giancarlo.paoletti@ifo.gov.it (G.P.); patrizia.vici@ifo.gov.it (P.V.)
2. Department of Clinical Pathology, IRCCS Regina Elena National Cancer Institute, Via Elio Chianesi 53, 00144 Rome, Italy; chiara.mandoj@ifo.gov.it (C.M.); laura.conti@ifo.gov.it (L.C.)
3. Medical Oncology Unit, Sant'Andrea Hospital, Via di Grottarossa, 1035/1039, 00189 Rome, Italy; danielemarinelli1@gmail.com (D.M.); paolo.marchetti@uniroma1.it (P.M.)
4. Department of Surgery, IRCCS Regina Elena National Cancer Institute, Via Elio Chianesi 53, 00144 Rome, Italy; claudio.botti@ifo.gov.it
5. Radiology Department, IRCCS Regina Elena National Cancer Institute, Via Elio Chianesi 53, 00144 Rome, Italy; ramy.kayal@ifo.gov.it (R.K.); francescaromana.ferranti@ifo.gov.it (F.R.F.)
6. Biostatistics Unit, IRCCS Regina Elena National Cancer Institute, Via Elio Chianesi 53, 00144 Rome, Italy; isabella.sperduti@ifo.gov.it
7. Pathology Department, IRCCS Regina Elena National Cancer Institute, Via Elio Chianesi 53, 00144 Rome, Italy; letizia.perracchio@ifo.gov.it
8. Department of Radiation Oncology, IRCCS Regina Elena National Cancer Institute, Via Elio Chianesi 53, 00144 Rome, Italy; giuseppe.sanguineti@ifo.gov.it
9. Scientific Direction, IRCCS Regina Elena National Cancer Institute, Via Elio Chianesi 53, 00144 Rome, Italy; gennaro.ciliberto@ifo.gov.it
10. Medical Oncology Unit, Ospedale dell'Angelo, Via Paccagnella 11, 30174 Mestre, Italy; giacomo.barchiesi88@gmail.com
* Correspondence: marcomazzotta88@gmail.com (M.M.); maddalena.barba@gmail.com (M.B.)
† These authors contributed equally.
‡ Equal contributors.

Received: 14 February 2020; Accepted: 30 March 2020; Published: 1 April 2020

Abstract: A hypercoagulable state may either underlie or frankly accompany cancer disease at its onset or emerge in course of cancer development. Whichever the case, hypercoagulation may severely limit administration of cancer therapies, impose integrative supporting treatments and finally have an impact on prognosis. Within a flourishing research pipeline, a recent study of stage I-IIA breast cancer patients has allowed the development of a prognostic model including biomarkers of coagulation activation, which efficiently stratified prognosis of patients in the study cohort. We are now validating our risk assessment tool in an independent cohort of 108 patients with locally advanced breast cancer with indication to neo-adjuvant therapy followed by breast surgery. Within this study population, we will use our tool for risk assessment and stratification in reference to 1. pathologic complete response rate at definitive surgery, intended as our primary endpoint, and 2. rate of thromboembolic events, intended as our secondary endpoint. Patients' screening and enrollment procedures are currently in place. The trial will be shortly enriched by experimental tasks centered on next-generation sequencing techniques for identifying additional molecular targets of treatments which may integrate current standards of therapy in high-risk patients.

Keywords: coagulation activation; locally advanced breast cancer; prognostic model; pCR; venous thromboembolism

1. Introduction

Large and consistent evidence supports the mutual association between cancer and coagulation abnormalities, with cancer being increasingly renowned as a predisposing factor for thromboembolic events [1]. Indeed, at the general population level, incidence rates for venous thromboembolism (VTE) approximate one to two cases per 1000 people/year, while cancer patients generally show a 4 to 10 times greater risk [2]. Consistently, VTE is associated with poor prognosis of disease in glioblastoma, ovarian, colorectal, lung and pancreatic cancer [3–5]. In strict regard to breast cancer, data are available in support of the prognostic relevance of coagulation activation on survival in both advanced and early disease [6].

Our research team has long and actively participated in initiatives led by the Cochrane collaboration, a global network of health professionals [7], with a focus on the design and update of systematic reviews (SR) and meta-analyses (MA) of anticoagulants use in cancer patients. In reference to our findings from a quite recently published work, which included data for a total of 1486 participants, we could not elicit a mortality benefit from the use of anticoagulants in cancer patients. However, when addressing the overall completeness and applicability of our study results, we pointed out that the greatest majority of the data analyzed were from randomized trials of lung cancer patients. On this basis, we underlined the need for further ad hoc studies focused on the effects of anticoagulants in patients with different types and stages of cancer [8]. In this view, given a prespecified type of cancer and stage at diagnosis, further steps of a well-focused research strategy are ideally aimed at clarifying the extent to which patient- and cancer-related features, along with differences in the activation state of the coagulation cascade, may affect health outcomes in reference to both cancer- and VTE-related endpoints.

Based on prior work performed in collaboration with the Cochrane network and supported by the expertise of scientists who have long operated in the management of thrombosis in cancer patients, we are now further extending our research pipeline on coagulation activation in breast cancer. We have previously moved our very first step within the early setting and carried out an observational study of 235 stage I-IIA patients with a 95-month follow up. Based on procedures whose details will be summarized in the methods section, we developed a prognostic model for the assessment and stratification of risk of death upon factors related to relevant clinic-pathologic characteristics and coagulation profile. This tool is shown in Table 1 and has proven efficacy in distinguishing patients' categories characterized by significantly different survival estimates [9]. On this basis, more recently, we have required and obtained formal approvals from the dedicated institutional bodies for the conduct of a validation study on an independent cohort of breast cancer patients consenting to participate and to be prospectively followed in a trial on the prognostic relevance of biomarkers of coagulation activation for risk assessment and stratification in reference to patients' important outcomes in breast cancer. This trial outline will be described across the following sections of the manuscript herein presented.

Table 1. Prognostic score assessment in the ARIAS trial participants.

Score Factors	Score Points		
	0	1	2
pT	T2	–	T3-4
FVIII	Normal	Abnormal	–
Age	≤ 70	> 70	–
DD	Low	–	High

pT, pathologic; T, Age in years; FVIII, factor VIII; normal range for the lab of reference, 50–150%; D, d-dimer; normal values for the lab of reference < 280 ng/mL.

Risk categories:

Score = 0-1 → High probability of pathologic complete response (pCR).
Score = 2 → Intermediate probability of pCR.
Score > 2 → Low probability of pCR.

2. Results

Results available at the time of writing are preliminary only. The Institutional Review Board (IRB) of the coordinating center, the IRCCS Regina Elena National Cancer Institute, has released formal approval for the ARIAS trial in January 2020 (Register code: RS1307/19_2303). The documents considered for IRB approval included a written consent form for patients' consultation and, eventually, signing prior to any study procedures.

The study Gantt chart is displayed in Figure 1. Patients' characteristics to be evaluated for study eligibility are summarized in the methods section. Thus far, within a time window of approximately 40 days, four patients have been identified as potentially suitable for inclusion based on the available clinical, instrumental and pathological records. The screened/enrolled ratio for patients' participation is currently equal to 1, i.e., 3/3. In more detail, three patients were invited to adhere and undersigned the written consent form, while the fourth will be contacted at the time of completion of the diagnostic workup.

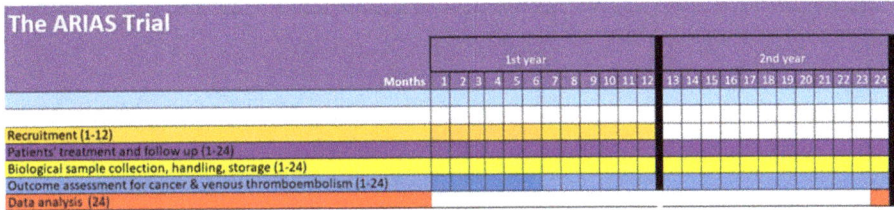

Figure 1. ARIAS Trial Gantt chart.

For patients enrolled, data concerning the variables of interest have been collected in a face-to-face interview carried out by specifically trained medical personnel involved in this trial conduct. Blood sample collection was performed according to highly standardized operative procedures (SOPs) previously set by dedicated personnel of our clinical pathology lab. Similarly, SOPs have been codified concerning blood sample handling, storage and biomarkers assessment as reported in more detail in the methods section. Patients' enrollment, data and baseline blood sample collection took place or will take place at the time of the first access to the oncology day hospital (DH) for chemotherapy administration. Thus far, no delays or, more generally, negative interferences were reported for the activities related to the therapeutic management of the patients enrolled. The ARIAS participants will be prospectively followed by dedicated personnel. Their profile will be updated in parallel with the DH accesses for chemotherapy administration. Blood sample collection will be repeated at the time of last chemotherapy, prior to breast surgery. Pathologic assessment of surgical breast samples will provide data related to the primary study endpoint, i.e., pathologic complete response (pCR) (yes/no). Data on thromboembolic events will be collected in course of therapy administration and following breast surgery, with the latest update being scheduled 6 months after surgery.

As specified in the Methods section, the ARIAS trial has been conceived as a multicentric initiative. Patients enrollment will shortly be active also at the four satellite centers. On average, based on the trial design, the estimated enrollment capacity of each of the centers involved is expected to broadly vary within a 1-to-3 patient/month range. Thus, the expected number of patients enrolled within a 12-month time window will be encompassed within a 60-to-180 range, which will fully address the minimum number of patients to be enrolled required based on the sample size calculations reported in the methods section. Over the course of the second year, therapy administration, biomarkers' assessment and patients follow up will inevitably overlap and converge towards the study closure and data analysis. Overall, a study length of about 2 years is foreseen, with a potential no-cost extension of about 6 months.

3. Discussion

We have herein outlined the main features of the ARIAS trial, a multicenter, observational study with prospective design focused on the prognostic role of biomarkers of coagulation activation in breast cancer patients undergoing neoadjuvant chemotherapy (NACT) and breast surgery in clinical practice. This trial is well placed within a research pipeline on coagulation and cancer. It is primarily aimed at validating the prognostic accuracy of our previously developed prognostic model in an independent cohort of breast cancer patients [9]. The ARIAS trial has received formal approval by the IRB of the coordinating center. The enrollment procedures have started. Results obtained thus far in terms of recruitment rate and study feasibility are extremely encouraging.

Our prior work was funded on the hypothesis that the activation state of the coagulation cascade significantly concurs to the definition of patients' important outcomes in breast cancer, along with patient- and cancer-related features. Breast cancer patients may thus be allocated to different risk categories for the outcomes of interest based on the use of the tool we developed. Upon validation, this prognostic model may help inform therapeutic decisions and favor the use of alternative or integrating treatments in patients for whom less favorable outcomes are foreseen.

In our prior study, we identified patient- and disease-related characteristics with prognostic relevance and included them into a prognostic model which proved accuracy in risk assessment and stratification in reference to the survival outcomes assessed in a cohort of 235 breast cancer patients diagnosed and treated at the IRCCS Regina Elena National Cancer Institute (IRE) between 2008 and 2010 [9]. Age, pathologic T (pT), baseline circulating levels of D-dimer (DD) and factor VIII (FVIII) proved prognostically relevant in multivariate models of overall survival (OS). The identified outcome predictors were then used for prognostic score assessment. The score including these factors proved efficacious in distinguishing risk categories in reference to OS, in that patients within the lowest risk category showed significantly longer OS compared to their counterparts ($p < 0.0001$). Based on our prior experience, we now expect significantly less favorable outcomes in the highest category of risk compared to the lowest as defined based on the prognostic model for risk assessment and stratification in course of validation. In strict referral to the single outcomes and related endpoints, this may translate into lower pCR rates and higher rates of VTE-related events for patients placed within the highest risk category. While conducting the ARIAS trial, some problems may emerge. Concerning the recruitment target of at least 108 patients in about 12 months defined upon ad hoc calculations, at the coordinating center, the average number of patients with an indication to NACT followed by breast surgery is of about 1–3 per month. This would allow the recruitment of 12–36 patients in 12 months. The remaining patients will be recruited at the collaborating centers, which will support our project working in kind and whose recruitment capacities are overall fairly comparable to ours.

Though statistically adequate in reference to our cancer-related endpoint, the sample size of our study population is relatively restricted. The overall number of deep vein thrombosis (DVT) and pulmonary embolism (PE) cases occurring within a 12-month time window in such a population may be relatively low. Indeed, based on literature data, the reported 1-year VTE incident rate (events per 100 patients per year) is about 0.9 [10]. However, literature data also support a relevant impact of several patient- and disease-related characteristics on VTE incident rates in cancer patients [11]. In more detail, VTE-related events are more often detected at the time of cancer diagnosis or within the first 6 months from diagnosis, as well as in patients with relevant disease burden, those with fast-growing tumors and those who receive anti-neoplastic agents [6,12–14]. In addition, an increased incidence of VTE is associated with the use of indwelling upper extremity and central venous catheters (CVC), with the incidence rates of clinically overt CVC-related DVT in cancer patients potentially rising to 28.3% [15]. All the previously mentioned patient- and disease-related features were considered at the time of our study conception and will be represented within the ARIAS cohort. This may considerably increase the VTE incident rates observed in the study under consideration. However, at the study closure, we intend to perform ad hoc power calculation to estimate the ARIAS power in reference to the VTE endpoint in light of our accomplishment in terms of number of patients enrolled and VTE events that occurred. It is also noteworthy to highlight the different stage of development of the prognostic model in reference to our primary and secondary endpoint. Indeed, the ARIAS was conceived with validation purposes in reference to our primary endpoint, i.e., pCR. Conversely, no VTE-related endpoints have been addressed in our prior study [9]. Thus, data from the ARIAS will be used to identify prognostically relevant factors in reference to VTE outcomes. This suggests the need of further validation of our model in reference to VTE outcomes in an independent cohort.

As previously stated, the ARIAS trial is intended as a validation study in reference to our primary endpoint, i.e., pCR rate following definitive breast surgery. In orienting our choice, we considered data from consistent literature in support of the predictive role of pCR on survival outcomes, with more favorable event-free and overall survival, particularly in patients diagnosed with the most aggressive breast cancer subtype [16,17]. These data support the correct use of pCR as a short-term surrogate of survival, offering the possibility to validate our previous risk model built on survival outcomes within a short follow-up framework. However, we are committed to also report on the accuracy of our model in predicting survival outcomes for the ARIAS participants when data from an adequately long follow up will be available. In these respects, an appropriate median length of follow up may be set at three years [16].

In the ARIAS trial, strengths and potentials for innovation come from the following key points: 1. the evidence elicited in our prior study in support of the role of coagulation activation in cancer will be now be validated in a study population which is homogeneous by primitive cancer site and setting at diagnosis; 2. The predefined sample size and prospective design confer an acceptable quality to our data. In addition, we are planning additional experimental tasks which will allow for the assessment of the burden of mutational events throughout a next-generation sequencing (NGS) approach in paraffin-embedded, formalin-fixed (PEFF) breast tissue samples collected at baseline. The presence of a higher mutational burden assessed by NGS in the highest risk category may further confirm our model in terms of accuracy.

4. Methods and Statistical Analysis

The ARIAS trial was conceived as a validation trial focused on a prognostic model developed in our prior study [9]. The tool we developed included patient- and disease-related features along with biomarkers of coagulation activation. In the herein proposed study, clinical–pathological data will be collected at baseline. Two tubes for citrate vacutainer and 3 EDTA will be collected at study entrance and before surgery, then centrifuged, aliquoted and stored at -80 °C for subsequent tests. The following components of the hemostatic systems will be immediately analyzed by coagulation, chromogenic and immunological methods on a fully automated ACLTOP analyzer using commercial HemosIL®kits

(Instrumentation Laboratory Company, Bedford, MA USA): PT, aPTT, Resistance (APCR) Fibrinogen, FVIII, DD, Protein C (PC), Protein S (PS), Antithrombin (AT) and Activated Protein C.

The accuracy of our prognostic model will be validated against the following endpoints: 1. Cancer-related endpoints, exemplified in this setting by pCR, defined as no residual invasive cancer, both in breast and axilla, i.e., ypT0/is ypN0. The assessment will be performed in tissue samples collected at the time of definitive surgery. Breast surgery will be performed within a time window of about 4 weeks from the end of the last cycle of NACT. 2. VTE-related endpoints, exemplified by symptomatic deep vein thrombosis (DVT), symptomatic pulmonary embolism (PE), central vein catheter (CVC) thrombosis and arm vein thrombosis. DVT will be confirmed by 1. compression ultrasonography (US) showing new or prior undocumented non-compressibility of one or more proximal venous segments, popliteal or higher of the legs; or 2. venography showing constant intraluminal filling defect in two or more vessels. PE will be confirmed by 1. spiral computed tomography (CT) identifying thrombus in pulmonary vessels or 2. ventilation/perfusion lung scan showing one or more perfusion mismatches. Arm vein thrombosis and CVC thrombosis will be assessed based on DD testing and US.

The ARIAS trial is being conducted in accordance with the Declaration of Helsinki.

Eligible participants are stage IIB-IIIC breast cancer patients undergoing NACT followed by breast surgery according to the current guidelines. The following inclusion criteria are to be met: age older than 18 years, normal range of kidney and liver function parameters, ECOG performance status ≤2, and a baseline left ventricular ejection fraction of at least 55 percent. At enrollment, participants must have no prophylactic or therapeutic indications to the use of anticoagulants. Reasons for exclusions are pregnancy, metastatic breast cancer, previous chemotherapy, prior hormonal therapy, prior radiotherapy, prior malignancies or contralateral breast cancer.

Study participants will be followed up at the Institute of reference over the course of NACT until breast surgery. Pathologic assessment of surgical breast tissues is planned to be performed in loco, with a central revision in a randomly selected 10% of the samples analyzed at the satellite institutes. Similarly, a second radiologist will perform an independent review of the ultrasound (US) and CT images for 10% of the cases assessed in reference to VTE-related endpoints. Biomarkers of coagulation activation will be centrally assessed.

Descriptive statistics will be computed for all the variables of interest. Means and standard deviations will be used to describe continuous variables. Categorical variables will be addressed by χ^2 test or Fisher's exact test. A receiver operating curve (ROC) approach will be used to evaluate the accuracy of the prognostic model in reference to pCR outcomes. VTE data will be analyzed according to a time-to-event approach using the product limit estimator to build Kaplan Meier survival curves according to the variables of interest and compare them by log-rank test. Cox regression models will be used to compute the effect of multiple factors on the VTE risk, and identify those relevant. The Harrell's concordance index will be used to calculate the risk scores. Statistical analysis will be performed by using the SPSS and MedCalc software.

5. Sample Size Calculations

The primary objective is the validation of the accuracy of the prognostic model developed in our prior study and inclusive of clinical–pathological factors, i.e., clinical T (cT), D Dimer and Factor VIII, in patients with locally advanced stage IIB-IIIC breast cancer, treated with NACT and breast surgery in clinical practice. To the purpose of our trial, we will enroll at least 108 patients with the previously defined characteristic features. This sample size has been defined by considering an AUC value of 0.95 as significant compared to a value of 0.84 (null hypothesis) and a low/high risk ratio, i.e., better/worse prognosis, equal to 2, at a level of significance or 0.05 and with a statistical power of 80%.

6. Conclusions

In summary, we have briefly provided the outline of the ARIAS trial, a multicenter, observational trial with prospective design, which has recently been granted with IRB approval for the coordinating center and has thus started the enrollment procedures with encouraging results. The ARIAS trial is a validation study in referral to our primary endpoint. As such, it is placed within a pre-existing research pipeline centered on the key role of coagulation activation in cancer, with a specific focus on breast cancer. The evidence we are currently producing throughout this trial conduct hold acceptable quality, since it stems from a study conducted with a prospective design, in which ad hoc sample size calculations were performed and study endpoints predefined. In addition, SOPs were applied to the collection, handling and assessment of the biomarkers of interest. Our study potentials will be shortly further enriched by additional tasks focused on the NGS assessment of key genes of relevant pathways related to coagulation activation as assessed in PEFF bioptic tissue samples collected at baseline.

Author Contributions: Conceptualization M.B., L.P. (Laura Pizzuti), E.K., C.M., L.C., P.V.; Methodology M.B., L.C.,P.V., I.S.; Writing Original Draft Preparation M.B., L.P (Laura Pizzuti)., E.K., D.M., M.M.; Writing Review & Editing D.S., E.C., G.P., C.B., R.K., F.R.F., L.P. (Letizia Perracchio), G.S., P.M., G.B., G.C.; Funding Acquisition, Not applicable. All authors have read and agreed to the published version of the manuscript.

Acknowledgments: We thank Ana Maria Edlisca and Federica Falcioni for the administrative support. We are also grateful to Alessandro Zennaro for the technical assistance.

Conflicts of Interest: The authors declare no conflict of interest.

References

1. Iorga, R.A.; Bratu, O.G.; Marcu, R.D.; Constantin, T.; Mischianu, D.L.D.; Socea, B.; Gaman, M.A.; Diaconu, C.C. Venous thromboembolism in cancer patients: Still looking for answers. *Exp. Ther. Med.* **2019**, *18*, 5026–5032. [CrossRef] [PubMed]
2. Chew, H.K.; Wun, T.; Harvey, D.; Zhou, H.; White, R.H. Incidence of venous thromboembolism and its effect on survival among patients with common cancers. *Arch. Intern. Med.* **2006**, *166*, 458–464. [CrossRef] [PubMed]
3. Cohen, A.; Lim, C.S.; Davies, A.H. Venous Thromboembolism in Gynecological Malignancy. *Int. J. Gynecol. Cancer* **2017**, *27*, 1970–1978. [CrossRef] [PubMed]
4. Barbarawi, M.; Zayed, Y.; Kheiri, B.; Gakhal, I.; Barbarawi, O.; Bala, A.; Alabdouh, A.; Abdalla, A.; Rizk, F.; Bachuwa, G.; et al. The role of anticoagulation in venous thromboembolism primary prophylaxis in patients with malignancy: A systematic review and meta-analysis of randomized controlled trials. *Thromb. Res.* **2019**, *181*, 36–45. [CrossRef] [PubMed]
5. Emoto, S.; Nozawa, H.; Kawai, K.; Hata, K.; Tanaka, T.; Shuno, Y.; Nishikawa, T.; Sasaki, K.; Kaneko, M.; Hiyoshi, M.; et al. Venous thromboembolism in colorectal surgery: Incidence, risk factors, and prophylaxis. *Asian J. Surg.* **2019**, *42*, 863–873. [CrossRef] [PubMed]
6. Chew, H.K.; Wun, T.; Harve, D.J.; Zhou, H.; White, R.H. Incidence of venous thromboembolism and the impact on survival in breast cancer patients. *J. Clin. Oncol.* **2007**, *25*, 70–76. [CrossRef] [PubMed]
7. Cochrane. Available online: http://www.cochrane.org/ (accessed on 1 April 2020).
8. Kahale, L.A.; Hakoum, M.B.; Tsolakian, I.G.; Matar, C.F.; Barba, M.; Yosuico, V.E.D.; Terrenato, I.; Sperati, F.; Schünemann, H.; Akl, E.A. Oral anticoagulation in people with cancer who have no therapeutic or prophylactic indication for anticoagulation. *Cochrane. Database Syst. Rev.* **2017**, *12*. [CrossRef] [PubMed]
9. Mandoj, C.; Pizzuti, L.; Sergi, D.; Sperduti, I.; Mazzotta, M.; Di Lauro, L.; Amodio, A.; Carpano, S.; Di Benedetto, A.; Botti, C.; et al. Observational study of coagulation activation in early breast cancer: development of a prognostic model based on data from the real world setting. *J. Transl. Med.* **2018**, *16*, 129. [CrossRef] [PubMed]
10. White, R.H.; Zhou, H.; Murin, S.; Harvey, D. Effect of ethnicity and gender on the incidence of venous thromboembolism in a diverse population in California in 1996. *Thromb. Haemost.* **2005**, *93*, 298–305. [PubMed]
11. Wun, T.; White, R.H. Venous Thromboembolism (VTE) in Patients with Cancer: Epidemiology and Risk Factors. *Cancer Investig.* **2009**, *27*, 63–74. [CrossRef] [PubMed]

12. Chew, H.K.; Davies, A.M.; Wun, T.; Harvey, D.; Zhou, H.; White, R.H. The incidence of venous thromboembolism among patients with primary lung cancer. *J. Thromb. Haemost.* **2008**, *6*, 601–608. [CrossRef] [PubMed]
13. Alcalay, A.; Wun, T.; Khatri, V.; Chew, H.K.; Harvey, D.; Zhou, H.; White, R.H. Venous thromboembolism in patients with colorectal cancer: incidence and effect on survival. *J. Clin. Oncol.* **2006**, *24*, 1112–1118. [CrossRef] [PubMed]
14. Haddad, T.C.; Greeno, E.W. Chemotherapy-induced thrombosis. *Thromb. Res.* **2006**, *118*, 555–568. [CrossRef] [PubMed]
15. Verso, M.; Agnelli, G. Venous thromboembolism associated with long-term use of central venous catheters in cancer patients. *J. Clin. Oncol.* **2003**, *21*, 3665–3675. [CrossRef] [PubMed]
16. Cortazar, P.; Zhang, L.; Untch, M.; Mehta, K.; Costantino, J.P.; Wolmark, N.; Bonnefoi, H.; Cameron, D.; Gianni, L.; Valagussa, P.; et al. Pathological complete response and long-term clinical benefit in breast cancer: The CTNeoBC pooled analysis. *Lancet* **2014**, *384*, 164–172. [CrossRef]
17. Von Minckwitz, G.; Untch, M.; Blohmer, J.U.; Costa, S.D.; Eidtmann, H.; Fasching, P.A.; Gerber, B.; Eiermann, W.; Hilfrich, J.; Huober, J.; et al. Definition and impact of pathologic complete response on prognosis after neoadjuvant chemotherapy in various intrinsic breast cancer subtypes. *J. Clin. Oncol.* **2012**, *30*, 1796–1804. [CrossRef] [PubMed]

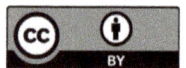

© 2020 by the authors. Licensee MDPI, Basel, Switzerland. This article is an open access article distributed under the terms and conditions of the Creative Commons Attribution (CC BY) license (http://creativecommons.org/licenses/by/4.0/).

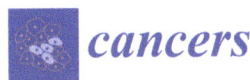

Review

Primary Thromboprophylaxis in Ambulatory Cancer Patients: Where Do We Stand?

Frits I. Mulder [1,2,*], Floris T. M. Bosch [1,2] and Nick van Es [1]

[1] Department of Vascular Medicine, Amsterdam Cardiovascular Science, Amsterdam UMC, University of Amsterdam, 1105 AZ Amsterdam, The Netherlands; f.t.bosch@amsterdamumc.nl (F.T.M.B.); n.vanes@amsterdamumc.nl (N.v.E.)
[2] Department of Internal Medicine, Tergooi Hospitals, 1213 XZ Hilversum, The Netherlands
* Correspondence: f.i.mulder@amsterdamumc.nl; Tel.: +31-20-566-1925; Fax: +31-20-566-9343

Received: 11 January 2020; Accepted: 2 February 2020; Published: 5 February 2020

Abstract: Venous thromboembolism (VTE), comprising deep-vein thrombosis and pulmonary embolism, is a frequent complication in ambulatory cancer patients. Despite the high risk, routine thromboprophylaxis is not recommended because of the high number needed to treat and the risk of bleeding. Two recent trials demonstrated that the number needed to treat can be reduced by selecting cancer patients at high risk for VTE with prediction scores, leading the latest guidelines to suggest such an approach in clinical practice. Yet, the interpretation of these trial results and the translation of the guideline recommendations to clinical practice may be less straightforward. In this clinically-oriented review, some of the controversies are addressed by focusing on the burden of VTE in cancer patients, discussing the performance of available risk assessment scores, and summarizing the findings of recent trials. This overview can help oncologists, hematologists, and vascular medicine specialists decide about thromboprophylaxis in ambulatory cancer patients.

Keywords: venous thromboembolism; cancer-associated venous thromboembolism; thrombosis; pulmonary embolism; neoplasms; anticoagulants; direct oral anticoagulants; coumarins; low molecular weight heparins

---

1. Background and Aim

Venous thromboembolism (VTE), comprising deep-vein thrombosis and pulmonary embolism, is a frequent complication in cancer patients. Overall, approximately 8% of patients develop VTE in the first year after their cancer diagnosis [1]. However, the risk of cancer-associated VTE heavily depends on tumor type, ranging from 1% in patients with low-risk tumors, such as breast or prostate cancer, to up to 20% in those with high-risk tumors, such as pancreatic cancer [2]. Other important risk factors include tumor stage and chemotherapy [3,4].

Despite the high risk, routine thromboprophylaxis for all ambulatory cancer patients is not recommended [5,6]. However, recent studies have brought new insights leading to changes in guidelines on primary VTE prevention in cancer patients [7,8]. Yet, the interpretation of these trial results and the translation of the guideline recommendations to clinical practice may be less straightforward. In this clinically-oriented review, we will address some of the controversies to help oncologists, hematologists, and vascular medicine specialists in making decisions about thromboprophylaxis in ambulatory cancer patients. We will focus on the burden of VTE in cancer patients, discuss several of the available risk scores, summarize the findings of recent trials, and provide potential directions for future research.

2. The Burden of Venous Thromboembolism in Cancer Patients

Cancer patients often experience complications during the course of their disease, including infections, side effects of chemotherapy, and symptoms directly related to the tumor. VTE is yet another frequently occurring complication. However, the decision to provide thromboprophylaxis to cancer patients has to depend on a careful assessment of the benefits (i.e., reduction in VTE and possibly arterial thromboembolism) and harms (i.e., bleeding). To be able to weigh the risks and benefits, clinicians need to be familiar with the burden of VTE in cancer patients. We will now summarize the available data on the short- and long-term consequences of VTE, which are listed in Table 1.

Table 1. Why VTE should be prevented in cancer patients.

Short Term Consequences
• Increased mortality [9]
• Morbidity caused by symptoms of pulmonary embolism or deep-vein thrombosis [10,11]
• Reduced quality of life [12]
• Interruption of cancer treatment [13,14]
• Financial consequences [15,16]
Long Term Consequences
• Post thrombotic syndrome [12]
• Chronic Thromboembolic pulmonary hypertension [17]
• Long-term bleeding risk [18]

2.1. Mortality

The primary goal of physicians treating cancer patients is to prevent death. It has been well recognized that VTE is strongly associated with worse survival, an association first shown by Sørensen and colleagues who analyzed data from more than 27,000 VTE patients in the Danish National Patient Registries [19]. Patients in whom cancer and VTE were diagnosed concurrently were compared to those with a cancer diagnosis without VTE, matched by cancer type, age, sex and year of diagnosis. Patients with VTE at the time of cancer diagnosis had a significantly higher 1-year mortality rate (HR 2.5, 95% CI 2.3–2.7). The association between VTE and mortality was also studied in the CATS cohort, a prospective observational cohort study comprising 1685 cancer patients [20]. During the 2-year study period, VTE occurred in 145 (9%) patients, of whom 79 (55%) died during follow-up, compared to 647 (38%) of those who did not develop VTE (HR 3.0, 95% CI 2.4–3.8). Although these studies showed that VTE is strongly correlated with mortality in cancer patients, it is unlikely that this association is causal. This is underscored by several randomized controlled trials which compared primary thromboprophylaxis to observation or placebo in cancer patients. These studies did show a reduction in VTE risk in those receiving thromboprophylaxis, but no significant difference in all-cause mortality (HR 0.93, 95% CI 0.8–1.1) [21,22]. Similarly, no difference in mortality was observed in studies evaluating LMWH in cancer without an indication for anticoagulation [23]. It is likely that the association between VTE and increased mortality risk merely reflects the prothrombotic state in patients with aggressive or progressive cancer, which can be caused by upregulation of procoagulant factors in tumor cells, such as tissue factor [24,25].

Nonetheless, VTE is often referred to as the second leading cause of death in cancer patients [26–30], which is mainly based on a study by Khorana and colleagues in which cause of death was assigned by treating physicians in 4466 cancer patients who had initiated chemotherapy [31]. However, the detailed breakdown of the study results shows that VTE may be less frequently fatal than often assumed. The most frequent cause of death was cancer progression ($n = 100$; 71%), followed by infection ($n = 13$; 9.2%), arterial thromboembolism (ATE) ($n = 8$; 5.6%), VTE ($n = 5$; 3.5%), unknown cause of death ($n = 5$, 3.5%), and death due to other causes ($n = 9$; 6.4%). The combined risk of arterial and venous thromboembolism is the second leading cause of death ($n = 13$; 9.2%), while the risk of fatal VTE, however, was lower than that of infectious disease, arterial thromboembolism, and death due to other causes. Moreover, the absolute risk of fatal VTE in this cohort was only 0.11%, which is in line with the fatal VTE rate of 0.5% and 0.6% in the control groups of the large FRAGMATIC and SAVE-ONCO trials [32,33].

Although there is a strong correlation between VTE and mortality in cancer patients, it remains unclear how often VTE directly results in death. Studies in which fatal VTE is ascertained by autopsy data are scant. Based on the currently available data, it appears that the absolute risk of fatal VTE might be not as high as often assumed. Consequently, the benefit of thromboprophylaxis will rely more on preventing VTE-related morbidity, decreased quality of life, and costs associated with VTE.

2.2. Morbidity and Quality of Life

When evaluating the impact of VTE on patients' morbidity or quality of life, it is important to note that there is a wide spread in the severity of VTE. The severity of complications in cancer patients are commonly described according to the Common Terminology Criteria for Adverse Events (CTCAE) published by the National Cancer Institute [34]. In this document, the severity of adverse events is graded according to standardized definitions ranging from grade 1 (mild) to 5 (death). The severity of deep-vein thrombosis is graded as moderate (grade 2). Pulmonary embolism is graded as severe (grade 3), as life-threatening (grade 4) in case of hemodynamic instability, or as fatal (grade 5) in case of a fatal pulmonary embolism. Since deep-vein thrombosis and the majority of pulmonary embolism (e.g. incidental or subsegmental) do not cause hemodynamic instability or result in death, most VTE cases are classified as a grade 3 adverse event or lower. Nonetheless, in the non-cancer population, it is well recognized that VTE of all grades of severity are associated with substantial morbidity and has a negative impact on quality of life [35].

Few studies have evaluated the impact of VTE on quality of life in cancer patients. Lloyd and colleagues assessed changes in quality of life associated with recurrent VTE in patients in the CATCH trial, a randomized controlled trial that compared the efficacy and safety of tinzaparin with warfarin in 900 cancer patients with acute VTE during seven months of follow-up [12]. Each month, patients were asked to fill in EQ-5D questionnaires, which assesses health in five domains: mobility, self-care, usual activities, pain/discomfort, and anxiety/depression [36]. The influence of recurrent VTE on quality of life was estimated in a model that compared quality of life in those with recurrent VTE to that of a reference case, i.e. a male from Western Europe with symptomatic deep-vein thrombosis, an ECOG score of 1, and no distant metastasis at baseline. In this model, patients with recurrent VTE had a significantly lower quality of life compared to the reference case (0.57 vs. 0.65, $p = 0.021$). Hence, recurrent VTE during anticoagulant treatment appears to negatively influence quality of life in cancer patients, although potential cancer relapse coinciding with recurrence was not taken into account in this model.

Marin-Barrera and colleagues evaluated the impact of primary VTE on the quality of life in a prospective cohort study comprising 128 cancer patients with VTE, and 297 cancer patients without VTE [37]. All patients completed general health-related and VTE-related questionnaires 1 month after inclusion, and indicated a significantly lower quality of life in cancer patients with VTE. These results should, however, be interpreted with caution since the groups were not matched, and substantial differences in baseline factors between the groups were observed which could be associated with quality of life, such as tumor type, performance score and cardiovascular disease history. In addition, several other factors associated with quality of life were not reported as time since cancer diagnosis, survival, specific cancer treatment, or whether patients received palliative or curative treatment.

Several small qualitative studies have been performed to assess patients' experience with cancer-associated VTE [10,11,38]. Seaman and colleagues interviewed fourteen patients with different types and stages of cancer who were previously diagnosed with pulmonary embolism or deep-vein thrombosis [10]. Patients mentioned that the diagnosis of VTE had a major impact on their lives, calling it "a distressing event with a profound impact on daily living", sometimes even more so than the cancer itself. The symptoms of pain in patients with deep-vein thrombosis and dyspnea in pulmonary embolism were experienced as very burdensome on a daily basis. In a comparable qualitative study by

Mockler and colleagues, ten cancer patients reported VTE as a significant setback during their cancer care and had difficulty coping with the event [11].

Overall, data on the influence of a first cancer-associated VTE on quality of life is limited. Findings from VTE patients without cancer cannot simply be extrapolated to cancer patients, because this latter group more often experiences anxiety, side effects of cancer treatment, and frequent hospitalizations. These factors make it complicated to estimate the impact of an additional VTE event on quality of life. More data on the physical and mental burden of VTE in cancer patients are needed to inform decision making about thromboprophylaxis, in which the harms of VTE and anticoagulation-related bleeding should be carefully balanced.

2.3. Risk of Bleeding and Recurrent Venous Thromboembolism

Cancer patients with VTE are at high risk of both recurrent VTE and bleeding during long-term anticoagulant treatment. The incidence of recurrent VTE during the 6 months after the initiation of anticoagulant therapy for cancer-associated VTE ranges from 7 to 9% in large RCTs, while the risk of major bleeding ranged from 3% to 6% [39–42]. These risks are approximately two to three fold higher, compared to patients without cancer [18].

The consequences of recurrent VTE and major bleeding can be serious. In a recent systematic review of 14 RCTs, the case-fatality rate was 17% (95% CI, 14–21%) for recurrent VTE and 11% (95% CI 3–18%) for bleeding [43]. Since international guidelines recommend to treat patients with anticoagulation for as long as the cancer is active [8], patients remain at risk of bleeding throughout the course of their disease. As primary thromboprophylaxis can prevent VTE in cancer patients, long-term anticoagulation therapy and the concurrent bleeding risk can be avoided.

2.4. Long-Term Sequelae

The long-term sequelae of VTE, including post-thrombotic syndrome in patients with deep-vein thrombosis and chronic thromboembolic pulmonary hypertension (CTEPH) in patients with pulmonary embolism, are also of clinical importance for cancer patients. Post-thrombotic syndrome is a common and burdensome syndrome that occurs in about 45% of non-cancer patients in the first 36 months after a deep-vein thrombosis [44]. It is associated with local pain, swelling, itching, cramps, or venous ulcers, and the severity can be assessed by using the Villalta score [45]. Compression stocking may reduce the risk of post-thrombotic syndrome, although there is controversy about their benefit [44]. Little evidence is available about post-thrombotic syndrome in cancer patients. A multicenter VTE registry in Japan, which included 3027 patients with VTE [46], showed that patients with active cancer had a higher risk of developing post-thrombotic syndrome (OR 3.6, 95% CI 2.3 to 5.8) than non-cancer patients, which might be due to the higher clot burden due to hypercoagulability in cancer patients. However, this increased risk of post-thrombotic syndrome in cancer patients was not observed in a large population-based study from the Netherlands including 1,668 patients (RR 0.8, 95% CI 0.4 to 1.4) [47]. Post-thrombotic syndrome was associated with a lower QoL in cancer patients enrolled in the CATCH trial [12].

CTEPH constitutes pulmonary hypertension caused by pulmonary embolism and can be associated with dyspnea, chest pain, and right-sided heart failure. The estimated incidence of CTEPH ranges from 0.5 to 5% in up to three years follow-up among different prospective studies in non-cancer patients [48,49], and the estimated three-year mortality is approximately 30% [48,50]. One small study assessed the incidence of CTEPH in 129 cancer patients, of whom only one (0.75%) was classified as "CTEPH likely" after six months. Although the presence of cancer could lower the threshold of suspicion for CTEPH, the low absolute risk probably does not justify routine screening for CTEPH in cancer patients. To our knowledge, no studies have been performed in quality of life in patients with CTEPH and cancer.

CTEPH and post-thrombotic syndrome are serious long-term disease complications after VTE. Due to the dramatic improvement in cancer survival over the last decades, clinicians should be aware that an increasing number of cancer patients and survivors will experience these long-term sequelae of VTE [51].

2.5. Interference with Cancer Treatment

Cancer-associated VTE can result in delays or interruptions of cancer treatment, which was demonstrated in a retrospective cohort study of 534 patients with esophageal cancer undergoing neoadjuvant chemoradiation [13]. Among the 75 patients (14%) who developed a thromboembolic event, the median time until surgery was 11 days longer compared to those without such an event (47 vs. 36 days, $p = 0.0004$), although this did not result in a difference in 30-day mortality (1% vs. 2%, $p = 0.9$). In a retrospective cohort study of 2047 patients who underwent pancreaticoduodenectomy for pancreatic cancer, VTE in the 30-day postoperative period was associated with omission of adjuvant chemotherapy, also after adjusting for potential confounders (adjusted OR 1.9; 95% CI 1.1 to 3.4) [14].

2.6. Financial Burden

Several studies assessed the economic burden of cancer-associated VTE. A retrospective study from the United States evaluated costs associated with VTE in 6732 patients with lung cancer starting chemotherapy [15].In the patients with VTE, the average unadjusted costs in the entire 12 months were 33% higher ($84,187) than in those without VTE ($56,818; $p < 0.0001$). This difference persisted after adjustment for demographic variables, medical history, insurance type, and cancer supportive care treatments. Similarly, another study from the United States including 529 patients with cancer and deep-vein thrombosis reported an average subsequent hospitalization of 11 days and associated costs of $20,000 per patient (corrected for inflation) [16]. The mean hospital stay and costs increased to 18 days and $43,000 respectively when patients experienced in-hospital bleeding due to anticoagulation. These findings indicate that the diagnostic and therapeutic management of VTE and the potential bleeding complications in cancer patients is costly. Hence, primary VTE prevention could be beneficial from a financial perspective.

2.7. Knowledge Gaps

Overall, it appears that little evidence is available concerning the burden of VTE in cancer patients. Although the increased risks of recurrence and bleeding during treatment are well-established, several knowledge gaps remain. More solid data are needed on the risk of fatal pulmonary embolism in cancer patients, the incidence of long-term VTE sequelae, and the impact of VTE on quality of life and on cancer treatment and whether this latter affects survival. Nonetheless, it is likely that VTE has at least similar negative consequences as in the general population, which should be taken into account when considering primary prevention of VTE in cancer patients.

3. Primary Thromboprophylaxis in Ambulatory Cancer Patients

The negative consequences of VTE in cancer patients can, at least in part, be avoided with primary thromboprophylaxis, a strategy that is already universally accepted in other settings with a high risk of VTE, such as following major surgery, in pregnant women with thrombophilia or previous VTE, or in high-risk patients during hospital admissions. Levine and colleagues presented the first evidence in 1994 for a potential clinical benefit of primary thromboprophylaxis. In a randomized controlled trial of 311 metastatic breast cancer patients, those assigned to low-dose warfarin with an INR target of 1.3 to 1.9 had a significant 3.7% absolute lower risk of VTE than those receiving placebo during approximately six months of follow-up [52]. It was not until fifteen years later, a period during which low-molecular-weight heparins (LMWH) was established as standard therapy for cancer-associated VTE [39], that the PROTECHT randomized, placebo-controlled trial was published. This study randomized 1150 ambulatory cancer patients who initiated chemotherapy to either prophylactic subcutaneous nadroparin (3800 IU daily) or to placebo once daily [53]. After a median follow-up of 3.5 months, 15 of 769 patients allocated to nadroparin had developed VTE (2.0%) compared to 15 of 381 patients (3.9%) receiving placebo (p = 0.02). Despite this 1.9% absolute lower VTE risk with nadroparin, the authors proposed to focus future studies on cancer patients at high risk of VTE to decrease the number needed to treat (NNT).

Following this pivotal study, several other randomized trials with comparable designs and treatment regimens followed. These were subsequently summarized in a comprehensive Cochrane systematic review meta-analysis by Di Nisio and colleagues [21]. The pooled results of nine randomized trials that compared LMWH with placebo or observation demonstrated a lower risk of symptomatic VTE with LMWH (7.1%) than with placebo or observation (3.9%), translating into a relative risk of 0.54 (95% confidence interval (CI), 0.38–0.75). Given the corresponding substantial NNT of 30 patients to prevent one VTE as well as the increased tendency for major bleeding with thromboprophylaxis (RR, 1.4; 95% CI, 0.98–2.1), the authors concluded that more data were needed before implementation of routine primary thromboprophylaxis in ambulatory cancer patients could be justified. They also advised future studies to include patients at high-risk of VTE only. Other drawbacks of primary thromboprophylaxis with LMWH that limited its widespread use in practice include the inconvenience associated with long-term daily subcutaneous injections and the substantial costs of this therapy [54]. Indeed, 36% of patients in the nadroparin group enrolled in the PROTECHT trial and 29% of those receiving subcutaneous placebo injections, prematurely discontinued treatment [53], possibly reflecting the burden of daily subcutaneous injections in a vulnerable population.

4. Prediction of Venous Thromboembolism in Cancer Patients

Several risk assessment tools for cancer-associated VTE have been introduced, which aim to reduce the NNT of primary thromboprophylaxis to prevent one VTE, by selecting high-risk patients only. The Khorana risk score, which was introduced in 2008, is currently the most widely known tool. It combines five clinically readily available variables to classify cancer patients initiating systemic anticancer treatment by their VTE risk [55]. Points are assigned for having a high or very high-risk primary tumor site (+1 or 2 points, respectively), pre-chemotherapy platelet count of 350×10^9/L or higher (+1 point), pre-chemotherapy hemoglobin concentration lower than 6.2 mmol/L or use of erythropoiesis-stimulating agents (+1 point), pre-chemotherapy leukocyte count lower than 11×10^9/L (+1 point), and a body mass index of 35 kg/m^2 or higher (+1 point, Table 2). Based on the sum score, patients are classified as low risk (0 points), intermediate risk (1 or 2 points), or high risk (3 points or more). Although the score has been endorsed by various guidelines [6,56], the performance of the score remains a matter of debate. Conflicting results have been reported about the positive predictive value, the sensitivity is only modest, and the performance varies substantially among cancer groups, with lower discrimination in patients with lung cancer [57,58]. Two large prospective cohort studies, initiated to validate and derive VTE risk scores in cancer patients, both independently concluded that only Khorana score variable 'primary tumor site' was significantly associated with cancer-associated VTE, but not the other items, i.e., hemoglobin level, white blood cell count, platelet count, and body mass index [59]. Therefore, the question arises whether the Khorana score is merely a complicated score that selects cancer types with the highest risk, instead of cancer patients with the highest risk.

Improvements to the Khorana score were suggested by assigning additional points for chemotherapy [60], patient performance status [61], the laboratory biomarkers soluble P-selectin and D-dimer [62], cancer stage, vascular compression by the tumor, and prior VTE [63]. Others proposed to use a fibrin generation test [64], genetic risk factors [65], cardiovascular risk factors, and the use of anti-hormonal therapy [66]. However, in general, most scores are not yet externally validated, only marginally improved prediction [57], or include biomarkers that are not readily available in each medical institute, which precludes their clinical use [59]. Consequently, Pabinger and colleagues proposed a new simplified prediction model based only on primary tumor site and D-dimer as variables [59]. Discrimination was significantly improved compared to the Khorana score in both the derivation and validation cohort. Future intervention studies are, however, needed to validate these results, demonstrate clinical feasibility of routine D-dimer testing, and evaluate clinical benefit of the model. Tumor-specific risk scores were recently developed for hematologic malignancies [67,68] and gynecological malignancies [69]. Because neither of these scores have been externally validated nor have been acknowledged by the current guidelines, we will not further discuss these risk assessment tools.

Table 2. Khorana risk score.

Patient Characteristics	Risk Score
Site of cancer	
Very high risk (stomach, pancreas, brain)	2
High risk (lung, lymphoma, gynecologic, bladder, myeloma, testicular or kidney)	1
Prechemotherapy platelet count $\geq 350 \times 10^9$/L	1
Prechemotherapy hemoglobin level < 6.2 mmol/L or use of red cell growth factors	1
Prechemotherapy leukocyte count > 11×10^9/L	1
Body mass index ≥ 35 kg/m^2	1

5. Primary Thromboprophylaxis in Selected Cancer Patients

The PHACS trial, published in 2017 by Khorana and colleagues, was the first to evaluate thromboprophylaxis in a selected cancer population based on a high risk of VTE. In this randomized controlled trial, performed at seven sites in the United States and 1 in Canada, 117 cancer patients with a Khorana score of 3 points or higher were randomly allocated either to prophylactic subcutaneous dalteparin at 5000 IU once daily for 12 weeks or observation. There was no significant difference in the rates of recurrent VTE or major bleeding between the groups. Unfortunately, no firm conclusions could be drawn as the trial was prematurely closed due to poor accrual after a five-year recruitment period, possibly as a result of aversion among patients against daily subcutaneous injections and competition of other studies in this population [70]. However, the design of this trial, and the introduction of direct oral anticoagulants as attractive treatment for cancer-associated VTE [41,42], provided the basis for two subsequent randomized trials.

CASSINI was a randomized, double-blind, placebo-controlled, multicenter trial that enrolled ambulatory cancer patients with a Khorana score of 2 or higher [71]. Of the 1080 potentially eligible patients, 49 (4.5%) were excluded because of (asymptomatic) deep-vein thrombosis detected by protocol-mandated screening with duplex compression ultrasonography of both legs at baseline, and 190 (18%) were excluded for other reasons. The remaining 841 patients without screen-detected deep-vein thrombosis at baseline were randomized to either rivaroxaban 10 mg once daily or placebo once daily for up to 180 days. Throughout the trial, patients were screened for asymptomatic deep-vein thrombosis by compression ultrasonography every eight weeks. The primary efficacy outcome was the composite of any proximal deep-vein thrombosis in a lower limb, non-fatal or fatal pulmonary embolism, symptomatic upper extremity deep-vein thrombosis, and symptomatic distal deep-vein thrombosis in a lower limb. The most common cancer types were pancreatic (33%), gastric/gastroesophageal junctional (21%), and lung cancer (16%). In the intention-to-treat analysis, there was no significant difference in the occurrence of the primary outcome between the groups during the complete follow-up period; VTE occurred in 25 of 420 patients (6.0%) randomized to rivaroxaban and in 37 of 421 patients (8.8%) randomized to placebo (hazard ratio (HR), 0.66; 95% CI, 0.40–1.1; NNT 36). Notably, the study drug was prematurely discontinued by 44% of the patients in the rivaroxaban group compared and by 50% of those randomized to placebo. In a secondary analysis confined to the on-treatment period, the primary outcome occurred in 2.6% of patients allocated to rivaroxaban and in 6.4% allocated to placebo, translating into a statistically significant 60% relative risk reduction in VTE (HR, 0.40; 95% CI, 0.20–0.80; NNT 26). A two-fold higher major bleeding rate was observed in patients in the rivaroxaban group (2.0%) as compared to the placebo group (1.0%) (HR 2.0, 95% CI 0.59–6.5, number needed to harm (NNH) 100). All-cause mortality was comparable between groups: 20% in the rivaroxaban group vs 24% in the placebo group (HR, 0.83; 95% CI, 0.62–1.1). The authors concluded that the trial provided information on VTE incidence in patients with a high Khorana score, but did not establish the benefit of prophylactic treatment with rivaroxaban, because the primary outcome during the 180-day trial period was not statistically significant. Ultrasound screening for asymptomatic deep-vein thrombosis resulted in exclusion of a substantial number of patients from the trial, while such screening during the trial identified 15 incidental proximal deep-vein thromboembolic events of the lower extremities during follow-up accounting for roughly 25% of the events in the primary outcome. This approach, which does not represent common daily clinical practice, hampers the interpretation of the findings because the clinical consequence of such asymptomatic deep-vein thrombosis is unclear [72].

In the AVERT trial, published by Carrier and coworkers, ambulatory cancer patients with a Khorana score of 2 points or higher were randomized to either apixaban 2.5 mg twice daily or to placebo [73]. The primary outcome was the occurrence of VTE in the 180-day study period, comprising incidental or symptomatic proximal deep-vein thrombosis of an upper-, or lower limb, pulmonary embolism, and pulmonary-related death. Although the design was similar to that of the CASSINI trial, no routine screening for VTE was performed throughout this study. The most frequent cancer types were gynecologic cancer (26%), lymphoma (25%), and pancreatic cancer (14%). Of the 288 patients randomized to apixaban, 12 (4.2%) had developed VTE after 180 days of follow-up compared to 28 of 275 patients (10.2%) in the placebo group (HR, 0.41; 95% CI, 0.26–0.65; NNT 17). Apixaban significantly increased the risk of major bleeding, which occurred in 10 patients (3.5%) in the intervention group and in five patients (1.8%) in the placebo group (HR 2.00; 95% CI 1.0–4.0; NNH 59). The risk of clinically relevant non-major bleeding was numerically higher in the group treated with apixaban (7.3%) compared to the placebo group (5.5%), though not statistically significant (HR, 1.3; 95% CI, 0.89–1.8; NNH, 56). A sensitivity analysis restricted to the on-treatment period, showed a stronger relative reduction in VTE, while the absolute risk reduction was similar; the incidence was 1% in those treated with apixaban in this period, compared to 7.3% in those receiving placebo (HR 0.14, 95% CI 0.05–0.42, NNT 16). All-cause mortality during the trial was not significantly different between the two treatment groups (12.2% in apixaban vs 9.8% in the placebo group; HR, 1.3; 95% CI, 0.98-1.7). The AVERT trial was the first trial that showed that selecting high-risk patients for thromboprophylaxis may be clinically beneficial. Although the NNT of 17 is encouraging, it remains a question whether the benefit-harm ratio of prophylactic apixaban in this setting is perceived positive enough by oncologists, who need to consider this in the context of other disease complications, survival, and patients' preference.

A recent systematic review aggregated data of the CASSINI and AVERT trial by performing a random effects meta-analysis of these two studies [22]. It is questionable whether a meta-analysis of just two studies is useful, also given the important differences in study design and cancer types included. Nonetheless, the summary risk ratio (RR) associated with the intervention in the intention-to-treat population during 6 months was 0.56 (95% CI, 0.35–0.89) for all VTE outcomes, and 0.58 (95% CI, 0.29–1.1) for symptomatic VTE. The summary RR for on-treatment major bleeding and CRNMB were 2.0 (0.80–4.8) and 1.3 (0.74–2.2), respectively.

It is important to emphasize that both trials considered patients with a Khorana score of 2 points or higher eligible for thromboprophylaxis, instead of the traditional threshold of 3 points or higher. A recent systematic review and meta-analysis, which evaluated the Khorana score in more than 34,000 cancer patients, estimated that 17% of all cancer patients have a Khorana score of 3 or higher and 47% a score of 2 or higher [58]. The estimated 6-month VTE incidence was lower in patients with a score of 2 or higher (8.9%; 95% CI 7.3–10.8) than in those with a score of 3 or higher (11%; 95% CI, 8.8–14). Hence, applying the lower threshold likely improved the feasibility of the CASSINI and AVERT trials, because more cancer patients were eligible for participation. However, this comes at the cost of a lower rate of VTE and higher NNT, as was confirmed in a pooled subgroup analysis of the AVERT and CASSINI trials; the pooled 6-month VTE incidence was 14.0% in patients with a Khorana score of 3 or higher receiving placebo versus 9.9% in the group with a score of 2 or higher [22]. The corresponding NNT was about 12 for cancer patients with a Khorana score of 3 or higher, but 17 for those with a score of 2 or higher. In the group of placebo recipients with a Khorana score of 2 points, the VTE incidence was 8.4% (NNT of 22). Whether thromboprophylaxis is justified for the latter group is debatable.

6. Where Do We Stand

Several international guidelines were recently updated after the publication of the CASSINI and AVERT trials. The guidance statement of the International Society on Thrombosis and Haemostasis (ISTH) now suggests the use of apixaban or rivaroxaban as primary thromboprophylaxis in ambulatory cancer patients starting chemotherapy with Khorana score ≥ 2 [7]. The guideline of the International Initiative on Thrombosis and Cancer (ITAC) recommends prophylactic rivaroxaban or apixaban for ambulatory cancer patients receiving systemic anticancer therapy at intermediate-to-high risk of VTE, identified by cancer type (i.e., pancreatic) or by a validated risk assessment model (i.e., a Khorana score ≥ 2) [74]. The latest guideline of the American Society of Clinical Oncologists (ASCO) is more prudent by stating that thromboprophylaxis with apixaban, rivaroxaban, or LMWH may be offered in cancer patients with Khorana score of 2 or higher [8]. All guidelines stress that the concomitant bleeding risk and patient preference should be taken into account.

The CASSINI and AVERT trials showed the potential of long-term thromboprophylaxis with DOACs in selected cancer patients. Whether the results from these trials should be translated directly to clinical practice remains unsure. Both used the Khorana score for patient selection for thromboprophylaxis. The role of this score merits careful consideration before the results can be implemented into clinical practice, since its performance directly relates to the number needed to screen, absolute risk reduction, and NNT.

Firstly, the sensitivity of the Khorana score is quite poor. When selecting patients with 3 points or more for thromboprophylaxis, 75% of all VTE events occur outside this high-risk group. When using a threshold of 2 points, approximately half of the total VTE events occur outside the high-risk group [58]. This means that the majority of cancer patients who will develop VTE do not benefit from risk stratification with the Khorana score, since they are not selected for thromboprophylaxis. The proportion of cancer patients classified as high-risk by a Khorana score cut-off value of 2 or 3 points, and the VTE incidence in these groups as observed in the AVERT trial, is graphically depicted in Figure 1.

Secondly, as the Khorana score is a pan-cancer prediction score, oncologists need to calculate the score for all their cancer patients to identify patients at high risk of VTE. This might be challenging given the daily time constraints experienced in the clinic, in particular for oncologists specialized in cancers at relatively low risk of VTE and a high number needed to screen, such as breast or prostate cancer. When a pan-cancer score is clinically used to select patients for primary thromboprophylaxis with DOACs, the premise is that the predictive performance of the score is similar for all cancer types. Previous studies, however, showed a substantial heterogeneity in the positive predictive value of the Khorana score across cancer groups [58]. Furthermore, a pan-cancer score should ideally have a similar benefit-risk trade-off of the treatment regimen for all cancer types. It has been acknowledged, however, that the efficacy and safety of DOACs in treatment of VTE may vary across cancer types [41,42,75,76]. For example, a substantial difference in the risk of VTE was observed between pancreatic and non-pancreatic cancer patients in the CASSINI trial. VTE incidence in the placebo group was 13% in those with pancreatic cancer and 6.7% in those with non-pancreatic cancer, resulting in a lower NNT for the former group. Conversely, the risk of bleeding may be greater for patients with gastrointestinal cancer than for those with other tumor types. For these reasons, an oncologist specialized in pancreatic cancer will likely be more interested in the safety and efficacy of thromboprophylaxis specifically for pancreatic cancer patients with a high-risk Khorana score than for other cancer types. However, other than for pancreatic cancer, data on safety and efficacy of primary thromboprophylaxis with DOACs are currently lacking for specific cancer types. More results of the CASSINI and AVERT trial stratified by cancer type are welcome, even if such analyses may be underpowered. More results of the CASSINI and AVERT trial stratified by cancer type are welcome, even if such analyses may be underpowered.

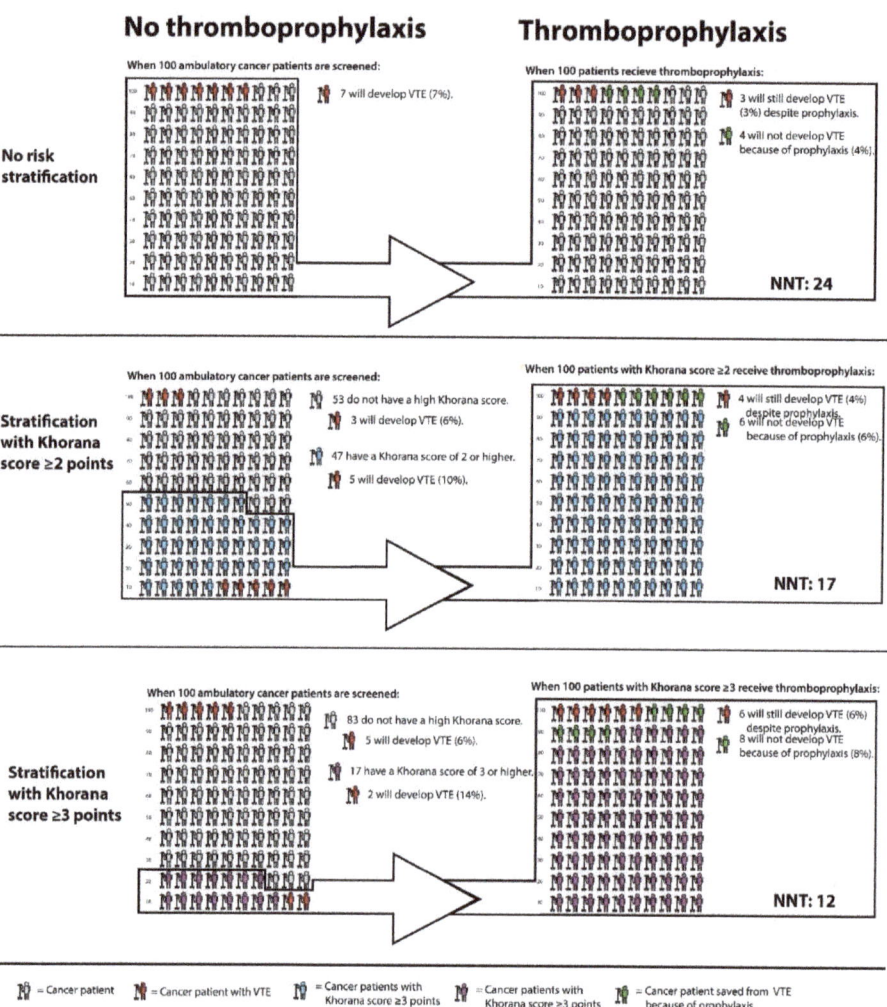

Figure 1. VTE incidence in cancer patients with and without thromboprophylaxis, stratified by Khorana score. Abbreviations: NNT, number needed to treat; VTE, venous thromboembolism. * Calculations based and extrapolated from Mulder et al; The Khorana Score For Prediction Of Venous Thromboembolism In Cancer Patients: A Systematic Review And Meta-Analysis [58], Carrier et al; Apixaban to Prevent Venous Thromboembolism in Patients with Cancer [73], and Li et al, Direct Oral Anticoagulant for the Prevention of Thrombosis in Ambulatory Patients with Cancer: A Systematic Review and Meta-Analysis [22].

Lastly, it remains questionable whether the observed benefit-harm ratio of prophylactic DOACs in cancer patients with Khorana score 2 or higher justifies the large-scale implementation of primary thromboprophylaxis. As mentioned previously, the protocol-mandated deep-vein thrombosis screening applied in the CASSINI trial makes it difficult to translate the results to clinical practice. The NNT of 17 to prevent one VTE as observed in the AVERT trial is encouraging. However, the combined risk of major bleeding and clinically relevant non-major bleeding was 3.5% higher in the apixaban arm compared to placebo, corresponding to a NNH of 29. The NNT of prophylactic apixaban in cancer patients with and without risk stratification with the Khorana score is graphically depicted in Figure 1. Further uncertainties associated with DOACs are potential drug-drug interactions with chemotherapeutic agents [77], risk of bleeding during periods of thrombocytopenia, the optimal duration of thromboprophylaxis, and the benefit-harm ratio in patients with specific cancer types. For participants in the AVERT trial, the anticipation of minimum three months of chemotherapy was required, which presumably excluded patients receiving curative cancer treatment. Hence, it is unclear whether the trial results can be extrapolated to cancer patients receiving neoadjuvant chemotherapy.

7. Future Directions

VTE is a frequent and potentially invalidating disease complication in cancer patients. Despite the recent and more remote advances (Figure 2), future steps in VTE prediction are needed to effectively reduce the burden associated with cancer-associated VTE. At present, we believe current evidence does not justify primary thromboprophylaxis in all cancer patients with a Khorana score of 2 or higher, which would have consequences for millions of patients worldwide. Additional randomized trials could strengthen the evidence and, when restricted to specific cancer types, address the uncertainty about the risk-benefit for specific cancer types. Improvements in VTE prediction in cancer patients are needed to lower the NNT to prevent one VTE associated with thromboprophylaxis. Most clinical prediction scores that were proposed as improvement to the Khorana score require further external validation. Several other clinical risk factors or biomarkers could ameliorate VTE prediction, such as serum platelet factor 4, citrullinated histone H3 as a marker for neutrophil extracellular traps, and extracellular vesicles bearing tissue factor, which showed promising results in smaller cohort studies [64,78,79]. Genetic risk factors for VTE have previously shown to be an important predictor for VTE in cancer patients [65], while specific tumor mutations also appeared to be associated with VTE [80,81]. This implies that genomic characterization of tumors could provide relevant information not only for cancer prognosis, but also for the risk of VTE. Repeated measurements of prediction scores should be explored to see whether continuously updated, dynamic risks are clinically helpful [82]. Machine learning could help in identifying new risk factors in large datasets to obtain accurate and precise personalized risk estimates [83]. From a pharmacological perspective, new agents for the treatment of VTE are currently explored, of which factor XI and XII inhibitors appear to be most promising [84–86]. If these agents prove to be safe and effective for the treatment of cancer-associated VTE, they could provide a basis for future thromboprophylactic strategies. More effort is needed in predicting the concurrent bleeding risk, which might help to reduce the NNH. Lastly, a cross-disciplinary discussion is needed to obtain consensus on an acceptable NNT and maximally tolerated bleeding risk.

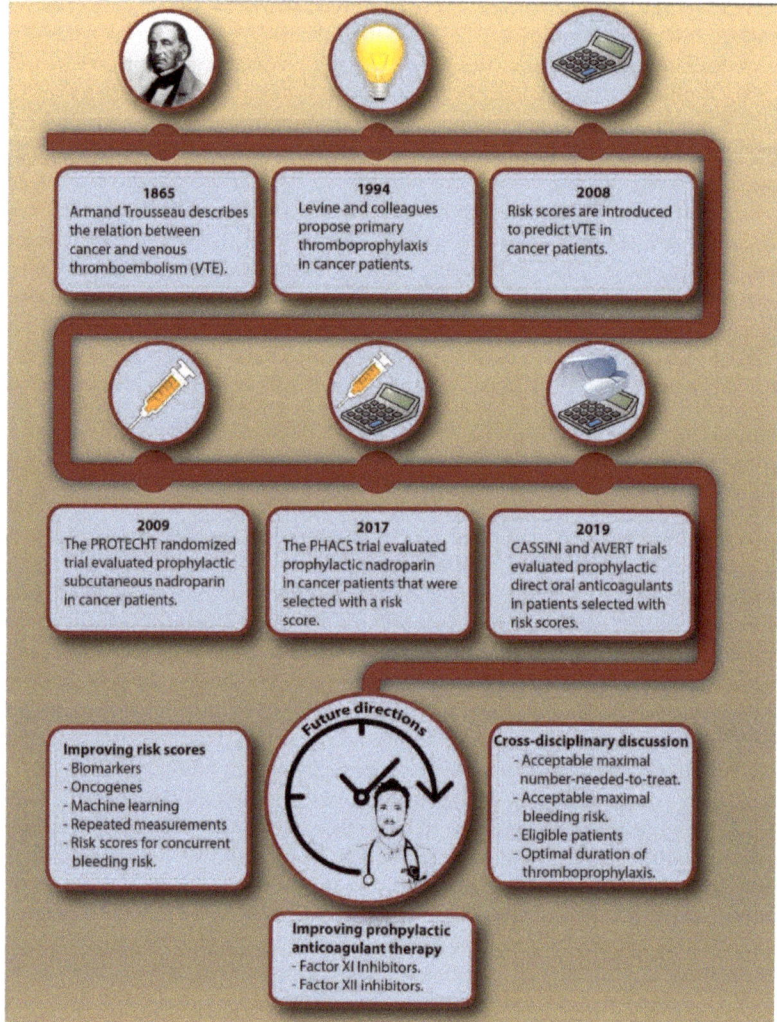

Figure 2. The chronological introduction of primary thromboprophylaxis in cancer patients and possible future directions. Abbreviations: NNT, number needed to treat; VTE, venous thromboembolism.

8. Conclusions

In a broader perspective, one could question whether the development of an efficient pan-cancer VTE prediction score is feasible, given the large heterogeneity across cancer types in tumor biology, cancer treatment, and thromboembolic and bleeding risk. Possibly, prediction scores should be developed for specific cancer types to help effectively individualize strategies for primary thromboprophylaxis in cancer patients. Until then, thromboprophylaxis with DOACs should probably be restricted to cancer patients at very high risk of VTE and low risk bleeding after an informed discussion with the patient.

Funding: This research received no external funding.

Conflicts of Interest: The authors declare no conflict of interest.

References

1. Timp, J.F.; Braekkan, S.K.; Versteeg, H.H.; Cannegieter, S.C. Epidemiology of cancer-associated venous thrombosis. *Blood* **2013**, *122*, 1712–1723. [CrossRef] [PubMed]
2. Cronin-Fenton, D.P.; Søndergaard, F.; Pedersen, L.A.; Fryzek, J.P.; Cetin, K.; Acquavella, J.; Baron, J.A.; Sørensen, H.T. Hospitalisation for venous thromboembolism in cancer patients and the general population: A population-based cohort study in Denmark, 1997–2006. *Br. J. Cancer* **2010**, *103*, 947–953. [CrossRef] [PubMed]
3. Di Nisio, M.; Candeloro, M.; Rutjes, A.W.S.; Porreca, E. Venous thromboembolism in cancer patients receiving neoadjuvant chemotherapy: A systematic review and meta-analysis. *J. Thromb. Haemost.* **2018**, *16*, 1336–1346. [CrossRef] [PubMed]
4. Khorana, A.A.; Connolly, G.C. Assessing Risk of Venous Thromboembolism in the Patient with Cancer. *J. Clin. Oncol.* **2009**, *27*, 4839–4847. [CrossRef] [PubMed]
5. Kahn, S.R.; Lim, W.; Dunn, A.S.; Cushman, M.; Dentali, F.; Akl, E.A.; Cook, D.J.; Balekian, A.A.; Klein, R.C.; Le, H.; et al. Prevention of VTE in Nonsurgical Patients. *Chest* **2012**, *141*, e195S–e226S. [CrossRef] [PubMed]
6. Lyman, G.H.; Bohlke, K.; Khorana, A.A.; Kuderer, N.M.; Lee, A.Y.; Arcelus, J.I.; Balaban, E.P.; Clarke, J.M.; Flowers, C.R.; Francis, C.W.; et al. Venous Thromboembolism Prophylaxis and Treatment in Patients With Cancer: American Society of Clinical Oncology Clinical Practice Guideline Update 2014. *J. Clin. Oncol.* **2015**, *33*, 654–656. [CrossRef]
7. Wang, T.; Zwicker, J.I.; Ay, C.; Pabinger, I.; Falanga, A.; Antic, D.; Noble, S.; Khorana, A.A.; Carrier, M.; Meyer, G. The use of direct oral anticoagulants for primary thromboprophylaxis in ambulatory cancer patients: Guidance from the SSC of the ISTH. *J. Thromb. Haemost.* **2019**, *17*, 1772–1778. [CrossRef]
8. Key, N.S.; Khorana, A.A.; Kuderer, N.M.; Bohlke, K.; Lee, A.Y.Y.; Arcelus, J.I.; Wong, S.L.; Balaban, E.P.; Flowers, C.R.; Francis, C.W.; et al. Venous Thromboembolism Prophylaxis and Treatment in Patients With Cancer: ASCO Clinical Practice Guideline Update. *J. Clin. Oncol.* **2020**. [CrossRef]
9. Krol, M.H.; Pemmaraju, N.; Oo, T.H.; Afshar-Kharghan, V.; Kroll, S. Mortality from Cancer-Associated Venous Thromboembolism. *Blood* **2014**, *124*, 4829. [CrossRef]
10. Seaman, S.; Nelson, A.; Noble, S. Cancer-associated thrombosis, low-molecular-weight heparin, and the patient experience: A qualitative study. *Patient Prefer. Adherence* **2014**, *8*, 453–461.
11. Mockler, A.; O'Brien, B.; Emed, J.; Ciccotosto, G. The Experience of Patients with Cancer Who Develop Venous Thromboembolism: An Exploratory Study. *Oncol. Nurs. Forum* **2012**, *39*, E233–E240. [CrossRef] [PubMed]
12. Lloyd, A.J.; Dewilde, S.; Noble, S.; Reimer, E.; Lee, A.Y.Y. What Impact Does Venous Thromboembolism and Bleeding Have on Cancer Patients' Quality of Life? *Value Health* **2018**, *21*, 449–455. [CrossRef] [PubMed]
13. Teman, N.R.; Silski, L.; Zhao, L.; Kober, M.; Urba, S.C.; Orringer, M.B.; Chang, A.C.; Lin, J.; Reddy, R.M. Thromboembolic Events Before Esophagectomy for Esophageal Cancer Do Not Result in Worse Outcomes. *Ann. Thorac. Surg.* **2012**, *94*, 1118–1125. [CrossRef] [PubMed]
14. Merkow, R.P.; Bilimoria, K.Y.; Tomlinson, J.S.; Paruch, J.L.; Fleming, J.B.; Talamonti, M.S.; Ko, C.Y.; Bentrem, D.J. Postoperative Complications Reduce Adjuvant Chemotherapy Use in Resectable Pancreatic Cancer. *Ann. Surg.* **2014**, *260*, 372–377. [CrossRef]
15. Connolly, G.C.; Dalal, M.; Lin, J.; Khorana, A.A. Incidence and predictors of venous thromboembolism (VTE) among ambulatory patients with lung cancer. *Lung Cancer* **2012**, *78*, 253–258. [CrossRef]
16. Elting, L.S.; Escalante, C.P.; Cooksley, C.; Avritscher, E.B.C.; Kurtin, D.; Hamblin, L.; Khosla, S.G.; Rivera, E. Outcomes and Cost of Deep Venous Thrombosis Among Patients With Cancer. *Arch. Intern. Med.* **2004**, *164*, 1653. [CrossRef]
17. Catella-Chatron, J.; Merah, A.; De Magalhaes, E.; Moulin, N.; Accassat, S.; Duvillard, C.; Mismetti, P.; Bertoletti, L. Frequency of chronic thromboembolic pulmonary hypertension screening after pulmonary embolism in cancer patients. *Eur. Respir. J.* **2018**, *52* (Suppl. 62), OA3804.
18. Prandoni, P.; Lensing, A.W.A.; Piccioli, A.; Bernardi, E.; Simioni, P.; Girolami, B.; Marchiori, A.; Sabbion, P.; Prins, M.H.; Noventa, F.; et al. Recurrent venous thromboembolism and bleeding complications during anticoagulant treatment in patients with cancer and venous thrombosis. *Blood* **2002**, *100*, 3484–3488. [CrossRef]

19. Sørensen, H.T.; Mellemkjær, L.; Olsen, J.H.; Baron, J.A. Prognosis of Cancers Associated with Venous Thromboembolism. *N. Engl. J. Med.* **2000**, *343*, 1846–1850. [CrossRef]
20. Posch, F.; Riedl, J.; Reitter, E.-M.; Kaider, A.; Zielinski, C.; Pabinger, I.; Ay, C. Hypercoagulabilty, venous thromboembolism, and death in patients with cancer. *Thromb. Haemost.* **2016**, *115*, 817–826. [CrossRef]
21. Di Nisio, M.; Porreca, E.; Candeloro, M.; De Tursi, M.; Russi, I.; Rutjes, A.W. Primary prophylaxis for venous thromboembolism in ambulatory cancer patients receiving chemotherapy. *Cochrane Database Syst. Rev.* **2016**. [CrossRef] [PubMed]
22. Li, A.; Kuderer, N.M.; Garcia, D.A.; Khorana, A.A.; Wells, P.S.; Carrier, M.; Lyman, G.H. Direct oral anticoagulant for the prevention of thrombosis in ambulatory patients with cancer: A systematic review and meta-analysis. *J. Thromb. Haemost.* **2019**, *17*, 2141–2151. [CrossRef] [PubMed]
23. Schunemann, H.; Ventresca, M.; Crowther, M.; Di Nisio, M.; Briel, M.; Zhou, Q.; Noble, S.; Macbeth, F.; Griffiths, G.; Garcia, D.; et al. An individual participant data meta-analysis of 13 randomized trials to evaluate the impact of prophylactic use of heparin in oncological patients. In Proceedings of the 59th ASH Annual Meeting and Exposition, Atlanta, GA, USA, 9–12 December 2017.
24. Uno, K.; Homma, S.; Satoh, T.; Nakanishi, K.; Abe, D.; Matsumoto, K.; Oki, A.; Tsunoda, H.; Yamaguchi, I.; Nagasawa, T.; et al. Tissue factor expression as a possible determinant of thromboembolism in ovarian cancer. *Br. J. Cancer* **2007**, *96*, 290–295. [CrossRef] [PubMed]
25. Kaźmierczak, M.; Lewandowski, K.; Wojtukiewicz, M.Z.; Turowiecka, Z.; Kołacz, E.; Łojko, A.; Skrzydlewska, E.; Zawilska, K.; Komarnicki, M. Cancer procoagulant in patients with adenocarcinomas. *Blood Coagul. Fibrinolysis* **2005**, *16*, 543–547. [CrossRef] [PubMed]
26. Farge, D.; Bounameaux, H.; Brenner, B.; Cajfinger, F.; Debourdeau, P.; Khorana, A.A.; Pabinger, I.; Solymoss, S.; Douketis, J.; Kakkar, A. International clinical practice guidelines including guidance for direct oral anticoagulants in the treatment and prophylaxis of venous thromboembolism in patients with cancer. *Lancet Oncol.* **2016**, *17*, e452–e466. [CrossRef]
27. Fernandes, C.J.; Morinaga, L.T.K.; Alves, J.L.; Castro, M.A.; Calderaro, D.; Jardim, C.V.P.; Souza, R. Cancer-associated thrombosis: The when, how and why. *Eur. Respir. Rev.* **2019**, *28*, 180119. [CrossRef] [PubMed]
28. Manly, D.A.; Wang, J.; Glover, S.L.; Kasthuri, R.; Liebman, H.A.; Key, N.S.; Mackman, N. Increased microparticle tissue factor activity in cancer patients with Venous Thromboembolism. *Thromb. Res.* **2010**, *125*, 511–512. [CrossRef]
29. Noble, S.; Prout, H.; Nelson, A. Patients' experiences of living with CANcer-associated thrombosis: The PELICAN study. *Patient Prefer. Adherence* **2015**, *9*, 337–345.
30. Sheth, R.A.; Niekamp, A.; Quencer, K.B.; Shamoun, F.; Knuttinen, M.-G.; Naidu, S.; Oklu, R. Thrombosis in cancer patients: Etiology, incidence, and management. *Cardiovasc. Diagn. Ther.* **2017**, *7*, S178–S185. [CrossRef]
31. Khorana, A.A.; Francis, C.W.; Culakova, E.; Kuderer, N.M.; Lyman, G.H. Thromboembolism is a leading cause of death in cancer patients receiving outpatient chemotherapy. *J. Thromb. Haemost.* **2007**, *5*, 632–634. [CrossRef]
32. Macbeth, F.; Noble, S.; Evans, J.; Ahmed, S.; Cohen, D.; Hood, K.; Knoyle, D.; Linnane, S.; Longo, M.; Moore, B.; et al. Randomized Phase III Trial of Standard Therapy Plus Low Molecular Weight Heparin in Patients With Lung Cancer: FRAGMATIC Trial. *J. Clin. Oncol.* **2016**, *34*, 488–494. [CrossRef] [PubMed]
33. Agnelli, G.; George, D.J.; Kakkar, A.K.; Fisher, W.; Lassen, M.R.; Mismetti, P.; Mouret, P.; Chaudhari, U.; Lawson, F.; Turpie, A.G.G. Semuloparin for Thromboprophylaxis in Patients Receiving Chemotherapy for Cancer. *N. Engl. J. Med.* **2012**, *366*, 601–609. [CrossRef] [PubMed]
34. Common Terminology Criteria for Adverse Events (CTCAE), USA Department of Health and Human Services. Available online: https://ctep.cancer.gov/protocoldevelopment/electronic_applications/docs/CTCAE_v5_Quick_Reference_8.5x11.pdf (accessed on 9 December 2019).
35. Marvig, C.L.; Verhoef, T.I.; de Boer, A.; Kamali, F.; Redekop, K.; Pirmohamed, M.; Daly, A.K.; Manolopoulos, V.G.; Wadelius, M.; Bouvy, M.; et al. Quality of life in patients with venous thromboembolism and atrial fibrillation treated with coumarin anticoagulants. *Thromb. Res.* **2015**, *136*, 69–75. [CrossRef] [PubMed]
36. Sullivan, P.W.; Ghushchyan, V. Preference-Based EQ-5D Index Scores for Chronic Conditions in the United States. *Med. Decis. Mak.* **2006**, *26*, 410–420. [CrossRef] [PubMed]

37. Marin-Barrera, L.; Muñoz-Martin, A.J.; Rios-Herranz, E.; Garcia-Escobar, I.; Beato, C.; Font, C.; Oncala-Sibajas, E.; Revuelta-Rodriguez, A.; Areses, M.C.; Rivas-Jimenez, V.; et al. A Case-Control Analysis of the Impact of Venous Thromboembolic Disease on Quality of Life of Patients with Cancer: Quality of Life in Cancer (Qca) Study. *Cancers* **2019**, *12*, 75. [CrossRef] [PubMed]
38. Noble, S.; Nelson, A.; Scott, J.; Berger, A.; Schmidt, K.; Swarnkar, P.; Lee, A. Patient Experience of Living With Cancer-Associated Thrombosis in Canada (PELICANADA). *Res. Pract. Thromb. Haemost.* **2019**, *4*, 154–160. [CrossRef] [PubMed]
39. Lee, A.Y.Y.; Levine, M.N.; Baker, R.I.; Bowden, C.; Kakkar, A.K.; Prins, M.; Rickles, F.R.; Julian, J.A.; Haley, S.; Kovacs, M.J.; et al. Low-Molecular-Weight Heparin versus a Coumarin for the Prevention of Recurrent Venous Thromboembolism in Patients with Cancer. *N. Engl. J. Med.* **2003**, *349*, 146–153. [CrossRef]
40. Lee, A.Y.Y.; Kamphuisen, P.W.; Meyer, G.; Bauersachs, R.; Janas, M.S.; Jarner, M.F.; Khorana, A.A. Tinzaparin vs Warfarin for Treatment of Acute Venous Thromboembolism in Patients With Active Cancer. *JAMA* **2015**, *314*, 677. [CrossRef]
41. Young, A.M.; Marshall, A.; Thirlwall, J.; Hale, D.; Lokare, A.; Hobbs, F.D.R.; Maraveyas, A.; Poole, C.J.; Lyman, G.H.; Petrou, S.; et al. Comparison of an Oral Factor Xa Inhibitor With Low Molecular Weight Heparin in Patients With Cancer With Venous Thromboembolism: Results of a Randomized Trial (SELECT-D). *J. Clin. Oncol.* **2018**, *36*, 2017–2023. [CrossRef]
42. Raskob, G.E.; van Es, N.; Verhamme, P.; Carrier, M.; Di Nisio, M.; Garcia, D.; Grosso, M.A.; Kakkar, A.K.; Kovacs, M.J.; Mercuri, M.F.; et al. Edoxaban for the Treatment of Cancer-Associated Venous Thromboembolism. *N. Engl. J. Med.* **2018**, *378*, 615–624. [CrossRef]
43. Abdulla, A.; Davis, W.; Ratnaweera, N.; Scott, B.; Lee, A.Y.Y. Case Fatality Rate of Recurrent Venous Thromboembolism and Major Bleeding Events Among Patients Treated for Cancer-Associated Venous Thromboembolism: A Systematic Review. *Blood* **2018**, *132*, 2528. [CrossRef]
44. Subbiah, R.; Aggarwal, V.; Zhao, H.; Kolluri, R.; Chatterjee, S.; Bashir, R. Effect of compression stockings on post thrombotic syndrome in patients with deep vein thrombosis: A meta-analysis of randomised controlled trials. *Lancet Haematol.* **2016**, *3*, e293–e300. [CrossRef]
45. Baldwin, M.J.; Moore, H.M.; Rudarakanchana, N.; Gohel, M.; Davies, A.H. Post-thrombotic syndrome: A clinical review. *J. Thromb. Haemost.* **2013**, *11*, 795–805. [CrossRef] [PubMed]
46. Nishimoto, Y.; Yamashita, Y.; Morimoto, T.; Saga, S.; Amano, H.; Takase, T.; Hiramori, S.; Kim, K.; Oi, M.; Akao, M.; et al. Risk factors for post-thrombotic syndrome in patients with deep vein thrombosis: From the COMMAND VTE registry. *Heart Vessels* **2019**, *34*, 669–677. [CrossRef] [PubMed]
47. Tick, L.W.; Kramer, M.H.H.; Rosendaal, F.R.; Faber, W.R.; Doggen, C.J.M. Risk factors for post-thrombotic syndrome in patients with a first deep venous thrombosis. *J. Thromb. Haemost.* **2008**, *6*, 2075–2081. [CrossRef] [PubMed]
48. Kim, N.H.; Delcroix, M.; Jais, X.; Madani, M.M.; Matsubara, H.; Mayer, E.; Ogo, T.; Tapson, V.F.; Ghofrani, H.-A.; Jenkins, D.P. Chronic thromboembolic pulmonary hypertension. *Eur. Respir. J.* **2019**, *53*, 1801915. [CrossRef]
49. Klok, F.A.; van Kralingen, K.W.; van Dijk, A.P.J.; Heyning, F.H.; Vliegen, H.W.; Huisman, M.V. Prospective cardiopulmonary screening program to detect chronic thromboembolic pulmonary hypertension in patients after acute pulmonary embolism. *Haematologica* **2010**, *95*, 970–975. [CrossRef]
50. Delcroix, M.; Lang, I.; Pepke-Zaba, J.; Jansa, P.; D'Armini, A.M.; Snijder, R.; Bresser, P.; Torbicki, A.; Mellemkjaer, S.; Lewczuk, J.; et al. Long-Term Outcome of Patients With Chronic Thromboembolic Pulmonary Hypertension. *Circulation* **2016**, *133*, 859–871. [CrossRef]
51. Jemal, A.; Ward, E.M.; Johnson, C.J.; Cronin, K.A.; Ma, J.; Ryerson, A.B.; Mariotto, A.; Lake, A.J.; Wilson, R.; Sherman, R.L.; et al. Annual Report to the Nation on the Status of Cancer, 1975–2014, Featuring Survival. *JNCI J. Natl. Cancer Inst.* **2017**, *109*. [CrossRef]
52. Levine, M.; Hirsh, J.; Arnold, A.; Gent, M.; Levine, M.; Arnold, A.; Bramwell, V.; Pritchard, K.I.; Stewart, D.; Warr, D.; et al. Double-blind randomised trial of very-low-dose warfarin for prevention of thromboembolism in stage IV breast cancer. *Lancet* **1994**, *343*, 886–889. [CrossRef]
53. Agnelli, G.; Gussoni, G.; Bianchini, C.; Verso, M.; Mandalà, M.; Cavanna, L.; Barni, S.; Labianca, R.; Buzzi, F.; Scambia, G.; et al. Nadroparin for the prevention of thromboembolic events in ambulatory patients with metastatic or locally advanced solid cancer receiving chemotherapy: A randomised, placebo-controlled, double-blind study. *Lancet. Oncol.* **2009**, *10*, 943–949. [CrossRef]

54. Schulman, S. Advantages and limitations of the new anticoagulants. *J. Intern. Med.* **2014**, *275*, 1–11. [CrossRef] [PubMed]
55. Khorana, A.A.; Kuderer, N.M.; Culakova, E.; Lyman, G.H.; Francis, C.W. Development and validation of a predictive model for chemotherapy-associated thrombosis. *Clin. Trials Obs.* **2008**, *111*, 4902–4908. [CrossRef] [PubMed]
56. Streiff, M.B.; Holmstrom, B.; Ashrani, A.; Bockenstedt, P.L.; Chesney, C.; Eby, C.; Fanikos, J.; Fenninger, R.B.; Fogerty, A.E.; Gao, S.; et al. Cancer-associated venous thromboembolic disease, version 1.2015: Featured updates to the NCCN Guidelines. *JNCCN J. Natl. Compr. Cancer Netw.* **2015**, *13*, 1079–1095. [CrossRef]
57. van Es, N.; Di Nisio, M.; Cesarman, G.; Kleinjan, A.; Otten, H.M.; Mahé, I.; Wilts, I.T.; Twint, D.C.; Porreca, E.; Arrieta, O.; et al. Comparison of risk prediction scores for venous thromboembolism in cancer patients: A prospective cohort study. *Haematologica* **2017**, *102*, 1494–1501. [CrossRef]
58. Mulder, F.I.; Candeloro, M.; Kamphuisen, P.W.; Di Nisio, M.; Bossuyt, P.M.; Guman, N.; Smit, K.; Büller, H.R.; van Es, N. The Khorana score for prediction of venous thromboembolism in cancer patients: A systematic review and meta-analysis. *Haematologica* **2019**, *104*, 1277–1287. [CrossRef]
59. Pabinger, I.; van Es, N.; Heinze, G.; Posch, F.; Riedl, J.; Reitter, E.M.; Di Nisio, M.; Cesarman-Maus, G.; Kraaijpoel, N.; Zielinski, C.C.; et al. A clinical prediction model for cancer-associated venous thromboembolism: A development and validation study in two independent prospective cohorts. *Lancet Haematol.* **2018**, *5*, e289–e298. [CrossRef]
60. Verso, M.; Agnelli, G.; Barni, S.; Gasparini, G.; LaBianca, R. A modified Khorana risk assessment score for venous thromboembolism in cancer patients receiving chemotherapy: The Protecht score. *Intern. Emerg. Med.* **2012**, *7*, 291–292. [CrossRef]
61. Pelzer, U.; Sinn, M.; Stieler, J.; Riess, H. Primäre medikamentöse Thromboembolieprophylaxe bei ambulanten Patienten mit fortgeschrittenem Pankreaskarzinom unter Chemotherapie? *Dtsch. Medizinische Wochenschrift* **2013**, *138*, 2084–2088. [CrossRef]
62. Ay, C.; Dunkler, D.; Marosi, C.; Chiriac, A.; Vormittag, R.; Simanek, R.; Quehenberger, P.; Zielinski, C.; Pabinger, I. Prediction of venous thromboembolism in cancer patients. *Blood* **2010**, *116*, 5377–5382. [CrossRef]
63. Cella, C.A.; Di Minno, G.; Carlomagno, C.; Arcopinto, M.; Cerbone, A.M.; Matano, E.; Tufano, A.; Lordick, F.; De Simone, B.; Muehlberg, K.S.; et al. Preventing Venous Thromboembolism in Ambulatory Cancer Patients: The ONKOTEV Study. *Oncologist* **2017**, *22*, 601–608. [CrossRef] [PubMed]
64. van Es, N.; Hisada, Y.; Di Nisio, M.; Cesarman, G.; Kleinjan, A.; Mahé, I.; Otten, H.M.; Kamphuisen, P.W.; Berckmans, R.J.; Büller, H.R.; et al. Extracellular vesicles exposing tissue factor for the prediction of venous thromboembolism in patients with cancer: A prospective cohort study. *Thromb. Res.* **2018**, *166*, 54–59. [CrossRef] [PubMed]
65. Muñoz Martín, A.J.; Ortega, I.; Font, C.; Pachón, V.; Castellón, V.; Martínez-Marín, V.; Salgado, M.; Martínez, E.; Calzas, J.; Rupérez, A.; et al. Multivariable clinical-genetic risk model for predicting venous thromboembolic events in patients with cancer. *Br. J. Cancer* **2018**, *118*, 1056–1061. [CrossRef] [PubMed]
66. Gerotziafas, G.T.; Taher, A.; Abdel-Razeq, H.; AboElnazar, E.; Spyropoulos, A.C.; El Shemmari, S.; Larsen, A.K.; Elalamy, I. A Predictive Score for Thrombosis Associated with Breast, Colorectal, Lung, or Ovarian Cancer: The Prospective COMPASS–Cancer-Associated Thrombosis Study. *Oncologist* **2017**, *22*, 1222–1231. [CrossRef] [PubMed]
67. Antic, D.; Milic, N.; Nikolovski, S.; Todorovic, M.; Bila, J.; Djurdjevic, P.; Andjelic, B.; Djurasinovic, V.; Sretenovic, A.; Vukovic, V.; et al. Development and validation of multivariable predictive model for thromboembolic events in lymphoma patients. *Am. J. Hematol.* **2016**, *91*, 1014–1019. [CrossRef] [PubMed]
68. Barbui, T.; Finazzi, G.; Carobbio, A.; Thiele, J.; Passamonti, F.; Rumi, E.; Ruggeri, M.; Rodeghiero, F.; Randi, M.L.; Bertozzi, I.; et al. Development and validation of an International Prognostic Score of thrombosis in World Health Organization–essential thrombocythemia (IPSET-thrombosis). *Blood* **2012**, *120*, 5128–5133. [CrossRef]
69. Norris, L.A.; Abu Saadeh, F.; Ward, M.; O'Toole, S.A.; Machocki, Z.; Ibrahim, N.; Gleeson, N. Development and validation of a risk model for prediction of venous thromboembolism in gynaecological cancer patients. *Thromb. Res.* **2018**, *164*, S183–S184. [CrossRef]
70. Khorana, A.A.; Francis, C.W.; Kuderer, N.M.; Carrier, M.; Ortel, T.L.; Wun, T.; Rubens, D.; Hobbs, S.; Iyer, R.; Peterson, D.; et al. Dalteparin thromboprophylaxis in cancer patients at high risk for venous thromboembolism: A randomized trial. *Thromb. Res.* **2017**, *151*, 89–95. [CrossRef]

71. Khorana, A.A.; Soff, G.A.; Kakkar, A.K.; Vadhan-Raj, S.; Riess, H.; Wun, T.; Streiff, M.B.; Garcia, D.A.; Liebman, H.A.; Belani, C.P.; et al. Rivaroxaban for Thromboprophylaxis in High-Risk Ambulatory Patients with Cancer. *N. Engl. J. Med.* **2019**, *380*, 720–728. [CrossRef]
72. Sandset, P.M.; Dahm, A.E.A. Is venous thromboembolism a problem in patients with cancer in palliative care? *Lancet Haematol.* **2019**, *6*, e61–e62. [CrossRef]
73. Carrier, M.; Abou-Nassar, K.; Mallick, R.; Tagalakis, V.; Shivakumar, S.; Schattner, A.; Kuruvilla, P.; Hill, D.; Spadafora, S.; Marquis, K.; et al. Apixaban to Prevent Venous Thromboembolism in Patients with Cancer. *N. Engl. J. Med.* **2019**, *380*, 711–719. [CrossRef] [PubMed]
74. Farge, D.; Frere, C.; Connors, J.M.; Ay, C.; Khorana, A.A.; Munoz, A.; Brenner, B.; Kakkar, A.; Rafii, H.; Solymoss, S.; et al. 2019 international clinical practice guidelines for the treatment and prophylaxis of venous thromboembolism in patients with cancer. *Lancet Oncol.* **2019**, *12*, 805–807. [CrossRef]
75. Kraaijpoel, N.; Di Nisio, M.; Mulder, F.I.; Van Es, N.; Beyer-Westendorf, J.; Carrier, M.; Garcia, D.; Grosso, M.; Kakkar, A.K.; Mercuri, M.F.; et al. Clinical Impact of Bleeding in Cancer-Associated Venous Thromboembolism: Results from the Hokusai VTE Cancer Study. *Thromb. Haemost.* **2018**, *118*, 1439–1449. [CrossRef] [PubMed]
76. Mulder, F.I.; van Es, N.; Kraaijpoel, N.; Di Nisio, M.; Carrier, M.; Duggal, A.; Gaddh, M.; Garcia, D.; Grosso, M.A.; Kakkar, A.K.; et al. Edoxaban for treatment of venous thromboembolism in patient groups with different types of cancer: Results from the Hokusai VTE Cancer study. *Thromb. Res.* **2020**, *185*, 13–19. [CrossRef]
77. Steffel, J.; Verhamme, P.; Potpara, T.S.; Albaladejo, P.; Antz, M.; Desteghe, L.; Haeusler, K.G.; Oldgren, J.; Reinecke, H.; Roldan-Schilling, V.; et al. The 2018 European Heart Rhythm AssociationPractical Guide on the use of non-vitamin Kantagonist oral anticoagulants in patients withatrial fibrillation: Executive summary. *Eur. Heart J.* **2018**, *39*, 1330–1393. [CrossRef]
78. Mauracher, L.-M.; Posch, F.; Martinod, K.; Grilz, E.; Däullary, T.; Hell, L.; Brostjan, C.; Zielinski, C.; Ay, C.; Wagner, D.D.; et al. Citrullinated histone H3, a biomarker of neutrophil extracellular trap formation, predicts the risk of venous thromboembolism in cancer patients. *J. Thromb. Haemost.* **2018**, *16*, 508–518. [CrossRef]
79. Poruk, K.E.; Firpo, M.A.; Huerter, L.M.; Scaife, C.L.; Emerson, L.L.; Boucher, K.M.; Jones, K.A.; Mulvihill, S.J. Serum platelet factor 4 is an independent predictor of survival and venous thromboembolism in patients with pancreatic adenocarcinoma. *Cancer Epidemiol. Biomarkers Prev.* **2010**, *19*, 2605–2610. [CrossRef]
80. Ades, S.; Kumar, S.; Alam, M.; Goodwin, A.; Weckstein, D.; Dugan, M.; Ashikaga, T.; Evans, M.; Verschraegen, C.; Holmes, C.E. Tumor oncogene (KRAS) status and risk of venous thrombosis in patients with metastatic colorectal cancer. *J. Thromb. Haemost.* **2015**, *13*, 998–1003. [CrossRef]
81. Ünlü, B.; van Es, N.; Arindrarto, W.; Kiełbasa, S.M.; Mei, H.; Westerga, J.; Middeldorp, S.; Kuppen, P.J.K.; Otten, J.M.M.B.; Cannegieter, S.; et al. Genes associated with venous thromboembolism in colorectal cancer patients. *J. Thromb. Haemost.* **2018**, *16*, 293–302. [CrossRef]
82. Di Nisio, M.; van Es, N.; Rotunno, L.; Anzoletti, N.; Falcone, L.; De Tursi, M.; Natoli, C.; Tinari, N.; Cavallo, I.; Valeriani, E.; et al. Long-term performance of risk scores for venous thromboembolism in ambulatory cancer patients. *J. Thromb. Thrombolysis* **2019**, *48*, 125–133. [CrossRef]
83. Ferroni, P.; Zanzotto, F.M.; Scarpato, N.; Riondino, S.; Guadagni, F.; Roselli, M. Validation of a Machine Learning Approach for Venous Thromboembolism Risk Prediction in Oncology. *Dis. Markers* **2017**, *2017*. [CrossRef] [PubMed]
84. Weitz, J.I.; Fredenburgh, J.C. Factors XI and XII as targets for new anticoagulants. *Front. Med.* **2017**, *4*, 19. [CrossRef] [PubMed]
85. Ramacciotti, E.; Myers, D.D.; Wrobleski, S.K.; Deatrick, K.B.; Londy, F.J.; Rectenwald, J.E.; Henke, P.K.; Schaub, R.G.; Wakefield, T.W. P-selectin/ PSGL-1 Inhibitors versus enoxaparin in the resolution of venous thrombosis: A meta-analysis. *Thromb. Res.* **2010**, *125*, 138–142. [CrossRef] [PubMed]
86. Büller, H.R.; Bethune, C.; Bhanot, S.; Gailani, D.; Monia, B.P.; Raskob, G.E.; Segers, A.; Verhamme, P.; Weitz, J.I. Factor XI antisense oligonucleotide for prevention of venous thrombosis. *N. Engl. J. Med.* **2015**, *372*, 232–240. [CrossRef] [PubMed]

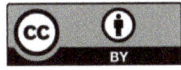
© 2020 by the authors. Licensee MDPI, Basel, Switzerland. This article is an open access article distributed under the terms and conditions of the Creative Commons Attribution (CC BY) license (http://creativecommons.org/licenses/by/4.0/).

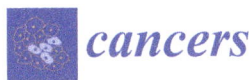

Review

Risk Prediction and New Prophylaxis Strategies for Thromboembolism in Cancer

Alice Labianca [1], Tommaso Bosetti [1], Alice Indini [2], Giorgia Negrini [1] and Roberto Francesco Labianca [1,*]

[1] Medical Oncology Unit, Department of Oncology and Haematology, ASST Papa Giovanni XXIII, 24121 Bergamo, Italy; alice.labiancadr@gmail.com (A.L.); tbosetti@asst-pg23.it (T.B.); gnegrini@asst-pg23.it (G.N.)

[2] Medical Oncology Unit, Fondazione IRCCS Ca' Granda Ospedale Maggiore Policlinico, 20019 Milano, Italy; alice.indini@gmail.com

* Correspondence: rlabian@tin.it

Received: 24 June 2020; Accepted: 23 July 2020; Published: 27 July 2020

Abstract: In the general population, the incidence of thromboembolic events is 117 cases/100,000 inhabitants/year, while in cancer patient incidence, it is four-fold higher, especially in patients who receive chemotherapy and who are affected by pancreatic, lung or gastric cancer. At the basis of venous thromboembolism (VTE) there is the so-called Virchow triad, but tumor cells can activate coagulation pathway by various direct and indirect mechanisms, and chemotherapy can contribute to VTE onset. For these reasons, several studies were conducted in order to assess efficacy and safety of the use of anticoagulant therapy in cancer patients, both in prophylaxis setting and in therapy setting. With this review, we aim to record principal findings and current guidelines about thromboprophylaxis in cancer patients, with particular attention to subjects with additional risk factors such as patients receiving chemotherapy or undergoing surgery, hospitalized patients for acute medical intercurrent event and patients with central venous catheters. Nonetheless we added a brief insight about acute and maintenance therapy of manifested venous thromboembolism in cancer patients.

Keywords: thromboprophylaxis; venous thromboembolism; chemotherapy; low-molecular-weight heparin (LMWH); VKA; UFH; DOACs

1. Introduction

The correlation between cancer and venous thromboembolism (VTE), which comprehends deep vein thrombosis (DVT) and pulmonary embolism (PE), is well known. In the general population incidence of thromboembolic events is 117 cases/100,000 inhabitants/year, while in cancer patient incidence is four-fold higher and in patients who receive chemotherapy is seven-fold higher [1]. In addition, thromboembolic risk is higher in patients who receive hormonotherapy, who have central venous catheter and who undergo surgery.

At the basis of VTE there is the so-called Virchow triad (see Table 1).

The first data about the incidence of venous thromboembolism in oncological patients on active anticancer treatment come from NSABP-14 and NSABP-20 trials; in these trials, estrogen and progesterone receptors positive-nodes negative breast cancer patients treated with tamoxifen and chemotherapy had a higher incidence of VTE compared with patients receiving tamoxifen alone or placebo (5 years incidence 4.3%, 0.9% and 0.2%, respectively) [2,3]. Association of chemotherapy and anti-VEGF antibodies worsens even more the risk of venous and arterial thrombosis. In addition, patients with malignant gastric, pancreatic, pulmonary cancers or glioblastomas have a higher risk of VTE (10–30%) [4].

For these reasons, VTE prophylaxis in oncological patients has been the subject of several studies in the last years.

Recent international guidelines provided updated recommendations for the management of VTE in cancer patients. Nonetheless, several reviews have been published in the last few years: Horsted et al. in 2012 conducted a systematic review about the incidence of VTE in cancer patients, in order to provide data about the risk of VTE in different cancer types, stratify patients and highlight which kind of patient should receive prophylaxis [5]. In 2014 Matzdorff and colleagues outlined pathophysiology of VTE in cancer patients and reported the most recent indications about VTE therapy and prophylaxis, as well as the use of new oral anticoagulants (but concluded that DOACs were not recommended according to 2014 international guidelines) [6]. Singh et al. in 2017 outlined pathophysiology and diagnosis of venous thromboembolism in patients with cancer, as well as pharmacological and mechanical prophylaxis [7]; Imberti and colleagues, the subsequent year, reported the most important findings about VTE treatment, focusing on the results of Hokusai VTE-cancer trial about the comparison between low-molecular-weight heparin (LMWH) and the direct oral anticoagulant edoxaban, which showed that edoxaban is non-inferior to dalteparin with a trend toward fewer recurrent venous thromboembolic events, but with higher major bleeding risk [8].

Still, some uncertainties remain, both for prophylaxis and treatment of VTE, due to the yet limited evidence available. With this review, we aim to summarize the latest evidence on VTE prophylaxis and treatment in patients with cancer, based on the newest guidelines and papers published in the last few months, as well as synthesize the major clinical trials and meta-analyses that have been conducted until now and highlight the most clinically relevant unmet needs.

Table 1. Virchow triad: factors contributing to thrombosis.

Virchow Triad
Blood stasis
Endothelial injury or vessel walls injury
Hypercoagulability

2. Thrombosis Pathophysiology in Cancer Patients

Tumor cells can activate coagulation pathway by a direct and an indirect mechanism: the direct mechanism involves the production of pro-coagulant factors such as the *tissue factor* which is constitutively expressed by tumor cells and which binds factor VII and activates coagulation pathway; and the *cancer procoagulant*, a cysteine protease expressed in tumor cells and in fetal tissues which activates factor X in absence of factor VII [9,10].

Among indirect mechanisms, we can enumerate production of cytokines such as IL-2, TNF and VEGF that activate monocytes, platelets and endothelial cells inducing procoagulant phenotype expression. In addition, tumor cells have superficial adhesion molecules that can bind monocytes, platelets and endothelial cells activating and stimulating fibrin production. Moreover, some predisposing factors can add prothrombotic risk such as hospitalization, systemic inflammatory status and tumor compression stasis.

Chemotherapy can contribute to VTE onset with various mechanisms, such as vessel walls acute damage, and this is the case of bleomycin, carmustine and vinca alkaloids or retarded damage for adriamycin; coagulation regulator factors reduction, such as reduction of protein C and S in the case of CMF scheme (cyclophosphamide, methotrexate and 5-fluorouracil) or reduction of antithrombin II by L-asparaginase.

3. VTE Risk Prediction in Cancer Patients

In order to assess VTE risk in cancer patients, various factors need to be considered. First of all, personal thrombophilic conditions such as advanced age, obesity, history of previous venous thromboembolism, prolonged immobility, prothrombotic blood alterations. Then, risk factors associated with the tumor itself, such as histology, grading, primary site, presence of metastasis, and factors associated with tumor treatment, such as ongoing or recent chemotherapy, hormonal therapy, anti-angiogenesis agents, immunotherapy, radiotherapy, recent surgery, presence of central venous catheters, hospitalization.

Some blood biomarkers have been studied and associated with elevated VTE risk, such as platelets and leucocytes count, D-dimer, soluble *P*-selectin and other markers of coagulation activation, markers of neutrophil extracellular trap formation, such as citrullinated histone H3 and many others [11–13].

Some risk models have been developed and proposed over the last few years. The most known and used is the Khorana risk score (Table 2) [14], published in 2008, validated in several subsequent studies and still used by clinicians. Some variations of the Khorana risk score have been published subsequently, such as the PROTECHT, CONKO and Vienna CATS score [15–17]. Thereafter, the COMPASS-CAT and the ONKOTEV56 models were developed, the first one for patients with breast, colorectal, lung and ovarian cancers, including variables such as cardiovascular risk factors, personal history of VTE, presence of central venous catheter, chemotherapy or hormonal therapy, tumor stage and platelet count; the second one based on Khorana risk score >2 associated with the presence of metastasis, vascular compression, previous VTE [18,19].

Table 2. Khorana score risk factors: predictive model for chemotherapy-associated venous thromboembolism (VTE) [14]. (from Khorana, A.A.; Kuderer, N.M. Development and validation of a predictive model for chemotherapy-associated thrombosis. Blood 2008, 111, 4902–4907).

Factors	Points
Primary cancer site	
Pancreas, stomach	2
Lung, renal, bladder, testicular, lymphoma, gynecologic	1
Hemoglobin < 10 g/dL or use of red cell growth factors	1
Leukocytes > 11.000/µL	1
Platelets ≥ 350.000/µL	1
BMI ≥ 35 kg/m^2	1
Interpretation:	
High-risk score	≥3 points
Intermediate-risk score	1–2 points
Low-risk score	0 points

4. VTE Prophylaxis in Patients Receiving Chemotherapy

Clinical studies about the use of thromboprophylaxis in outpatients receiving systemic treatment for cancer were conducted in two moments; the first moment saw clinical trials evaluating safety and efficacy of low-molecular-weight heparin (LMWH) in this setting of patients, the second one evaluated safety and efficacy of direct oral anticoagulants (DOACs) in high risk patients.

Analyzing literature, five meta-analyses and two recent randomized trials investigated thromboprophylaxis in cancer patients. The five meta-analyses primarily analyzed LMWH use: in a meta-analysis published in 2012, Di Nisio et al. outlined how LMWH significantly reduces asymptomatic VTE (HR 0.54, CI 95% 0.38–0.75) with a non-statistically significant higher risk of major bleeding (HR 1.44, CI 95% 0.98–2.11) [20]. The 2014 meta-analysis of Ben-Aharon et al. showed similar results [21].

Two meta-analyses (Thein et al. and Fuentes et al.) [22,23] analyzed lung cancer setting; LMWH reduced the risk of VTE of about half, but it did not significantly affect OS. In Thein et al. meta-analysis, the use of LMWH significantly increased the risk of non-major, but clinically relevant bleeding (RR 3.35, CI 95% 2.09–5.06), while it did not affect the risk of major bleeding. In Fuentes et al. meta-analysis the use of LMWH did not significantly affect the risk of total bleedings.

The meta-analysis by Tun et al. analyzed only patients with advanced pancreatic cancer, demonstrating how the use of LMWH reduces the risk of symptomatic VTE (RR 0.18, 95% CI 0.08–0.39) without significantly increasing the rate of major bleeding (RR 1.25, 95% CI 0.48–3.31) [24].

Two randomized controlled trials were conducted in the last years to analyze the use of DOACs in patients receiving active treatment for cancer and with Khorana score ≥2 (see Table 2) [25,26].

The AVERT study, a double-blind, randomized, placebo-controlled clinical trial, evaluated the efficacy and safety of apixaban at a dosage of 2.5 mg twice/daily in the primary prevention of VTE in 574 ambulatory patients with Khorana score ≥2 receiving chemotherapy. Apixaban significantly reduced limbs deep vein thrombosis, pulmonary embolism and VTE-related death compared to placebo (4.2% vs. 10.2% with apixaban vs. placebo, respectively, HR 0.41, 95% CI 0.26–0.65). However, apixaban prophylaxis was associated with an increased risk of major bleedings (3.5% vs. 1.8% with apixaban vs. placebo, HR 2.00 CI 95% 1.01–3.95) [25].

The second clinical trial that assessed the efficacy and safety of a DOAC in the primary prevention of VTE was the CASSINI study, a randomized, double-blind clinical trial with rivaroxaban 10 mg/day vs. placebo, in 841 outpatients affected by stage III or IV tumors and Khorana score ≥2 which were about to start systemic chemotherapy. In this study, patients were screened with venous ultrasound before randomization and every eight weeks afterwards. The use of rivaroxaban was associated with a statistically insignificant decrease in the primary outcome in ITT (intention-to-treat) population (deep vein thrombosis of the limbs 6.0% vs. 8.8% with rivaroxaban vs. placebo, HR 0.66, CI 95% 0.4–1.9), while in a prespecified analysis of all randomized patients the primary VTE endpoint on treatment occurred in 2.6% of 420 and in 6.4% of 421 patients in the rivaroxaban and placebo arms, respectively (HR0.40, 95% CI 0.2–0.8); also, the use of rivaroxaban was associated with a statistically insignificant increase in the risk of major bleeding (2% vs. 1%, rivaroxaban vs. placebo arm, HR 1.96, CI 95% 0.59–6.49) [26].

In a recent meta-analysis published by Becattini et al. including Avert study, Cassini study and a phase II study with apixaban, thromboprophylaxis reduced the incidence of VTE of about 50% (49%, CI 95% 0.43–0.61) in particular in patients with lung cancer, pancreatic cancer and in the so-called high-risk patients, without observing a significant increase in the risk of major bleeding (OR 1.3, 95% CI 0.98–1.73) [27].

Some ad hoc studies evaluated the impact of VTE prophylaxis in patients affected by multiple myeloma in therapy with thalidomide or lenalidomide, and it was found that prophylactic dosage of LMWH, warfarin or aspirin reduced the risk of VTE; moreover, there was a lower effect of warfarin compared to LMWH in patients over 65 years [28,29].

In late 2019, an update of clinical practice guidelines from the International Initiative on Thrombosis and Cancer working group has been published. According to these guidelines, thromboprophylaxis with rivaroxaban or apixaban is recommended in ambulatory intermediate/high risk patients receiving chemotherapy and who do not have active bleeding or high bleeding risk. In particular, VTE prophylaxis is recommended in patients treated with immunomodulatory drugs, chemotherapy and steroids, due to the high risk of VTE in this setting of patients [30].

Thromboprophylaxis with LMWH is suggested in ambulatory patients with metastatic or locally advanced pancreatic cancer receiving chemotherapy and without major bleeding risk [31,32].

The American Society of Clinical Oncology (ASCO) recently updated its clinical practice guidelines. Among this update, the introduction of DOACs in the treatment strategy and in the prophylaxis of VTE in cancer patients represents one of the most important novelty [33,34].

A systematic review and meta-analysis which includes 30 randomized controlled trials and determines the efficacy and safety of thromboprophylaxis in patients with cancer has recently been published [35]. In this meta-analysis no significant difference in all-cause mortality has been observed in patients who did and did not receive thromboprophylaxis. Thromboprophylaxis can reduce VTE events in patients with cancer undergoing surgery or chemotherapy and does not increase major bleeding events or the incidence of thrombocytopenia. Limitations of this review are different cancer types and staging, different anticoagulants and dosage administered and potential interactions between antithrombotic drugs and patients' concomitant medications.

A careful analysis of international guidelines allows us to summarize the following recommendations [34,36]:

- Anti-thrombotic prophylaxis should not be offered routinely in all unselected cancer patients on active oncological therapy;
- In high-risk patients with multiple myeloma and in therapy with lenalidomide or thalidomide, prophylaxis with LMWH should always be practiced unless specific clinical contraindications. In patients in this setting, but at low risk of VTE, aspirin prophylaxis can be practiced instead of LMWH;
- In general, prophylaxis with LMWH, apixaban or rivaroxaban should be considered for cancer outpatients who receive chemotherapy and who are at high thromboembolic risk.

Prospective randomized ad hoc trials evaluating thromboprophylaxis in different types of neoplasia and cancer therapy are needed. More studies are also necessary to evaluate the risk of bleeding in patients taking DOACs and suffering from gastrointestinal or genitourinary cancers, as well as studies assessing possible drug interactions with immunotherapy and with tyrosine kinase inhibitors [37]. Development of new risk models as well as refinement of already in use models are needed in order to provide a more accurate risk stratification for cancer patients receiving chemotherapy or new anticancer therapies.

5. Prophylaxis of Central Venous Catheter Thromboembolism

Upper limbs venous thrombosis related to the insertion of central venous catheter in patients on active cancer therapy has long been debated. There are controversial studies about the benefit of thromboprophylaxis: in past decades, some studies showed a statistically significant reduction of VTE with the use of warfarin or LMWH, with an incidence of events in patients non receiving prophylaxis of even 14%. Most recent studies have resized the problem, limiting the incidence of VTE without prophylaxis to 4–5% and attesting a non-statistically significant difference between patients who received thromboprophylaxis and those who received placebo [38]; this is maybe due to greater expertise in the insertion of venous catheters and new less thrombogenic materials. Moreover, the ETHIC study demonstrated a statistically insignificant reduction in thromboembolic events between patients treated with enoxaparin 40 mg and patients treated with placebo [39].

To be noted that at least two meta-analyses highlighted a higher incidence of VTE with peripherally inserted central catheter (PICC line) than with central venous catheter (CVC) [40].

Based on this evidences, a routine thromboprophylaxis with LMWH in patients with central venous catheter is not currently indicated.

6. Thromboprophylaxis in Hospitalized Patients with Acute Medical Condition

Oncological diseases, hospital immobilization, sepsis, advanced age, exacerbations of chronic obstructive pulmonary disease (COPD) are risk factors for the development of VTE in hospitalized patients, as well as personal history of previous VTE. Without thromboprophylaxis, incidence of VTE in hospitalized patients ranges from 10% to 40%, with most of the events occurring after discharge [41].

Three clinical studies assessed the efficacy of primary thromboembolic prophylaxis in hospitalized cancer patients confined to bed with an acute medical complication: the MEDENOX [42] and the PREVENT [43] study evaluated the use of enoxaparin and dalteparin, the ARTEMIS study [44] the use of fondaparinux, with a percentage of cancer patients in these studies of about 10–15%.

In the MEDENOX study, prophylaxis with enoxaparin 40 mg/die reduced the incidence of VTE to 5.5% compared to 15% of patients treated with placebo or enoxaparin 20 mg/die. A subgroup analysis showed that in cancer patients the use of enoxaparin 40 mg/die reduces VTE events by 60%.

The CERTIFY study compared LMWH vs. unfractionated heparin (UFH) in VTE prevention in hospitalized cancer patients with acute medical event, highlighting equal effectiveness and safety [45].

A recent meta-analysis by Carrier et al. showed discordant results, demonstrating that a thromboprophylaxis with LMWH does not statistically reduce the risk of VTE (RR 0.91, 95% CI 0.21–4.0), despite some limitations such as the heterogeneity of the studies and the low sample size [46].

In contrast, another recent meta-analysis showed that in hospitalized cancer patients with other risk factors, the use of LMWH significantly reduced VTE risk (RR 0.32, 95% CI 0.14–0.71) [47].

In conclusion, current guidelines recommend preventive use of LMWH or fondaparinux in hospitalized cancer patients with an acute medical complication. Currently, there is no strong data to support the use of DOACs and the duration of prophylaxis is also an unsolved hot topic.

7. Post-Surgical Thromboprophylaxis

In the literature, patients with active cancer undergoing surgery have been reported to have almost twice the risk of experiencing VTE compared to non-cancer patients (37% vs. 20% using fibrinogen uptake test in a study published in 1970) with a quadrupled risk of fatal pulmonary embolism [48,49]; more recently, the risk of VTE following surgery in oncological patients has been resized, thanks to new surgical techniques, new detection methods, and especially to the introduction of pharmacological and mechanical VTE prophylaxis [50]. Various studies compared the safety and efficacy of unfractionated heparin with LMWH in this setting of patients, demonstrating equal efficacy and greater manageability for LMWH [51–55]; particularly a randomized multicenter trial of patients undergoing elective pelvic or abdominal oncological surgery [56] showed that enoxaparin 40 mg/die vs. UFH at low dosage were equivalent in terms of safety and efficacy in reducing the incidence of VTE.

Therefore, in patients undergoing oncological surgery, thromboprophylaxis with LMWH, UFH or fondaparinux, associated with the use of graduated compression stockings, should be taken into account, with LMWH as first choice thanks to the greater manageability (once-daily administration) and the lower risk of heparin-induced thrombocytopenia. There are currently no data on the use of DOACs in this setting of patients.

For what concerns the duration of treatment, ENOXACAN II study evaluated efficacy of enoxaparin 40 mg/die for one week vs. the same dose for four weeks after surgery, in patients undergoing abdominal or pelvic oncological surgery. Results showed that prolonging thromboprophylaxis reduces the risk of VTE from 12% to 4.8% (RR 60%, 95% CI 0.1–0.82) [56,57]. Further studies with different LMWH confirmed these data [58–60].

A recent meta-analysis by Bottaro et al. showed that a 4–5 weeks prophylaxis reduces the risk of deep vein thrombosis of 53% compared to one week prophylaxis, with a similar hemorrhagic risk [61].

In conclusion, current guidelines recommend thromboprophylaxis of the duration of at least 7–10 days after both laparotomic and laparoscopic cancer surgery, to be extended up to four weeks especially in case of additional risk factors such as prolonged immobility, advanced age, obesity or previous personal history of VTE [34,62,63].

8. VTE Therapy

For what concerns the treatment of VTE in cancer patients, it is important to distinguish two phases of the disease: an acute phase, with the initial treatment and a late phase, with the maintenance treatment.

The initial treatment of the acute phase of VTE in oncological patients (first 5–10 days of therapy) involves the administration of LMWH in single-dose or in double-daily administration based on body weight or UFH in initial bolus of 5000 IU followed by continuous infusion, modulated in order to obtain a PTT ratio of 1.5–2.5 times the basal value. LMWH demonstrated the same efficacy as UFH in the initial treatment of VTE in both non-oncological and oncological patients [64–66]. In addition, a recent meta-analysis showed that LMWH is associated with a 3-month reduction in mortality compared to UFH [67–69].

Fondaparinux can also be used for the initial treatment of established VTE in patients with cancer. Among the advantages of this drug, its administration contributes to an increased manageability for possibly long-lasting outpatient therapies.

In conclusion, LMWH can be considered the standard of care in the initial treatment of VTE in oncological patients, also thanks to its manageability, while UFH and fondaparinux represent valid second line alternatives.

To be remembered is that LMWH is contraindicated in patients with severe renal failure (i.e., with creatinine clearance <30 mL/min); in those cases, UFH is preferred.

The select-D study verified how rivaroxaban is a good alternative in the treatment of the acute phase of VTE in most oncological patients, while leading to an increased risk of gastrointestinal and genitourinary bleeding which must be balanced and evaluated with each patient based on its advantages (i.e., oral intake, etc.) [65].

For patients who do not have a high risk of gastrointestinal or genitourinary bleeding, rivaroxaban or edoxaban (the last one after at least five days of parenteral anticoagulation) can be used for the initial treatment of established VTE in patients with cancer [30].

A frequent problem in oncological patients is represented by the thrombocytopenia which can be due to chemotherapy, radiation therapy, bone marrow invasion or disseminated intravascular coagulation. The presence of thrombocytopenia is associated with an increased bleeding risk but does not appear to be protective towards thromboembolic events [9].

Therefore, the decision to start heparin in thrombocytopenic patients must take into account several factors including platelet count, recurrence risk, additional hemorrhagic risk factors (liver or renal function alterations, brain metastases, etc.). Based on retrospective analyses and case series, a full-dose treatment with platelet count $>50 \times 10^9$ L is generally suggested, thus considering the suspension for values $<25 \times 10^9$ L [70,71]. Among patients with platelet count ranging from 25×10^9 L to 50×10^9 L, the decision to administer heparin should consider other bleeding risk factors. Overall, it is usually suggested to administer anticoagulants without reaching the full expected dose.

For what concerns the treatment of the maintenance phase, numerous studies evaluated the efficacy and safety of vitamin K antagonists (VKAs) and DOACs vs. LMWH. In cancer patients undergoing chemotherapy, the use of VKAs is associated with a greater bleeding risk and a greater risk of thromboembolism recurrence. LMWH remains the first choice in the 3–6 months treatment of VTE in oncological patients, also thanks to its lower half-life that allows rapid dose adjustments (for example in case of bleeding or invasive maneuvers); the VKAs are not easy to handle also due to interactions with chemotherapy that can make it difficult to keep international normalized ratio (INR) in range.

DOACs demonstrated the same efficacy and a better safety profile as VKAs in the prolonged treatment of VTE in some randomized clinical trials; in these studies, however, cancer patients were a small minority. Two studies evaluating the use of DOACs versus LMWH in cancer patients with VTE have recently been published: the Select-D study (rivaroxaban vs. dalteparin) and the HOKUSAI VTE-cancer study (edoxaban vs. dalteparin) [72,73]. In addition, recently a review has been conducted assessing the efficacy and safety of DOACs, LMWH and VKAs in cancer patients affected by VTE [74]. From these studies emerged that DOACs are effective in preventing VTE recurrence but are associated with an increased risk of bleeding compared to LMWH. Therefore, the choice of the anti-coagulant therapy must be modulated for each patient also on the basis of the primary tumor site (for example gastrointestinal or genitourinary) and of patients' preferences.

Another study has recently been published about the comparison of apixaban vs. dalteparin in cancer patients with acute venous thromboembolism: in the Caravaggio study, a prospective, randomized, non-inferiority clinical trial, patients were randomized to receive oral apixaban or subcutaneous dalteparin for six months. Apixaban was administered at a dosage of 10 mg twice daily for the first week and then five milligrams twice daily, while dalteparin was given at a dosage of 200 IU/kg for the first month and then 150 IU/kg once daily. The primary endpoint of the study was recurrent VTE and the primary safety outcome was major bleeding. Recurrent venous thromboembolism occurred in 5.6% of patients in the apixaban group and in 7.9% of patients in the dalteparin group (HR 0.63, 95% CI 0.37–1.07, $p < 0.001$). Major bleeding occurred in 3.8% of patients in the apixaban group and in 4% of patients in the dalteparin group (HR 0.82, 95% CI 0.40–1.69, $p = 0.60$). In conclusion, apixaban was found to be non-inferior to dalteparin for the treatment of venous thromboembolism in cancer patients without an increased risk of major bleeding [75,76].

Results concerning major bleeding risk are in contrast with other recent studies, where it was found a higher incidence of major bleeding in patients taking DOACs than LMWH. On the other hand, episodes of nonmajor bleeding were numerically higher in the apixaban group, consistently with previous studies (see also Table 3).

The updated ASCO guidelines recommend the use of LMWH, UFH, fondaparinux or rivaroxaban as initial treatments of VTE in cancer patients, while LMWH, edoxaban or rivaroxaban are preferred for the maintenance phase; however, the use of DOACs should be balanced considering the bleeding risk especially in patients with gastrointestinal cancers and in patients with important polypharmacy, due to the risk of drugs interactions [33,34].

In late 2019, an update of clinical practice guidelines from International Initiative on Thrombosis and Cancer working group have been published. The most important novelty is that DOACs are recommended for the maintenance treatment of VTE in cancer patients with creatinine clearance ≥30 mL/min. To keep in mind is the risk of drug interactions and the bleeding risk, which is higher than with LMWH, so caution must be used with patients with gastrointestinal tract malignancies, especially because of data suggesting increased bleeding risk in patients treated with edoxaban and rivaroxaban [30].

There is much debate about the optimal duration of anticoagulant treatment after a first episode of VTE in oncological patients as well as in the general population. Usually it is advised to continue the anticoagulation for the entire duration of cancer treatment unless there are contraindications, with frequent re-evaluations of each patient case in order to ensure that the risk-benefit ratio is still favorable (see also Table 4).

In conclusion, in oncological patients affected by venous thromboembolism, long term therapy (6 months) with LMWH or apixaban/edoxaban/rivaroxaban should be evaluated, and this therapy should be preferred to VKAs.

Regarding patients with recurrent VTE during anticoagulation treatment, a possible approach may be switching from one drug to another (i.e., switch from LMWH to DOACs, from DOACs to LMWH, from AVK to LMWH or DOACs) or increasing dosage of low molecular weight heparin by 20–25% [30].

However, ad hoc prospective studies are needed in the setting of oncological patients on active treatment experiencing VTE, in order to evaluate the use of anticoagulants beyond six months and the interactions in terms of major bleeding, impact on recurrence of VTE and mortality.

Table 3. Summary of characteristics and results of the main clinical trials cited in the text on prevention and treatment of VTE in cancer patients.

Trial	Study Design	Setting	Patients' Disease Characteristics	Anticoagulant Drug	Duration (Months)	Number of Patients	Thromboembolic Events	Major Bleeding
Carrier et al. (2019) [25]	Randomized Double blind	Prevention	Khorana score ≥2 cancer patients starting chemotherapy	Apixaban 2.5 mg BID vs. placebo	6	288/275	4.2% apixaban 10.2% placebo	3.5% apixaban 1.8% placebo
Khorana et al. (2019) [26]	Randomized Double blind	Prevention	Khorana score ≥2 cancer patients starting chemotherapy	Rivaroxaban 10 mg OD vs. placebo	6	420/421	6% rivaroxaban 8.8% placebo	2% rivaroxaban 1% placebo
Agnelli et al. (2009) [77]	Randomised Double blind	Prevention	Metastatic or locally advanced solid cancer patients receiving chemotherapy	Nadroparin 3800 IU OD vs. placebo	4	779/387	2% nadroparin group 3.9% placebo group	0.7% nadroparin group 0% placebo group
Haas et al. (2012) [78]	Two randomised Double blind	Prevention	Metastatic breast cancer or stage III/IV lung cancer patients	Certoparin 3000 IU OD vs. placebo	6	447/453	TOPIC-1: 4% certoparin 4% placebo TOPIC-2: 4.5% certoparin 8.3% placebo	TOPIC-1: 1.7% certoparin 0% placebo TOPIC-2: 3.7% certoparin 2.2% placebo
Agnelli et al. (2020) [76]	Randomized Open label	Treatment	Cancer patients with VTE	Apixaban 10 mg BID for the first 7 days, then 5 mg bid vs. dalteparin 200 IU/kg OD for the first month, then 150 IU/kg OD	6	576/579	5.6% apixaban 7.9% dalteparin	3.8% apixaban 4% dalteparin
Young et al. (2018) [72]	Randomized Open label	Treatment	Cancer patients with VTE	Dalteparin 200 IU/kg OD for 1 month, then 150 IU/kg OD vs. rivaroxaban 15 mg BID for 3 weeks then 20 mg OD	6	203/203	11% dalteparin 4% rivaroxaban	4% dalteparin 6% rivaroxaban
Raskob et al. (2018) [73]	Randomized Open label	Treatment	Cancer patients with VTE	LMWH for at least 5 days then edoxaban 60 mg OD vs. dalteparin 200 IU/kg OD for 1 month then dalteparin 150 IU/kg OD	6–12	522/524	7.9% edoxaban 11.3% dalteparin	6.9% edoxaban 4% dalteparin

VTE = venous thromboembolism, BID = twice daily, OD = once daily, IU = international unit, VTE = venous thromboembolism.

Table 4. Recommendations from international guidelines on anticoagulant treatment of established VTE in cancer patients.

Guidelines	Initial Treatment	Maintenance Treatment	Duration
ESMO 2011	Weight-adjusted LMWH or UFH. Monitor anti-Xa activity if creatinine clearance is <25–30 mL/min.	LMWH or VKA.	≥3–6 months; the optimal duration should be individually assessed. In palliative setting, an indefinite treatment should be proposed.
NCCN 2011	Weight-adjusted LMWH, UFH or fondaparinux.	LMWH (preferred for the first six months as monotherapy) or VKA.	3–6 months for DVT and 6–12 months for PE. In patients with active cancer or persistent risk factors, indefinite treatment.
ASCO 2015	LMWH is recommended for the initial 5–10 days.	LMWH.	six months.
ACCP 2016	LMWH is suggested over VKA or DOAC.	LMWH is suggested over VKA or DOAC.	For at least three months, but extended anticoagulation is recommended in patients with active cancer.
ITAC 2019	First 10 days: LMWH is recommended; UFH, fondaparinux, DOAC can be also used.	LMWHs is preferred over VKA. DOAC can be considered.	three to six months, then termination or continuation should be based on individual benefit-to-risk ratio.
ASCO 2019	LMWH, UFH, fondaparinux or rivaroxaban can be used.	LMWH, edoxaban or rivaroxaban are preferred options.	≥six months. Continuing anticoagulation beyond six months should be considered for selected patients.

ESMO—European Society for Medical Oncology; NCCN—National Comprehensive Cancer Network; ASCO—American Society of Clinical Oncology; ITAC—International Initiative on Thrombosis and Cancer; ACCP—American College of Chest Physicians; LMWH—low molecular weight heparin; UFH—unfractioned heparin; VKA—vitamin K antagonist; DOAC—direct oral anticoagulant.

9. Anticoagulant Therapy and Impact on Disease Prognosis

In the last few years, some retrospective studies assessed the impact of anticoagulant therapy on the prognosis of cancer patients. Two systematic reviews of the studies in the literature provided nonunivocal results [79,80]. On the contrary, a meta-analysis of the studies that investigated the efficacy of UFH and LMWH in patients affected by VTE showed a reduction in mortality in patients treated with LMWH [81].

Three ad hoc prospective studies (MALT, FAMOUS and a study by Altinbas et al. on SCLC patients) support this hypothesis [77,78,82]. The CLOT study also highlighted that the use of LMWH in secondary thrombosis prophylaxis improves the prognosis of patients with initial stage disease compared to VKAs [21]. On the contrary, the IMPACT study did not demonstrate any benefit from the use of LMWH [83].

An overall evaluation of these studies seems to support the hypothesis that the use of LMWH can improve the outcome of patients, in particular those with non-advanced disease.

However, there are numerous critical issues regarding these trials (different doses of LMWH in the various studies, different chemotherapy schemes, nonuniformity in patient selection), and therefore at the present time the predictive role of LMWH in this setting remains to be defined.

10. Observations and Future Research Perspectives

Several meta-analyses and reviews have been conducted about VTE prophylaxis and treatment in the last decades. Important limitations of these studies are heterogeneity of cancer types and staging, variability in cancer treatments, different antithrombotic drugs and doses, potential interactions with other patients' drugs, presence of comorbidities. Due to these limitations, data can result weak and poorly consistent between different meta-analyses.

The use of VTE prophylaxis is currently recommended in cancer patients admitted to hospital for an acute medical condition, but we still do not have sufficient information about the risk of bleeding during thromboprophylaxis. Concerning the thromboprophylaxis in ambulatory cancer patients receiving oncological treatment, refinement of existing VTE risk models or development of new models are needed in order to improve risk stratification of these patients.

The latest guidelines have introduced recommendations about the use of edoxaban and rivaroxaban for treatment of VTE in patients with cancer, but we still need information and experience about real-world use of DOACs in cancer patients, especially for what concerns drug interactions and bleeding risk.

Hence, the management of venous thromboembolism in patients with cancer remains a challenge. Further studies about cancer-associated thromboembolism are ongoing, in order to refine our knowledge concerning the management of VTE therapy and prophylaxis in this delicate setting of patients.

11. Conclusions

Cancer patients have a higher risk of developing venous thromboembolism compared to general population, and this is due to several factors such as production of procoagulant factors by tumor cells, administration of chemotherapy and hormonotherapy, hospitalization, systemic inflammatory status and tumor compression stasis.

Several clinical studies about thromboprophylaxis in outpatients receiving systemic treatment for cancer were conducted. Anti-thrombotic prophylaxis seems to be not necessary in all unselected cancer patients on active oncological therapy, whereas prophylaxis with LMWH, apixaban or rivaroxaban should be considered for cancer outpatients who receive chemotherapy and who are at high thromboembolic risk. Current guidelines also recommend preventive use of LMWH or fondaparinux in hospitalized cancer patients with an acute medical complication. Differently, routine thromboprophylaxis with LMWH in patients with venous central catheter is not indicated, but a thromboprophylaxis of at least 7–10 days should be administered after cancer surgery, to be extended up to four weeks especially in presence of additional risk factors.

For what concerns the therapy of manifested VTE in cancer patients, several studies have been conducted; in oncological patients affected by venous thromboembolism, long term therapy (6 months) with LMWH or edoxaban/rivaroxaban/apixaban should be evaluated, and this therapy should be preferred to VKAs. There is much debate about the optimal duration of anticoagulant treatment, and usually it is advised to continue it for the entire duration of cancer treatment unless contraindications.

However, ad hoc prospective studies are needed in the setting of thromboprophylaxis and of therapy of manifested VTE in oncological patients, in order to evaluate safety and efficacy of different anticoagulants, optimal duration of therapy and possible interactions with chemotherapy, immunotherapy and targeted therapy, as well as correlation with patients' outcome.

Funding: This research received no external funding.

Conflicts of Interest: The authors declare no conflict of interest.

References

1. Silverstein, M.D.; Heith, J.A. Trends in the incidence of deep vein thrombosis and pulmonary embolism: A 25-year population-based study. *Arch. Intern. Med.* **1998**, *158*, 585–593. [CrossRef] [PubMed]
2. Fisher, B.; Dignam, J. Tamoxifen and chemotherapy for lymph node-negative, estrogen receptor-positive breast cancer. *J. Natl. Cancer Inst.* **1997**, *89*, 1673–1682. [CrossRef] [PubMed]
3. Fisher, B.; Costantino, J. A randomized clinical trial evaluating tamoxifen in the treatment of patients with node-negative breast cancer who have estrogen-receptor-positive tumors. *N. Engl. J. Med.* **1989**, *320*, 479–484. [CrossRef] [PubMed]
4. Chew, H.K.; Wun, T. Incidence of venous thromboembolism and its effect on survival among patients with common cancers. *Arch. Intern. Med.* **2006**, *166*, 458–464. [CrossRef]

5. Horsted, F.; West, J. Risk of Venous Thromboembolism in Patients with Cancer: A Systematic Review and Meta-Analysis. *PLoS Med.* **2012**, *9*, e1001275. [CrossRef] [PubMed]
6. Matzdorff, A.C.; Green, D. Management of venous thromboembolism in cancer patients. *Rev. Vasc. Med.* **2014**, *2*, 24–36. [CrossRef]
7. Singh, G.; Rathi, A.K. Venous thromboembolism in cancer patients—Magnitude of problem, approach, and management. *Indian J. Cancer* **2017**, *54*, 308–312. [CrossRef] [PubMed]
8. Imberti, D.; Cimminiello, C. Antithrombotic therapy for venous thromboembolism in patients with cancer: Expert guidance. *Expert Opin. Pharm.* **2018**, *19*, 1177–1185. [CrossRef]
9. Falanga, A.; Schieppati, F. Pathophysiology 1. Mechanisms of Thrombosis in Cancer Patients. *Cancer Treat. Res.* **2019**, *179*, 11–36.
10. Falanga, A.; Russo, L. Mechanisms and risk factors of thrombosis in cancer. *Crit. Rev. Oncol. Hematol.* **2017**, *118*, 79–83. [CrossRef]
11. Pabinger, I.; Thaler, J. Biomarkers for prediction of venous thromboembolism in cancer. *Blood* **2013**, *122*, 2011–2018. [CrossRef] [PubMed]
12. Mauracher, L.M.; Posch, F. Citrullinated histone H3, a biomarker of neutrophil extracellular trap formation, predicts the risk of venous thromboembolism in cancer patients. *J. Thromb. Haemost.* **2018**, *16*, 508–518. [CrossRef] [PubMed]
13. Riedl, J.; Preusser, M. Podoplanin expression in primary brain tumors induces platelet aggregation and increases risk of venous thromboembolism. *Blood* **2017**, *129*, 1831–1839. [CrossRef] [PubMed]
14. Khorana, A.A.; Kuderer, N.M. Development and validation of a predictive model for chemotherapy-associated thrombosis. *Blood* **2008**, *111*, 4902–4907. [CrossRef]
15. Verso, M.; Agnelli, G. A modified Khorana risk assessment score for venous thromboembolism in cancer patients receiving chemotherapy: The Protecht score. *Intern. Emerg. Med.* **2012**, *7*, 291–292. [CrossRef]
16. Pelzer, U.; Sinn, M. Primary pharmacological prevention of thromboembolic events in ambulatory patients with advanced pancreatic cancer treated with chemotherapy? *Dtsch. Med. Wochenschr.* **2013**, *138*, 2084–2088. (In German)
17. Ay, C.; Dunkler, D. Prediction of venous thromboembolism in cancer patients. *Blood* **2010**, *116*, 5377–5382. [CrossRef]
18. Gerotziafas, G.T.; Taher, A. A predictive score for thrombosis associated with breast, colorectal, lung, or ovarian cancer: The prospective COMPASS-cancer-associated thrombosis study. *Oncologist* **2017**, *22*, 1222–1231. [CrossRef]
19. Cella, C.A.; Di Minno, G. Preventing venous thromboembolism in ambulatory cancer patients: The ONKOTEV study. *Oncologist* **2017**, *22*, 601–608. [CrossRef]
20. Di Nisio, M.; Porreca, E. Primary prophylaxis for venous thromboembolism in ambulatory cancer patients receiving chemotherapy. *Cochrane Database Syst. Rev.* **2016**, *12*, CD008500. [CrossRef]
21. Ben-Aharon, I.; Stemmer, S.M. Low molecular weight heparin (LMWH) for primary thrombo-prophylaxis in patients with solid malignancies-systematic review and meta-analysis. *Acta Oncol.* **2014**, *53*, 1230–1237. [CrossRef] [PubMed]
22. Thein, K.Z.; Yeung, S.J. Primary thromboprophylaxis (PTP) in ambulatory patients with lung cancer receiving chemotherapy: A systematic review and meta-analysis of randomized controlled trials (RCTs). *Asia Pac. J. Clin. Oncol.* **2018**, *14*, 210–216. [CrossRef] [PubMed]
23. Fuentes, H.E.; Oramas, D.M. Meta-analysis on anticoagulation and prevention of thrombosis and mortality among patients with lung cancer. *Thromb. Res.* **2017**, *154*, 28–34. [CrossRef] [PubMed]
24. Tun, N.M.; Guevara, E. Benefit and risk of primary thromboprophylaxis in ambulatory patients with advanced pancreatic cancer receiving chemotherapy: A systematic review and meta-analysis of randomized controlled trials. *Blood Coagul. Fibrinolysis* **2016**, *27*, 270–274. [CrossRef]
25. Carrier, M.; Abou-Nassar, K. Apixaban to prevent Venous Thromboembolism in patients with Cancer. *N. Engl. J. Med.* **2019**, *380*, 711–719. [CrossRef]
26. Khorana, A.A.; Soff, G.A. Rivaroxaba for Thromboprophylaxis in High-Risk Ambulatory Patients with Cancer. *N. Engl. J. Med.* **2019**, *380*, 720–728. [CrossRef]
27. Becattini, C.; Verso, M. Updated meta-analysis on prevention of venous thromboembolism in ambulatory cancer patients. *Haematology* **2019**, *105*, 838–848. [CrossRef]

28. Larocca, A.; Cavallo, F. Aspirin or enoxaparin thromboprophylaxis for patients with newly diagnosed multiple myeloma treated with lenalidomide. *Blood* **2012**, *119*, 933–939. [CrossRef]
29. Palumbo, A.; Cavo, M. Aspirin, warfarin, or enoxaparin thromboprophylaxis in patients with multiple myeloma treated with thalidomide: A phase III, open-label, randomized trial. *J. Clin. Oncol.* **2011**, *29*, 986–993. [CrossRef]
30. Farge, D.; Frere, C. 2019 international clinical practice guidelines for the treatment and prophylaxis of venous thromboembolism in patients with cancer. *Lancet Oncol.* **2019**, *20*, 566–581. [CrossRef]
31. Pelzer, U.; Opitz, B. Efficacy of prophylactic low-molecular weight heparin for ambulatory patients with advanced pancreatic cancer: Outcomes from the CONKO-004 trial. *J. Clin. Oncol.* **2015**, *33*, 2028–2034. [CrossRef] [PubMed]
32. Maraveyas, A.; Waters, J. Gemcitabine versus gemcitabine plus dalteparin thromboprophylaxis in pancreatic cancer. *Eur. J. Cancer* **2012**, *48*, 1283–1292. [CrossRef]
33. Verso, M.; Di Nisio, M. Management of venous thromboembolism in cancer patients: Considerations about the clinical practice guideline update of the American society of clinical oncology. *Eur. J. Intern. Med.* **2020**, *71*, 4–7. [CrossRef]
34. Key, N.S.; Khorana, A.A. Venous thromboembolism prophylaxis and treatment in patients with cancer: ASCO clinical practice guideline update. *J. Clin. Oncol.* **2019**, *38*, 496–520. [CrossRef]
35. Liu, M.; Wang, G. Efficacy and safety of thromboprophylaxis in cancer patients: A systematic review and meta-analysis. *Adv. Med. Oncol.* **2020**, *12*. [CrossRef] [PubMed]
36. Chen, H.; Tao, R. Prevention of venous thromboembolism in patients with cancer with direct oral anticoagulants. A systematic review and meta-analysis. *Medicine* **2020**, *99*, e19000. [CrossRef]
37. Mandalà, M.; Petrella, M.C. *AIOM Guidelines: Line Guida sul Tromboembolismo Venoso nei Pazienti con Tumori Solidi*; AIOM: Milan, Italy, 2019.
38. D'Ambrosio, L.; Aglietta, M. Anticoagulation for central venous catheters in patients with cancer. *N. Engl. J. Med.* **2014**, *371*, 1362–1363. [CrossRef] [PubMed]
39. Verso, M.; Agnelli, G. Enoxaparin for the prevention of venous thromboembolism associated with central vein catheter: A double-blind, placebo controlled, randomized study in cancer patients. *J. Clin. Oncol.* **2005**, *23*, 4057–4062. [CrossRef]
40. Chopra, V.; Anand, S. Risk of venous thromboembolism associated with peripherally inserted central catheters: A systematic review and meta-analysis. *Lancet* **2013**, *382*, 311–325. [CrossRef]
41. Allaert, F.A.; Benzenine, E. Hospital incidence and annual rates of hospitalization for venous thromboembolic disease in France and the USA. *Phlebology* **2017**, *32*, 443–447. [CrossRef]
42. Samama, M.M.; Cohen, A.T. A comparison of enoxaparin with placebo for the prevention of venous thromboembolism in acutely ill medical patients: Prophylaxis in medical patients with enoxaparin study group. *N. Engl. J. Med.* **1999**, *341*, 793–800. [CrossRef] [PubMed]
43. Leizorovicz, A.; Cohen, A.T.; PREVENT Medical Thromboprophylaxis Study Group. Randomized, placebo-controlled trial of dalteparin for the prevention of venous thromboembolism in acutely ill medical patients. *Circulation* **2004**, *110*, 874–879. [CrossRef] [PubMed]
44. Cohen, A.T.; Davidson, B.L. Efficacy and safety of fondaparinux for the prevention of venous thromboembolism in older acute medical patients: Randomised placebo controlled trial. *BMJ* **2006**, *332*, 325–329. [CrossRef] [PubMed]
45. Haas, S.; Shewllong, S.M. Heparin based prophylaxis to prevent venous thromboembolic events and death in patients with cancer: A subgroup analysis of CERTIFY. *BMC* **2011**, *11*, 316. [CrossRef] [PubMed]
46. Carrier, M.; Khorana, A.A. Lack of evidence to support thromboprophylaxis in hospitalized medical patients with cancer. *Am. J. Med.* **2014**, *127*, 82–86. [CrossRef]
47. Barbar, S.; Rossetto, V. Thromboprophylaxis in medical inpatients with cancer. *Am. J. Med.* **2014**, *127*, 10–11. [CrossRef]
48. Kakkar, V.V.; Howe, C.T. Deep-vein thrombosis of the leg. Is there a "high risk" group? *Am. J. Surg.* **1970**, *120*, 527–530. [CrossRef]
49. Kakkar, A.K.; Williamson, R.C. Prevention of venous thromboembolism in cancer patients. *Semin. Thromb. Hemost.* **1999**, *25*, 239–243. [CrossRef]
50. Clagett, G.P.; Reisch, J.S. Prevention of venous thromboembolism in general surgical patients. Results of meta-analysis. *Ann. Surg.* **1988**, *208*, 227–240. [CrossRef]

51. Bergqvist, D.; Burmark, U.S. Low molecular weight heparin once daily compared with conventional low-dose heparin twice daily. A prospective double-blind multicentre trial on prevention of postoperative thrombosis. *Br. J. Surg.* **1986**, *73*, 204–208. [CrossRef]
52. Bergqvist, D.; Matzsch, T. Low molecular weight heparin given in the evening before surgery compared with conventional low-dose heparin in the prevention of thrombosis. *Br. J. Surg.* **1988**, *75*, 888–891. [CrossRef] [PubMed]
53. Samama, M.; Bernard, P. Low molecular weight heparin compared with unfractionated heparin in the prevention of postoperative thrombosis. *Br. J. Surg.* **1988**, *75*, 128–131. [CrossRef] [PubMed]
54. Leizorovicz, A.; Picolet, H. Prevention of postoperative deep vein thrombosis in general surgery: A multicenter double-blind study comparing two doses of logiparin and standard heparin. *Br. J. Surg.* **1991**, *78*, 412–416. [CrossRef] [PubMed]
55. Boneu, B. An international multicenter study: Clivarin in the prevention of venous thromboembolism in patients undergoing general surgery. *Blood Coagul. Fibrinolysis* **1993**, *4*, S21–S22. [PubMed]
56. ENOXACAN Study Group. Efficacy and safety of enoxaparin versus unfractionated heparin for prevention of deep vein thrombosis in elective cancer surgery: A double-blind randomized multicentre trial with venographic assessment. *Br. J. Surg.* **1997**, *84*, 1099–1103. [CrossRef]
57. Bergqvist, D.; Agnelli, G. Duration of prophylaxis against venous thromboembolism with enoxaparin after surgery for cancer. *N. Engl. J. Med.* **2002**, *346*, 975–980. [CrossRef]
58. Rasmussen, M.S.; Jorgensen, L.N. Prolonged prophylaxis with dalteparin to prevent late thromboembolic complications in patients undergoing major abdominal surgery: A multicenter randomized open-label study. *J. Thromb. Haemost.* **2006**, *4*, 2384–2390. [CrossRef]
59. Lausen, I.; Jensen, R. Incidence and prevention of deep vein thrombosis occurring late after general surgery: Randomized controlled study of prolonged prophylaxis. *Eur. J. Surg.* **1998**, *164*, 657–663. [CrossRef]
60. Kakkar, V.V.; Balibrea, J.L.; CANBESURE Study Group. Extendend prophylaxis with bemiparin for the prevention of venous thromboembolism after abdominal or pelvic surgery for cancer: The CANBESURE randomized study. *J. Thromb. Haemost.* **2010**, *8*, 1223–1229. [CrossRef]
61. Bottaro, F.J.; Elizondo, M.C. Efficacy of estended thrombo-prophylaxis in major abdominal surgery: What does the evidence show? A meta-analysis. *Throm. Haemost.* **2008**, *99*, 1104–1111.
62. Mandalà, M.; Falanga, A. Management of venous thromboembolism (VTE) in cancer patients: ESMO Clinical Practice Guidelines. *Ann. Oncol.* **2011**, *22*, 85–92. [CrossRef] [PubMed]
63. Lyman, G.H.; Khorana, A.A. American Society of Clinical Oncology guideline: Recommendations for venous thromboembolism prophylaxis and treatment in patients with cancer. *J. Clin. Oncol.* **2007**, *25*, 5490–5505. [CrossRef] [PubMed]
64. Lyman, G.H.; Khorana, A.A. Venous Thromboembolism Prophylaxis and Treatment in Patients with Cancer: American Society of Clinical Oncology Clinical Practice Guideline Update. *J. Clin. Oncol.* **2013**, *31*, 2189–2204. [CrossRef] [PubMed]
65. Levine, M.; Gent, M. A comparison of low molecular weight heparin administered at home with unfractioned heparin administered in the hospital for proximal deep vein thrombosis. *N. Engl. J. Med.* **1996**, *334*, 677–681. [CrossRef]
66. Koopman, M.M.W.; Prandoni, P. Treatment of venous thrombosis with intravenous infractioned heparin administered in the hospital as compared with subcutaneous low molecular weight heparin administered at home. *N. Engl. J. Med.* **1996**, *334*, 682–687. [CrossRef]
67. The Columbus Investigators. Low molecular weight heparin in the treatment of patients with venous thromboembolism. *N. Engl. J. Med.* **1997**, *337*, 657–662. [CrossRef]
68. Hakoum, M.B.; Kahale, L.A. Anticoagulation for the initial treatment of venous thromboembolism in people with cancer. *Cochrane Database Syst. Rev.* **2018**, *1*, CD006649. [CrossRef]
69. Carrier, M.; Cameron, C. Efficacy and safety of anticoagulant therapy for the treatment of acute cancer-associated thrombosis: A systematic review and meta-analysis. *Thromb. Res.* **2014**, *134*, 1214–1219. [CrossRef]
70. Kopolovic, I.; Lee, A.Y. Manangement and outcomes of cancer-associated venous thromboembolism in patients with concomigant thrombocytopenia: A retrospective cohort study. *Ann. Hematol.* **2015**, *94*, 329–336. [CrossRef]

71. Campbell, P.M.; Ippoliti, C. Safety of anticoagulation in thrombocytopenic patients with hematologic malignancies: A case series. *J. Oncol. Pharm. Pract.* **2017**, *23*, 220–225. [CrossRef]
72. Young, A.M.; Marshall, A. Comparison of an oral factor Xa inhibitor with low molecular weight heparin in patients with cancer with venous thromboembolism: Results of a randomized trial (SELECT-D). *J. Clin. Oncol.* **2018**, *36*, 2017–2023. [CrossRef] [PubMed]
73. Raskob, G.E.; van Es, N. Edoxaban for the treatment of cancer-associated venous thromboembolism. *N. Engl. J. Med.* **2018**, *378*, 615–624. [CrossRef]
74. Rossel, A.; Robert-Ebadi, H. Anticoagulant therapy for acute venous thrombo-embolism in cancer patients: A systematic review and network meta-analysis. *PLoS ONE* **2019**, *14*, e0213960. [CrossRef]
75. Agnelli, G.; Becattini, C. Apixaban versus dalteparin for the treatment of acute venous thromboembolism in patients with cancer: The Caravaggio Study. *Thromb. Haemost.* **2018**, *118*, 1668–1678. [CrossRef] [PubMed]
76. Agnelli, G.; Becattini, C. Apixaban for the treatment of venous thromboembolism associated with cancer. *N. Engl. J. Med.* **2020**, *382*, 1599–1607. [CrossRef] [PubMed]
77. Agnelli, G.; Gussoni, G. Nadroparin for the prevention of thromboembolic events in ambulatory patients with metastatic or locally advanced solid cancer receiving chemotherapy: A randomised, placebo controlled, double-blind study. *Lancet Oncol.* **2009**, *10*, 943–949. [CrossRef]
78. Haas, S.K.; Freund, M. Low-molecular-weight heparin versus placebo for the prevention of venous thromboembolism in metastatic breast cancer or stage III/IV lung cancer. *Clin. Appl. Thromb. Hemost.* **2012**, *18*, 159–165. [CrossRef]
79. Smorenburg, S.M.; Hettiarachchi, R.J. The effects of unfractioned heparin on survival in patients with malignancy: A systematic review. *Thromb. Haemost.* **1999**, *82*, 947–952.
80. Altinbas, M.; Coskun, H.S. A randomized clinical trial of combination chemotherapy with and without low molecular heparin in small cell lung cancer. *J. Thromb. Haemost.* **2004**, *2*, 1266–1271. [CrossRef]
81. Hettiarachchi, R.J.; Smorenburg, S.M. Do Heparins do more than just treat thrombosis? The influence of heparins on cancer spread. *Thromb. Haemost.* **1999**, *82*, 947–952. [CrossRef]
82. Meyer, G.; Marjanovic, Z. Comparison of low-molecular-weight heparin and warfarin for the secondary prevention of venous thromboembolism in patients with cancer: A randomized controlled study. *Arch. Intern. Med.* **2002**, *162*, 1729–1735. [CrossRef] [PubMed]
83. Van, E.S. Edoxaban for treatment of venous thromboembolism in patients with cancer. Rationale and design of the Hokusai VTE-cancer study. *Thromb. Haemost.* **2015**, *114*, 1268–1276.

© 2020 by the authors. Licensee MDPI, Basel, Switzerland. This article is an open access article distributed under the terms and conditions of the Creative Commons Attribution (CC BY) license (http://creativecommons.org/licenses/by/4.0/).

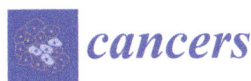

Review

Preventing Venous Thromboembolism in Ambulatory Patients with Cancer: A Narrative Review

Anne Rossel [1,2,*], Helia Robert-Ebadi [2,3] and Christophe Marti [1,2]

1 Division of General Internal Medicine, University Hospitals of Geneva, 1205 Geneva, Switzerland; christophe.marti@hcuge.ch
2 Faculty of Medicine, University of Geneva, 1205 Geneva, Switzerland; helia.robert-ebadi@hcuge.ch
3 Division of Angiology and Haemostasis, University Hospitals of Geneva, 1205 Geneva, Switzerland
* Correspondence: anne.rossel@hcuge.ch

Received: 2 February 2020; Accepted: 4 March 2020; Published: 6 March 2020

Abstract: Venous thromboembolism (VTE) is frequent among patients with cancer. Ambulatory cancer patients starting chemotherapy have a 5% to 10% risk of cancer associated thrombosis (CAT) within the first year after cancer diagnosis. This risk may vary according to patient characteristics, cancer location, cancer stage, or the type of chemotherapeutic regimen. Landmark studies evaluating thrombophrophylaxis with low molecular weight heparin (LMWH) for ambulatory cancer patients have shown a relative reduction in the rate of symptomatic VTE of about one half. However, the absolute risk reduction is modest among unselected patients given a rather low risk of events resulting in a number needed to treat (NNT) of 40 to 50. Moreover, this modest benefit is mitigated by a trend towards an increased risk of bleeding, and the economic and patient burden due to daily injections of LMWH. For these reasons, routine thromboprophylaxis is not recommended by expert societies. Advances in VTE risk stratification among cancer patients, and growing evidence regarding efficacy and safety of direct oral anticoagulants (DOACs) for the treatment and prevention of CAT have led to reconsider the paradigms of this risk–benefit assessment. This narrative review aims to summarize the recent evidence provided by randomized trials comparing DOACs to placebo in ambulatory cancer patients and its impact on expert recommendations and clinical practice.

Keywords: cancer associated thrombosis; VTE; venous thromboembolism; malignancy; low molecular weight heparin; direct oral anticoagulant

1. Introduction

Cancer is a major risk factor for venous thromboembolism (VTE). Approximately 20% of all VTE events are attributable to cancer [1], and an active cancer increases the risk to develop VTE up to seven times [2]. The burden of cancer associated thrombosis (CAT) is high, as the risk of mortality can be increased fourfold, depending on the type and stage of cancer [3]. Morbidity is also considerable, with an increased rate of hospitalization, home care, and decreased quality of life.

Nevertheless, the incidence of VTE in patients with cancer varies widely, ranging from 1.4% yearly [4] to over 10% [5] in high-risk patients. Among patients with pancreatic cancer receiving chemotherapy, this rate can rise as high as 20% at one year [6,7]. The relative risk for high-risk tumors is provided in Table 1. Moreover, a trend towards an increasing incidence of VTE has been observed [8], due to longer survival of patients with cancer, administration of prothrombotic chemotherapies, and improvement in the diagnosis of CAT [8].

Table 1. Relative risk of thromboembolism according to cancer type, compared to general population (based on [5]).

Cancer Site	Incidence Rate Ratio (IRR) (95%CI)
Overall	3.96 (3.66–4.27)
Pancreas	15.56 (10.50–23.06)
Hematological	12.65 (10.04–15.94)
Brain	10.40 (5.48–18.08)
Lung	7.27 (5.93–8.91)

Many factors influence the risk of developing CAT. In the presence of major transient risk factors, such as hospitalization for an acute medical illness, surgery, or reduced mobility, thromboprophylaxis is usually recommended, and these particular situations will not be discussed in this review [9]. However, the vast majority of CAT occur in the ambulatory setting, notably during the first 6 months following cancer diagnosis [2]. The primary location and type of cancer are important determinants of CAT risk. Breast and prostate cancer, for example, are associated with lower rates of VTE compared to pancreatic or hematologic malignancies [5]. The stage of cancer also impacts the risk of VTE [3], as well as the type of chemotherapy [10] and other supportive treatments such as red cell growth factors [11]. Metastatic disease is associated with an increased VTE risk and some treatments such as anti-EGFR molecules increase the rate of venous thromboembolic events [12,13]. As all these contributors influence the risk of VTE, the so-called "cancer population" represents in fact a highly heterogeneous population with a wide range of individual risks.

The benefits of thromboprophylaxis using low molecular weight heparins (LMWH) in cancer patients have been largely studied in the past. Despite a reduction of the rate of VTE in various randomized controlled trials (RCTs) and meta-analyses [14–16], the number needed to treat (NNT) was shown to be high (40 to 50), due to the overall low rate of events. As bleeding risk is also increased in patients with cancer [17], the benefit–risk ratio of primary prophylaxis of VTE with LMWH remained uncertain. Moreover, LMWH is expensive, and subcutaneous injections are burdensome and probably more difficult for the patient to tolerate in the setting of prevention than treatment, further altering the quality of life in a population where this is a particularly important issue.

Selecting high-VTE-risk subgroups of cancer patients with a potentially more favorable benefit–risk ratio expected from thromboprophylaxis has been one of the priorities of research in this setting during the last decade [18]. In the meantime, direct oral anticoagulants (DOAC) have emerged as a potential alternative for the treatment and prevention of CAT [19–21]. Two recently published randomized placebo-controlled trials, AVERT [22] and CASSINI [23], evaluated rivaroxaban and apixaban for the prevention of CAT in outpatients with cancer selected as being at increased risk of VTE.

In this narrative review, we will summarize the available evidence on VTE prevention in ambulatory cancer patients, and the impact of the recent trials' results on the latest recommendations and clinical practice.

2. Identification of Patients at Higher Risk of VTE

As previously discussed, thromboprophylaxis in ambulatory cancer patients is associated with a 50% reduction of VTE rate. However, the low absolute rate of events among unselected cancer patients, and treatment associated costs and potential harms result in an uncertain benefit–risk balance. Routine thromboprophylaxis is therefore not recommended in all cancer patients. Identification of cancer patients at high risk of VTE, who would thus have the highest potential benefit from thromboprophylaxis, has been the subject of active research over the last decade.

The best known risk stratification tool was derived by Khorana et al. in 2008 [18] in a cohort of 4000 ambulatory cancer patients. Two-thirds of the patients were assigned to the derivation cohort, whereas the remaining represented the validation cohort. The overall rate of VTE was low (2.2%), and the median duration of follow-up was relatively short (73 days). The multivariable regression analysis identified five predictors of VTE, which were included in the model: site of tumor (stratified by very high risk and high risk), body mass index (BMI), pre-chemotherapy hemoglobin or use of red cell growth factors, leucocyte and platelet count (Table 2). Patients with a score ≥3 were considered at high risk, corresponding to a VTE incidence of 7.1%. Of note, gastric and pancreatic cancers represented only 2% of the overall cohort.

This risk assessment model has been further validated in over 50 cohorts of ambulatory cancer patients. A recent meta-analysis identified 53 studies including more than 34,000 patients evaluating the Khorana score [24]. The reported incidence of VTE in the first 6 months was 5.0% among patients with a low-risk Khorana score (0 points), 6.6% in those with an intermediate-risk (1 or 2 points), and 11.0% in those with a high-risk Khorana score (≥3 points). The authors concluded that the Khorana score was a reliable tool to identify ambulatory cancer patients at high risk of VTE. However, only 17% of patients were classified at high risk, and most events (77%) occurred in non-high-risk patients. Using a threshold of ≥2 points to define high-risk patients, 47% of patients were classified at high risk and the incidence of VTE in this group was 8.9%. The proportion of VTE events occurring in the high-risk group was 55%, rather than 23% for a threshold of ≥3 points. Of note, the incidence of VTE in patients with a score of 0 or 1 remained substantial (5.5%). Therefore, the strength of the Khorana score lies mainly in the identification of patients with an increased risk of VTE but a low-risk score cannot put aside the occurrence of VTE.

Table 2. Risk assessment scores.

Patients Characteristics	Khorana Score [18]	CATS Score [25]	PROTECHT Score [26]	CONKO Score [27]	ONKOTEV Score [28]
Pancreatic or gastric cancer	+2	+2	+2	+2	-
Lung, gynecologic, or genitourinary cancer (except prostate), or lymphoma	+1	+1	+1	+1	-
Hemoglobin < 10 g/dL* or use of red cell growth factors	+1	+1	+1	+1	-
White blood cell count > 11×10^9/L*	+1	+1	+1	+1	-
Platelet count ≥ 350×10^9/L*	+1	+1	+1	+1	-
Body mass index > 35 kg/m^2	+1	+1	+1	-	-
D-dimers ≥ 1.44 µg/mL*	-	+1	-	-	-
P-selectin ≥ 53.1 ng/mL*	-	+1	-	-	-
Gemcitabine or platinum chemotherapy	-	-	+1	-	-
WHO performance status ≥ 2	-	-	-	+1	-
Khorana score ≥ 2 points	-	-	-	-	+1
Metastatic disease	-	-	-	-	+1
Previous venous thromboembolism	-	-	-	-	+1
Vascular/lymphatic macroscopic compression	-	-	-	-	+1
	High risk ≥3 Intermediate risk 1–2 Low risk 0				

* values measured before the beginning of chemotherapy.

Several adaptations of the Khorana score have been proposed and will be briefly presented below. The modifications included adding additional variables such as D-dimers and P-selectin [25]; treatment by gemcitabine or platinum [26]; replacing BMI by functional status [27], or adding metastatic disease, vascular compression, or previous VTE [28] (Table 2). In addition, novel scores have also been proposed including other predictive factors [29]. The proportion of patients classified as high risk by these different scores and the corresponding VTE incidence are summarized in Table 3.

Table 3. Incidence of venous thromboembolism (VTE) in patients classified as high risk according to different prediction models.

Score and Threshold for Defining High Risk	Incidence of VTE in the High-Risk Category	Proportion of Patients Classified in the High-Risk Category	Follow-Up
Khorana ≥ 3	11% [24]	17%	6 months
CATS ≥ 3	17.7% [25]	25.7%	6 months
PROTECHT ≥ 3	8.1% [26]	32%	12 months
COMPASS ≥ 7	13.3% [29]	50.5%	12 months
ONKOTEV ≥ 2	33.9% [28]	7%	12 months
Khorana ≥ 2	8.9% [24]	47%	6 months

After having shown that high levels of D-dimer and P-selectin [30,31] were associated with an increased risk of VTE, Ay et al. elaborated a VTE-risk assessment tool including these biomarkers, in the Vienna-Cancer And Thrombosis study (Vienna-CATS) cohort. The six-month VTE risk was 17.7% in the high-risk group (≥3 points). Although the positive predictive value of this score appeared higher than the Khorana score, its widespread clinical use is hampered by requirement of specific biomarkers, such as P-selectin. More recently, the same group elaborated a new score with only two items: tumor site and of D-dimer levels before chemotherapy, and reported [32] better c-indexes than the Khorana score in both the derivation (0.66 vs. 0.61) and validation (0.68 vs. 0.56) cohorts.

Based on data from the PROTECHT study [10], Verso et al. proposed to add gemcitabine, cisplatine, or carboplatin as additional risk factors [26]. Pelzer et al. suggested an adaptation of the Khorana score by replacing BMI with performance status in the CONKO004 study [27] evaluating LMWH prophylaxis in patients with pancreatic cancer [33]. This score has, to date, not been externally validated.

The ONKOTEV score [28] includes the presence of metastatic disease, the compression of vascular structures, and history of previous VTE (Table 2). In the validation study, the 12-months probability of VTE (including incidentally diagnosed VTE) was 33.9% among patients with a score of 3 or more, 19.4% among patients with a score of 2, 9.7% among patients with a score of 1, and 3.7% among patients with a score of 0. The AUC was reported as higher for ONKOTEV than Khorana score at 6 months (0.75 vs. 0.59) in this cohort. This score has been further validated on a retrospective cohort of patients with pancreatic cancer [34].

The COMPASS-CAT score was elaborated to improve the assessment of VTE risk for patients with lung, colon, breast, and ovarian cancers [29]. This score includes patient-related (cardiovascular risk factors, history of VTE, platelet count, recent hospitalization), cancer-related (stage, time since diagnosis), and treatment-related items (anthracycline or anti-hormonal therapy, central venous catheter). The risk of VTE was 1.7% in the low/intermediate-risk group, and 13.3% in the high-risk group. The score had a good discriminatory capacity (AUC 0.85), but external prospective validation is lacking.

A comparative analysis of the performance of these predictive models (with the exception of the Vienna-CATS and COMPASS-CAT score due to the lack of biomarker measurement and cardiovascular risk assessment) has been performed in a cohort of 776 ambulatory patients receiving chemotherapy [24]. Overall, the discriminatory power of the scores was low, with a c-index of approximately 0.60 for all scores. A positivity threshold of 2 points improved performance of all scores and captured a higher proportion of VTE. Another comparison of several scores [35] was conducted on a prospective multinational cohort of 876 patients with various cancers. C-statistics of the scores were again low, ranging from 0.52 for Khorana to 0.59 for PROTECHT.

In conclusion, although some alternative risk assessment models have a superior reported positive predictive value or overall accuracy in the studied cohorts, the Khorana score remains the most widely validated prediction score to date. Using a threshold of 2 or more, the Khorana score allows identifying a subgroup of cancer patients at high risk of VTE (expected 6-months VTE incidence of around 9%), representing potential candidates for thromboprophylaxis with a potentially favorable risk–benefit ratio.

3. Evidence Regarding Primary Prophylaxis

Many studies have been conducted on the use of anticoagulants for primary prevention of VTE in patients with cancer. Most studies used LMWH in this setting as this class of anticoagulants has been shown to be superior to Vitamin K antagonists (VKA) for the treatment of cancer associated thrombosis [21]. LMWH enhance antithrombin action to inhibit factor Xa. Their pharmacokinetic is better predictable than unfractionated heparin but their renal metabolism precludes their use in renal insufficiency. A few studies evaluated the use of vitamin K antagonists as prophylactic treatment. These molecules inhibit the synthesis of vitamin K-dependent coagulation factors, and their efficacy may be subject to important variations depending on vitamin K intake, especially in cancer patients receiving chemotherapy often resulting in reduced oral intake and/or nausea and vomiting. A selection of randomized studies using LMWH is reported in Table 4.

The primary outcome of earlier studies was the effect of LMWH on survival, after some encouraging in vitro and in vivo results [36]. However, the hoped benefit of LMWH on survival in cancer patients could not be demonstrated in large scale studies [37,38]. Thereafter, VTE incidence was the main outcome.

The SAVE-ONCO study [15] randomized 3212 patients with metastatic or locally advanced solid cancers to receive semuloparin or placebo, regardless of their thrombotic risk. Almost 70% had metastatic disease. Patients who received semuloparin presented fewer thrombotic events (HR 0.36; 95%CI 0.21–0.60), without a significant difference in the rate of major bleeding (HR 1.05; 95%CI 0.55–1.99). The benefit was particularly important among patients with lung and pancreatic cancers, with a relative VTE risk reduction of 64% (RR 0.36, 95% CI 0.17–0.76) and 78% (RR 0.22, 95% CI 0.06–0.74), respectively. However, the absolute risk reduction in the overall population of patients was low (2.2%).

The PROTECHT study [14] compared nadroparin to placebo in 1150 patients with metastatic or locally advanced cancer of various origins, without cerebral metastasis. Treatment was initiated for the duration of chemotherapy or 4 months. The primary efficacy outcome was a composite including VTE, arterial events (acute myocardial infarction, ischemic stroke, acute arterial thromboembolism), and VTE-related death. Whereas nadroparin significantly decreased the incidence of the composite outcome, the effect on VTE incidence was non-significant. (RR 0.50; 95%CI 0.22–1.13) and there was a trend towards more bleeding events (RR 5.46; 95%CI 0.30–98.43). Despite an inclusive definition of thromboembolism, the overall number of events was low, even in the placebo group where the occurrence of VTE was lower than the rate reported observational studies among patients treated by chemotherapy [7] (2.9% vs. 7.3% at 3.5 months). A possible explanation could be that the treatment duration and follow-up were relatively short, (median 112 days). Moreover, mortality at the end of treatment was low (4.3% vs. 4.2%), reflecting the selection of patients with a better prognosis than the general oncologic population.

Haas et al. [39] compared certoparin to placebo over 6 months in patients with metastatic breast cancer or stage III/IV non-small cell lung carcinoma. No significant difference was found in the rate of VTE (RR 0.57; 95%CI 0.24–1.35) or major bleeding (1.12; 95% CI 0.52–2.38).

The FRAGMATIC trial was conducted among patients with primary bronchial carcinoma of any stage [40], comparing dalteparin to placebo. VTE was less frequent in the LMWH group (RR 0.57; 95%CI 0.42–0.77), without an increase in major bleeding (RR 1.50; 95%CI 0.62–3.66). However, only 18.4% of patients were fully compliant, and 39% received half of the planned syringes or less.

In patients receiving gemcitabine for pancreatic cancer, adding primary prophylaxis with therapeutic doses of dalteparin significantly reduced VTE or arterial events (RR 0.15, 0.04–0.61) [41]. Despite therapeutic doses, the rate of bleeding events was low without a significant difference between groups (3.4% vs. 3.2%). In this study, VTE was a significant predictor of mortality (HR 1.93, 95% CI 1.23–3.03) but LMWH had no effect on mortality. Another randomized controlled study comparing enoxaparin added as primary prophylaxis to chemotherapy versus chemotherapy alone in patients with advanced pancreatic cancer (CONK004) [33] also showed a 3 month decrease in VTE risk with enoxaparin (HR 0.12; 95% CI 0.03–0.52). The rate of VTE in the control group (15% at 3 months) was remarkably high in this study. There was no significant increase in major bleeding (HR 1.4, 0.35–3.72).

LMWH primary prophylaxis trials in the setting of cancer are thus highly heterogeneous in terms of study populations, as some included unselected populations of cancer patients and others a very specific subgroup of patients with high-risk advanced cancer. This heterogeneity is well reflected by the event rates in the placebo (or no anticoagulation) arms (Table 4). In the two large placebo-controlled randomized SAVE-ONCO and PROTECHT studies of unselected cancer patients, the VTE rate in the placebo arm was 3.4% and 2.9%, respectively, indicating a low VTE risk cancer population.

Khorana et al. [42] aimed to assess LMWH prophylaxis in a selected population of patients with high risk of thrombotic event, defined by a Khorana score of ≥ 3 points. This study terminated prematurely (98 patients) because of a poor accrual. A non-significant reduction of the rate of VTE was observed (12% in dalteparin group vs. 21% in control arm; HR 0.69, 95% CI 0.23–1.89). In a phase II study, Zwicker et al. [43] stratified patients depending of their level of circulating tissue factor-bearing micro particles (TFMP) and randomized those at higher risk to enoxaparin or standard treatment. In this small study ($n = 34$), the rate of VTE at 2 months was particularly high in the control group (27.3%) and was significantly decreased in the enoxaparin arm (HR 0.15; 95% CI 0.03–0.97).

Several studies also evaluated Vitamin K Antagonists (VKA) prophylaxis in patients with cancer. The impact on VTE and survival were inconstant while some increase in bleeding risk was reported [44–47]. Finally, several studies evaluated thromboprophylaxis in specific subgroups of cancers such as multiple myeloma patients receiving thalidomide and derivatives. Among these patients, the one-year VTE risk may increase over 20% and may be reduced by the administration of aspirin LMWH or VKA [48,49].

Table 4. Randomized studies on VTE prevention with low molecular weight heparin (LMWH).

Author (Year)	Type of Cancer	Stage of Cancer (Proportion Metastatic)	Drug	Patient Number	Treatment Duration	Outcome Definition	VTE Relative Risk (95%CI)	Major Bleeding RR (95%CI)	Event Rate in Control Group
Agnelli (2012) [15]	Lung, pancreas, stomach, colon, rectum, bladder, ovary	Metastatic (68%) or locally advanced	Semuloplasmin 20 mg/d	3214	3 m	VTE or VTE death	0.36 (0.21–0.60)	1.05 (0.55–1.99)	3.4%
Agnelli (2009) [14]	Lung, GI, pancreatic, breast, ovarian, head, neck No brain metastasis	Metastatic (unknown) or locally advanced	Nadroparin 3800 UI sc/d	1150	120 d	Composite including VTE, arterial TE or VTE death Objectively confirmed	0.5 (0.22–1.13)	5.46 (0.30–98.4)	2.9%
Haas (2012) [39]	Breast or non-small cell lung cancer No brain metastasis	Metastatic breast cancer, stage III–IV lung cancer	Certoparin 3000 IU sc/d	883	6m	symptomatic or asymptomatic VTE	0.57 (0.24–1.35)	2.19 (0.89–5.70)	3.1%
Kakkar (2004) [37]	Breast, lung, GI, pancreas, liver, genitourinary	Metastatic (84%) or locally advanced	Dalteparin 5000 UI sc/d	374	1 y	Symptomatic confirmed VTE*	0.77 (0.21–2.84)	2.91 (0.12–70.9)	2.7%
Klerk (2005) [36]	Solid tumor	Metastatic (91%) or locally advanced	Nadroparin bid over 14d, then od	302	6w	NA	NA	5.20 (0.62–44.0)	NA
Macbeth (2016) [40]	Bronchial carcinoma	All stages, metastatic (61%)	Dalteparin 5000IU sc/d	2202	6m	NA	0.57 (0.42–0.77)	1.50 (0.62–3.66)	9.7%
Maraveyas (2012) [41]	Pancreatic cancer	Metastatic (54%) or locally advanced	Dalteparin 200 UI/kg sc od for 4w, then 150 UI/kg	123	12w	VTE or arterial event	0.15 (0.04–0.61)	1.05 (0.15–7.22)	18.3%
Pelzer (2015) [33]	Pancreatic cancer	Metastatic (76%) or locally advanced	Enoxaparin 1 mg/kg od	312	3 m	VTE or arterial event	0.12 (0.03–0.52)	1.4 (0.35–3.72)	14.5%
Perry (2010) [51]	Stage 3 or 4 glioma	Locally advanced	Dalteparin 5000 IU sc/d	186	6 m	VTE or arterial event	0.51 (0.19–1.4)	4.2 (0.48–36)	14.9%
Van Doormaal (2011) [38]	Stage IIIb non-small cell pulmonary carcinoma, prostate, pancreatic cancer	Metastatic (32%)	Nadroparin bid over 14d, then half therapeutic dose	503	Median duration: 12.6w	VTE	1.12 (NA)	1.18 (0.49–2.85)	6.5%

GI: gastro-intestinal, sc: subcutaneous, od: once daily, bid: Bi-daily, d: days, w: weeks, m: months, VTE: venous thromboembolism, NA: not available.

A Cochrane meta-analysis [16] published in 2016 included all randomized controlled trials comparing any anticoagulant to placebo or other anticoagulant, in outpatients receiving chemotherapy. Overall, primary thromboprophylaxis with LMWH significantly reduced the incidence of symptomatic VTE in outpatients treated with chemotherapy (RR 0.54; 95%CI 0.38–0.75). There was a trend towards increased major bleeding with LMWH, but this result did not achieve statistical significance (RR 1.44; 95%CI 0.98–2.11). Despite the clear benefit in terms of VTE risk reduction, and the relative safety regarding adverse bleeding events, the systematic use of LMWH as a prophylactic treatment has not been recommended, mainly because the absolute risk reduction remains limited in unselected populations of cancer patients. Moreover, the burden of daily subcutaneous injections is substantial, and premature treatment interruptions occurred in a large proportion of participants even in the setting of RCTs [40,49].

4. Use of DOAC for VTE Prevention

DOAC act by direct inhibition of factor Xa (rivaroxaban, apixaban, edoxaban) or factor IIa (dabigatran). Their major advantage is oral administration without requiring monitoring. However, because of their cytochrome-dependent metabolism, they are subject to potential drug–drug interactions. Andexanet alfa, a recombinant variant of human factor Xa, competes with endogenous factor Xa and has been shown efficient to decrease anti-factor Xa activity and restore hemostasis. Andexanet alfa is usually administered using a 400 mg bolus administered in 15 min followed by a 480 mg infusion over 2 h for patients receiving apixaban (800 mg bolus over 30 min followed by a 960 mg infusion for those receiving edoxaban or rivaroxaban) [52].

Two major phase III trials have recently been published, assessing apixaban [22] and rivaroxaban [23] for preventing VTE in ambulatory patients with cancer at high risk of VTE (Khorana score ≥ 2).

In the AVERT study [22], 574 ambulatory cancer patients from 13 centers starting a new course of chemotherapy with a Khorana score ≥ 2 were randomized to apixaban 2.5mg twice daily or placebo for 180 days. Around 25% of patients had lymphoma, 25% a gynecologic cancer, whereas pancreatic cancer was present in 13% (Table 5). Among solid cancers, one quarter were metastatic. Two thirds of the participants had a Khorana score of 2, and the remaining were ≥3. The primary efficacy outcome was VTE, including proximal DVT of upper or lower extremities, PE (symptomatic or incidental), or VTE-related death at 210 days. VTE occurred in 12/488 (4.2%) patients allocated to apixaban and 28/275 (10.2%) patients allocated to placebo (HR 0.41; 95% CI 0.26–0.65). Major bleeding occurred in 10/288 (3.5%) patients allocated to apixaban and 5/275 (1.8%) in the control group (HR 2.00; 95%CI 1.01–3.95). The increase in major bleeding was mainly due to higher rates of mucous bleedings, especially in the gastro-intestinal (GI), urinary, and gynecological tracts, and most events occurred in patients who entered the study with cancers in these locations. There was no significant difference in clinically relevant non-major bleeding (CRNMB).

Table 5. Characteristics of the AVERT and CASSINI trials.

Study Characteristics	AVERT	CASSINI
Intervention	Apixaban 2 × 2.5 mg/d	Rivaroxaban 10 mg/d
Type of cancer	Lymphoma 25%, gynecologic 26%, pancreas 13%, lung 10%	Pancreas 33%, upper GI 21%, lung 15%, lymphoma 7%
Outcome definition	Symptomatic or incidental VTE	Symptomatic or incidental VTE or VTE death *
VTE rate in control group	10.2%	8.8%
Mortality in control group	9.8%	23.8%

* Systematic DVT screening, VTE: venous thromboembolism.

In the CASSINI study [23], 841 ambulatory cancer patients from 11 countries with a solid tumor or lymphoma starting a new chemotherapy with a Khorana score ≥ 2 were randomized to rivaroxaban 10mg daily versus placebo over 180 days. The study population included patients with advanced metastatic cancers of different origins. Patients with primary brain cancer or cerebral metastases, and patients with hematological malignancies were excluded. One third of patients had pancreatic cancer, 21% an upper GI tract cancer, 15% lung cancer, 8% gynecological cancers, and 7% lymphomas. Among those with solid cancers, 54.5% had a metastatic disease.

Systematic screening for lower limb deep vein thrombosis (DVT) was performed with compression ultrasound (CUS) and only patients without DVT were included. Of note, 4.5% of patients screened with CUS had DVT and were excluded. Systematic lower limb CUS was repeated at 8, 16, and 24 weeks. The primary outcome was the composite of symptomatic or screen-detected proximal lower extremity DVT, symptomatic or incidental PE, symptomatic DVT in upper limb, distal DVT in lower limb, or VTE-related death. The primary outcome occurred in 25 of 420 patients (6.0%) in the rivaroxaban group and 37 of 421 (8.8%) in the control group (HR 0.66, 95%CI 0.40–1.09). A secondary analysis restricted to the on-treatment period showed a VTE rate of 2.6% on rivaroxaban versus 6.4% on placebo (HR 0.40, 95%CI 0.20–0.80). Major bleeding occurred in eight of 405 patients (2%) in the rivaroxaban group and in four of 404 (1%) in the control group (HR 1.96; 95%CI 0.59–6.49). There was no significant difference in clinically relevant non-major bleeding (CRNMB).

In summary, in AVERT, apixaban reduces VTE at the expense of increased major bleeding. In CASSINI, rivaroxaban does not significantly reduce VTE but does not significantly increase major bleeding. The differences in interventions, outcome definitions, and populations (Table 5) impact the direct comparison of results from AVERT and CASSINI trials.

A pooled analysis of the two studies has nevertheless been performed and showed a 6-month VTE risk reduction of 0.56 (95%CI 0.35–0.89) on DOACs, with a non-significant increase in major bleeding (1.96; 95%CI 0.80–4.82) [53]. In terms of absolute difference, this corresponded to a VTE risk reduction of 4% (95%CI 0.01–0.07, NNT 25) at the cost of a 1% (95%CI 0.0–0.02) increase (albeit statistically non-significant) in major bleeding (NNH 100). This risk–benefit ratio compares favorably with previous studies using LMWH, and all the more so when taking into account the lower cost and easier route of administration of DOACs compared to LMWH. However, this more favorable balance seems mainly to be due to the selection of patients with an higher basal VTE risk as the observed VTE relative risk reduction is very similar in studies using DOACs (0.56; 95%CI 0.35–0.89) [53] or LMWH (0.54; 95%CI 0.38–0.75) [16].

Based on these studies, thromboprophylaxis using apixaban or rivaroxaban has been endorsed in recent recommendations by expert societies. The American Society for Clinical Oncology (ASCO) recommends thromboprophylaxis in ambulatory cancer patients with a Khorana score ≥ 2 (moderate strength of recommendation) [54]. The International Initiative on Thrombosis and Cancer (ITAC) and International Society for Thrombosis and Hemostasis (ISTH) recently recommended thromboprophylaxis using apixaban or rivaroxaban in ambulatory patients receiving chemotherapy at intermediate-to-high risk of VTE based on cancer type or a validated risk assessment model [55]. According to these guidelines, patients with locally advanced or metastatic pancreatic cancer are considered at high risk of VTE, regardless of their score and thromboprophylaxis is recommended in these patients in the absence of a high risk of bleeding. ASCO and ISTH-ITAC guidelines are provided in Table 6.

Table 6. Recommendations for thromboprophylaxis in ambulatory patients with cancer.

ASCO [54]	ISTH-ITAC [55]
Routine thromboprophylaxis should not be offered to all outpatients with cancer	Primary prophylaxis in ambulatory patients receiving systemic cancer therapy is not recommended routinely
High-risk patients with cancer and Khorana score ≥ 2 may be offered thromboprophylaxis with apixaban, rivaroxaban, or LMWH in the absence of risk factors for bleeding	Primary prophylaxis with LMWH is indicated in ambulatory patients with locally advanced or metastatic pancreatic cancer treated with systemic cancer therapy and who have a low risk of bleeding
Patients with multiple myeloma receiving thalidomide or lenalidomide should receive thromboprophylaxis with AAS or LMWH for lower-risk patients and LMWH for higher-risk patients	Primary prophylaxis with DOAC (rivaroxaban or apixaban) is recommended in outpatients receiving systemic anticancer therapy at intermediate-to-high risk of VTE, identified by cancer type (i.e., pancreatic) or by a validated risk assessment model (i.e., a Khorana score ≥2), and not at a high risk of bleeding

AAS: aspirin, LMWH: low-molecular weight heparin, DOACS: direct anticoagulants.

Several issues remain to be highlighted. First, selection of patients using the Khorana score ≥ 2 resulted in a higher rate of VTE (10% in the placebo arm in AVERT and 9% in CASSINI) compared to unselected series of patients, which confirms that this score can be used as a prediction tool in this setting. Second, the tendency of DOAC to be associated with higher risk of mucosal bleeding seems once again to be confirmed and these molecules should be used with caution in patients with GI cancer. Third, VTE events in AVERT and CASSINI trials included incidentally diagnosed VTE (incidental PE represented one fourth of all events in both studies), whereas the necessity to treat these events is not fully elucidated. Fourth, systematic screening for DVT was performed before inclusion in the CASSINI study; this "pre-selection" of patients without DVT may have influenced the results. Moreover, systematic CUS was also performed in CASSINI, and asymptomatic proximal DVTs contributed to 29% of all events in the placebo arm. As the evolution of these DVTs, had they been undiagnosed, is unknown, the influence on the primary outcome is uncertain. Finally, an important point to highlight is the very high rate of discontinuation of treatment (37% in AVERT and 47% in CASSINI) reflecting the complexity of care in patients with active cancer on chemotherapy.

5. Conclusions

Thromboprophylaxis in ambulatory cancer patients using LMWH or DOACs (apixaban or rivaroxaban) reduces VTE events by about one half, but with a potential increase in major bleeding. DOAC represent an interesting option because of their oral administration and lower costs compared to LMWH. Large scale thromboprophylaxis prescription in ambulatory cancer patients is however not advised, and selection of the patients at high VTE risk without being at high risk of bleeding remains the main challenge. Patients with cancers at very high VTE risk (e.g., pancreas) are most likely to benefit most from primary prophylaxis with DOACs, whereas caution is needed in patients with GI and genitourinary cancers. Further studies based on specific cancers populations or alternative risk assessment models may allow to further improve patient selection. In the complex setting of patients with active cancer on chemotherapy, the decision to initiate thromboprophylaxis should be discussed individually, taking into account tumor site, concomitant treatments, bleeding risk, and most importantly patient's values and preferences.

Author Contributions: A.R. wrote the first draft of the manuscript and contributed to concept, design, and critical writing of the intellectual content. C.M. and H.R.-E. contributed to concept, design, and critical revising of the manuscript. All authors have read and agreed to the published version of the manuscript.

Funding: This research received no external funding.

Conflicts of Interest: C.M. reports participation to an advisory board for Daichii Sankyo. H.R.-E. reports speakers honoria to her institution (Daichii Sankyo) and travel grants (Bayer), A.R. declares no conflict of interest.

References

1. Heit, J.A.; O'Fallon, W.M.; Petterson, T.M.; Lohse, C.M.; Silverstein, M.D.; Mohr, D.N.; Melton, L.J., 3rd. Relative impact of risk factors for deep vein thrombosis and pulmonary embolism: A population-based study. *Arch. Intern. Med.* **2002**, *162*, 1245–1248. [CrossRef] [PubMed]
2. Blom, J.W.; Doggen, C.J.; Osanto, S.; Rosendaal, F.R. Malignancies, prothrombotic mutations, and the risk of venous thrombosis. *JAMA* **2005**, *293*, 715–722. [CrossRef] [PubMed]
3. Chew, H.K.; Wun, T.; Harvey, D.; Zhou, H.; White, R.H. Incidence of venous thromboembolism and its effect on survival among patients with common cancers. *Arch. Intern. Med.* **2006**, *166*, 458–464. [CrossRef]
4. Walker, A.J.; Card, T.R.; West, J.; Crooks, C.; Grainge, M.J. Incidence of venous thromboembolism in patients with cancer–a cohort study using linked United Kingdom databases. *Eur. J. Cancer* **2013**, *49*, 1404–1413. [CrossRef] [PubMed]
5. Horsted, F.; West, J.; Grainge, M.J. Risk of venous thromboembolism in patients with cancer: A systematic review and meta-analysis. *PLoS Med.* **2012**, *9*, e1001275. [CrossRef] [PubMed]
6. Frere, C.; Bournet, B.; Gourgou, S.; Fraisse, J.; Canivet, C.; Connors, J.M.; Buscail, L.; Farge, D.; Consortium, B. Incidence of Venous Thromboembolism in Patients with Newly Diagnosed Pancreatic Cancer and Factors Associated With Outcomes. *Gastroenterology* **2019**. [CrossRef]
7. Lyman, G.H.; Eckert, L.; Wang, Y.; Wang, H.; Cohen, A. Venous thromboembolism risk in patients with cancer receiving chemotherapy: A real-world analysis. *Oncologist* **2013**, *18*, 1321–1329. [CrossRef]
8. Khorana, A.A.; Francis, C.W.; Culakova, E.; Kuderer, N.M.; Lyman, G.H. Frequency, risk factors, and trends for venous thromboembolism among hospitalized cancer patients. *Cancer* **2007**, *110*, 2339–2346. [CrossRef]
9. Lyman, G.H.; Bohlke, K.; Khorana, A.A.; Kuderer, N.M.; Lee, A.Y.; Arcelus, J.I.; Balaban, E.P.; Clarke, J.M.; Flowers, C.R.; Francis, C.W.; et al. Venous thromboembolism prophylaxis and treatment in patients with cancer: American society of clinical oncology clinical practice guideline update 2014. *J. Clin. Oncol.* **2015**, *33*, 654–656. [CrossRef]
10. Barni, S.; Labianca, R.; Agnelli, G.; Bonizzoni, E.; Verso, M.; Mandala, M.; Brighenti, M.; Petrelli, F.; Bianchini, C.; Perrone, T.; et al. Chemotherapy-associated thromboembolic risk in cancer outpatients and effect of nadroparin thromboprophylaxis: Results of a retrospective analysis of the PROTECHT study. *J. Transl. Med.* **2011**, *9*, 179. [CrossRef]
11. Bennett, C.L.; Silver, S.M.; Djulbegovic, B.; Samaras, A.T.; Blau, C.A.; Gleason, K.J.; Barnato, S.E.; Elverman, K.M.; Courtney, D.M.; McKoy, J.M.; et al. Venous thromboembolism and mortality associated with recombinant erythropoietin and darbepoetin administration for the treatment of cancer-associated anemia. *JAMA* **2008**, *299*, 914–924. [CrossRef] [PubMed]
12. Choueiri, T.K.; Schutz, F.A.; Je, Y.; Rosenberg, J.E.; Bellmunt, J. Risk of arterial thromboembolic events with sunitinib and sorafenib: A systematic review and meta-analysis of clinical trials. *J. Clin. Oncol.* **2010**, *28*, 2280–2285. [CrossRef]
13. Petrelli, F.; Cabiddu, M.; Borgonovo, K.; Barni, S. Risk of venous and arterial thromboembolic events associated with anti-EGFR agents: A meta-analysis of randomized clinical trials. *Ann. Oncol.* **2012**, *23*, 1672–1679. [CrossRef] [PubMed]
14. Agnelli, G.; Gussoni, G.; Bianchini, C.; Verso, M.; Mandala, M.; Cavanna, L.; Barni, S.; Labianca, R.; Buzzi, F.; Scambia, G.; et al. Nadroparin for the prevention of thromboembolic events in ambulatory patients with metastatic or locally advanced solid cancer receiving chemotherapy: A randomised, placebo-controlled, double-blind study. *Lancet Oncol.* **2009**, *10*, 943–949. [CrossRef]
15. Agnelli, G.; George, D.J.; Kakkar, A.K.; Fisher, W.; Lassen, M.R.; Mismetti, P.; Mouret, P.; Chaudhari, U.; Lawson, F.; Turpie, A.G.; et al. Semuloparin for thromboprophylaxis in patients receiving chemotherapy for cancer. *New Engl. J. Med.* **2012**, *366*, 601–609. [CrossRef]
16. Di Nisio, M.; Porreca, E.; Candeloro, M.; De Tursi, M.; Russi, I.; Rutjes, A.W. Primary prophylaxis for venous thromboembolism in ambulatory cancer patients receiving chemotherapy. *Cochrane Database Syst. Rev.* **2016**, *12*, CD008500. [CrossRef]

17. Prandoni, P.; Lensing, A.W.; Piccioli, A.; Bernardi, E.; Simioni, P.; Girolami, B.; Marchiori, A.; Sabbion, P.; Prins, M.H.; Noventa, F.; et al. Recurrent venous thromboembolism and bleeding complications during anticoagulant treatment in patients with cancer and venous thrombosis. *Blood* **2002**, *100*, 3484–3488. [CrossRef] [PubMed]
18. Khorana, A.A.; Kuderer, N.M.; Culakova, E.; Lyman, G.H.; Francis, C.W. Development and validation of a predictive model for chemotherapy-associated thrombosis. *Blood* **2008**, *111*, 4902–4907. [CrossRef] [PubMed]
19. Raskob, G.E.; van Es, N.; Verhamme, P.; Carrier, M.; Di Nisio, M.; Garcia, D.; Grosso, M.A.; Kakkar, A.K.; Kovacs, M.J.; Mercuri, M.F.; et al. Edoxaban for the Treatment of Cancer-Associated Venous Thromboembolism. *New Engl. J. Med.* **2018**, *378*, 615–624. [CrossRef]
20. Young, A.M.; Marshall, A.; Thirlwall, J.; Chapman, O.; Lokare, A.; Hill, C.; Hale, D.; Dunn, J.A.; Lyman, G.H.; Hutchinson, C.; et al. Comparison of an Oral Factor Xa Inhibitor With Low Molecular Weight Heparin in Patients With Cancer With Venous Thromboembolism: Results of a Randomized Trial (SELECT-D). *J. Clin. Oncol.* **2018**, *36*, 2017–2023. [CrossRef] [PubMed]
21. Rossel, A.; Robert-Ebadi, H.; Combescure, C.; Grosgurin, O.; Stirnemann, J.; Addeo, A.; Garin, N.; Agoritsas, T.; Reny, J.L.; Marti, C. Anticoagulant therapy for acute venous thrombo-embolism in cancer patients: A systematic review and network meta-analysis. *PLoS ONE* **2019**, *14*, e0213940. [CrossRef] [PubMed]
22. Carrier, M.; Abou-Nassar, K.; Mallick, R.; Tagalakis, V.; Shivakumar, S.; Schattner, A.; Kuruvilla, P.; Hill, D.; Spadafora, S.; Marquis, K.; et al. Apixaban to Prevent Venous Thromboembolism in Patients with Cancer. *New Engl. J. Med.* **2019**, *380*, 711–719. [CrossRef] [PubMed]
23. Khorana, A.A.; Soff, G.A.; Kakkar, A.K.; Vadhan-Raj, S.; Riess, H.; Wun, T.; Streiff, M.B.; Garcia, D.A.; Liebman, H.A.; Belani, C.P.; et al. Rivaroxaban for Thromboprophylaxis in High-Risk Ambulatory Patients with Cancer. *New Engl. J. Med.* **2019**, *380*, 720–728. [CrossRef] [PubMed]
24. Mulder, F.I.; Candeloro, M.; Kamphuisen, P.W.; Di Nisio, M.; Bossuyt, P.M.; Guman, N.; Smit, K.; Buller, H.R.; van Es, N.; collaborators, C.A.-P. The Khorana score for prediction of venous thromboembolism in cancer patients: A systematic review and meta-analysis. *Haematologica* **2019**, *104*, 1277–1287. [CrossRef]
25. Ay, C.; Dunkler, D.; Marosi, C.; Chiriac, A.L.; Vormittag, R.; Simanek, R.; Quehenberger, P.; Zielinski, C.; Pabinger, I. Prediction of venous thromboembolism in cancer patients. *Blood* **2010**, *116*, 5377–5382. [CrossRef]
26. Verso, M.; Agnelli, G.; Barni, S.; Gasparini, G.; LaBianca, R. A modified Khorana risk assessment score for venous thromboembolism in cancer patients receiving chemotherapy: The Protecht score. *Intern. Emerg. Med.* **2012**, *7*, 291–292. [CrossRef]
27. Pelzer, U.; Sinn, M.; Stieler, J.; Riess, H. Primary pharmacological prevention of thromboembolic events in ambulatory patients with advanced pancreatic cancer treated with chemotherapy? *Dtsch. Med. Wochenschr.* **2013**, *138*, 2084–2088. [CrossRef]
28. Cella, C.A.; Di Minno, G.; Carlomagno, C.; Arcopinto, M.; Cerbone, A.M.; Matano, E.; Tufano, A.; Lordick, F.; De Simone, B.; Muehlberg, K.S.; et al. Preventing Venous Thromboembolism in Ambulatory Cancer Patients: The ONKOTEV Study. *Oncologist* **2017**, *22*, 601–608. [CrossRef]
29. Gerotziafas, G.T.; Taher, A.; Abdel-Razeq, H.; AboElnazar, E.; Spyropoulos, A.C.; El Shemmari, S.; Larsen, A.K.; Elalamy, I.; Group, C.-C.W. A Predictive Score for Thrombosis Associated with Breast, Colorectal, Lung, or Ovarian Cancer: The Prospective COMPASS-Cancer-Associated Thrombosis Study. *Oncologist* **2017**, *22*, 1222–1231. [CrossRef]
30. Ay, C.; Simanek, R.; Vormittag, R.; Dunkler, D.; Alguel, G.; Koder, S.; Kornek, G.; Marosi, C.; Wagner, O.; Zielinski, C.; et al. High plasma levels of soluble P-selectin are predictive of venous thromboembolism in cancer patients: Results from the Vienna Cancer and Thrombosis Study (CATS). *Blood* **2008**, *112*, 2703–2708. [CrossRef]
31. Sato, Y.; Kamura, T.; Shirata, N.; Murata, T.; Kudoh, A.; Iwahori, S.; Nakayama, S.; Isomura, H.; Nishiyama, Y.; Tsurumi, T. Degradation of phosphorylated p53 by viral protein-ECS E3 ligase complex. *PLoS Pathog.* **2009**, *5*, e1000530. [CrossRef] [PubMed]
32. Pabinger, I.; van Es, N.; Heinze, G.; Posch, F.; Riedl, J.; Reitter, E.M.; Di Nisio, M.; Cesarman-Maus, G.; Kraaijpoel, N.; Zielinski, C.C.; et al. A clinical prediction model for cancer-associated venous thromboembolism: A development and validation study in two independent prospective cohorts. *Lancet Haematol.* **2018**, *5*, e289–e298. [CrossRef]

33. Pelzer, U.; Opitz, B.; Deutschinoff, G.; Stauch, M.; Reitzig, P.C.; Hahnfeld, S.; Muller, L.; Grunewald, M.; Stieler, J.M.; Sinn, M.; et al. Efficacy of Prophylactic Low-Molecular Weight Heparin for Ambulatory Patients With Advanced Pancreatic Cancer: Outcomes From the CONKO-004 Trial. *J. Clin. Oncol.* **2015**, *33*, 2028–2034. [CrossRef] [PubMed]
34. Godinho, J.; Casa-Nova, M.; Moreira-Pinto, J.; Simoes, P.; Paralta Branco, F.; Leal-Costa, L.; Faria, A.; Lopes, F.; Teixeira, J.A.; Passos-Coelho, J.L. ONKOTEV Score as a Predictive Tool for Thromboembolic Events in Pancreatic Cancer-A Retrospective Analysis. *Oncologist* **2019**. [CrossRef]
35. Van Es, N.; Di Nisio, M.; Cesarman, G.; Kleinjan, A.; Otten, H.M.; Mahe, I.; Wilts, I.T.; Twint, D.C.; Porreca, E.; Arrieta, O.; et al. Comparison of risk prediction scores for venous thromboembolism in cancer patients: A prospective cohort study. *Haematologica* **2017**, *102*, 1494–1501. [CrossRef]
36. Lazo-Langner, A.; Goss, G.D.; Spaans, J.N.; Rodger, M.A. The effect of low-molecular-weight heparin on cancer survival. A systematic review and meta-analysis of randomized trials. *J. Thromb. Haemost.* **2007**, *5*, 729–737. [CrossRef]
37. Kakkar, A.K.; Levine, M.N.; Kadziola, Z.; Lemoine, N.R.; Low, V.; Patel, H.K.; Rustin, G.; Thomas, M.; Quigley, M.; Williamson, R.C. Low molecular weight heparin, therapy with dalteparin, and survival in advanced cancer: The fragmin advanced malignancy outcome study (FAMOUS). *J. Clin. Oncol.* **2004**, *22*, 1944–1948. [CrossRef]
38. Van Doormaal, F.F.; Di Nisio, M.; Otten, H.M.; Richel, D.J.; Prins, M.; Buller, H.R. Randomized trial of the effect of the low molecular weight heparin nadroparin on survival in patients with cancer. *J. Clin. Oncol.* **2011**, *29*, 2071–2076. [CrossRef]
39. Haas, S.K.; Freund, M.; Heigener, D.; Heilmann, L.; Kemkes-Matthes, B.; von Tempelhoff, G.F.; Melzer, N.; Kakkar, A.K.; Investigators, T. Low-molecular-weight heparin versus placebo for the prevention of venous thromboembolism in metastatic breast cancer or stage III/IV lung cancer. *Clin. Appl. Thromb. Hemost.* **2012**, *18*, 159–165. [CrossRef]
40. Macbeth, F.; Noble, S.; Evans, J.; Ahmed, S.; Cohen, D.; Hood, K.; Knoyle, D.; Linnane, S.; Longo, M.; Moore, B.; et al. Randomized Phase III Trial of Standard Therapy Plus Low Molecular Weight Heparin in Patients With Lung Cancer: FRAGMATIC Trial. *J. Clin. Oncol.* **2016**, *34*, 488–494. [CrossRef]
41. Maraveyas, A.; Waters, J.; Roy, R.; Fyfe, D.; Propper, D.; Lofts, F.; Sgouros, J.; Gardiner, E.; Wedgwood, K.; Ettelaie, C.; et al. Gemcitabine versus gemcitabine plus dalteparin thromboprophylaxis in pancreatic cancer. *Eur. J. Cancer* **2012**, *48*, 1283–1292. [CrossRef] [PubMed]
42. Khorana, A.A.; Francis, C.W.; Kuderer, N.M.; Carrier, M.; Ortel, T.L.; Wun, T.; Rubens, D.; Hobbs, S.; Iyer, R.; Peterson, D.; et al. Dalteparin thromboprophylaxis in cancer patients at high risk for venous thromboembolism: A randomized trial. *Thromb. Res.* **2017**, *151*, 89–95. [CrossRef] [PubMed]
43. Zwicker, J.I.; Liebman, H.A.; Bauer, K.A.; Caughey, T.; Campigotto, F.; Rosovsky, R.; Mantha, S.; Kessler, C.M.; Eneman, J.; Raghavan, V.; et al. Prediction and prevention of thromboembolic events with enoxaparin in cancer patients with elevated tissue factor-bearing microparticles: A randomized-controlled phase II trial (the Microtec study). *Br. J. Haematol.* **2013**, *160*, 530–537. [CrossRef] [PubMed]
44. Chahinian, A.P.; Propert, K.J.; Ware, J.H.; Zimmer, B.; Perry, M.C.; Hirsh, V.; Skarin, A.; Kopel, S.; Holland, J.F.; Comis, R.L.; et al. A randomized trial of anticoagulation with warfarin and of alternating chemotherapy in extensive small-cell lung cancer by the Cancer and Leukemia Group B. *J. Clin. Oncol.* **1989**, *7*, 993–1002. [CrossRef] [PubMed]
45. Zacharski, L.R.; Henderson, W.G.; Rickles, F.R.; Forman, W.B.; Cornell, C.J., Jr.; Forcier, R.J.; Edwards, R.; Headley, E.; Kim, S.H.; O'Donnell, J.R.; et al. Effect of warfarin on survival in small cell carcinoma of the lung. Veterans Administration Study No. 75. *JAMA* **1981**, *245*, 831–835. [CrossRef] [PubMed]
46. Maurer, L.H.; Herndon, J.E., 2nd; Hollis, D.R.; Aisner, J.; Carey, R.W.; Skarin, A.T.; Perry, M.C.; Eaton, W.L.; Zacharski, L.L.; Hammond, S.; et al. Randomized trial of chemotherapy and radiation therapy with or without warfarin for limited-stage small-cell lung cancer: A Cancer and Leukemia Group B study. *J. Clin. Oncol.* **1997**, *15*, 3378–3387. [CrossRef]
47. Levine, M.; Hirsh, J.; Gent, M.; Arnold, A.; Warr, D.; Falanga, A.; Samosh, M.; Bramwell, V.; Pritchard, K.I.; Stewart, D.; et al. Double-blind randomised trial of a very-low-dose warfarin for prevention of thromboembolism in stage IV breast cancer. *Lancet* **1994**, *343*, 886–889. [CrossRef]

48. Larocca, A.; Cavallo, F.; Bringhen, S.; Di Raimondo, F.; Falanga, A.; Evangelista, A.; Cavalli, M.; Stanevsky, A.; Corradini, P.; Pezzatti, S.; et al. Aspirin or enoxaparin thromboprophylaxis for patients with newly diagnosed multiple myeloma treated with lenalidomide. *Blood* **2012**, *119*, 933–939. [CrossRef]
49. Palumbo, A.; Cavo, M.; Bringhen, S.; Zamagni, E.; Romano, A.; Patriarca, F.; Rossi, D.; Gentilini, F.; Crippa, C.; Galli, M.; et al. Aspirin, warfarin, or enoxaparin thromboprophylaxis in patients with multiple myeloma treated with thalidomide: A phase III, open-label, randomized trial. *J. Clin. Oncol.* **2011**, *29*, 986–993. [CrossRef]
50. Klerk, C.P.; Smorenburg, S.M.; Otten, H.M.; Lensing, A.W.; Prins, M.H.; Piovella, F.; Prandoni, P.; Bos, M.M.; Richel, D.J.; van Tienhoven, G.; et al. The effect of low molecular weight heparin on survival in patients with advanced malignancy. *J. Clin. Oncol.* **2005**, *23*, 2130–2135. [CrossRef]
51. Perry, J.R.; Julian, J.A.; Laperriere, N.J.; Geerts, W.; Agnelli, G.; Rogers, L.R.; Malkin, M.G.; Sawaya, R.; Baker, R.; Falanga, A.; et al. PRODIGE: A randomized placebo-controlled trial of dalteparin low-molecular-weight heparin thromboprophylaxis in patients with newly diagnosed malignant glioma. *J. Thromb. Haemost.* **2010**, *8*, 1959–1965. [CrossRef] [PubMed]
52. Connolly, S.J.; Crowther, M.; Eikelboom, J.W.; Gibson, C.M.; Curnutte, J.T.; Lawrence, J.H.; Yue, P.; Bronson, M.D.; Lu, G.; Conley, P.B.; et al. Full Study Report of Andexanet Alfa for Bleeding Associated with Factor Xa Inhibitors. *New Engl. J. Med.* **2019**, *380*, 1326–1335. [CrossRef] [PubMed]
53. Li, A.; Kuderer, N.M.; Garcia, D.A.; Khorana, A.A.; Wells, P.S.; Carrier, M.; Lyman, G.H. Direct oral anticoagulant for the prevention of thrombosis in ambulatory patients with cancer: A systematic review and meta-analysis. *J. Thromb. Haemost.* **2019**, *17*, 2141–2151. [CrossRef] [PubMed]
54. Key, N.S.; Khorana, A.A.; Kuderer, N.M.; Bohlke, K.; Lee, A.Y.Y.; Arcelus, J.I.; Wong, S.L.; Balaban, E.P.; Flowers, C.R.; Francis, C.W.; et al. Venous Thromboembolism Prophylaxis and Treatment in Patients With Cancer: ASCO Clinical Practice Guideline Update. *J. Clin. Oncol.* **2019**. [CrossRef] [PubMed]
55. Farge, D.; Frere, C.; Connors, J.M.; Ay, C.; Khorana, A.A.; Munoz, A.; Brenner, B.; Kakkar, A.; Rafii, H.; Solymoss, S.; et al. 2019 International clinical practice guidelines for the treatment and prophylaxis of venous thromboembolism in patients with cancer. *Lancet Oncol.* **2019**, *20*, e566–e581. [CrossRef]

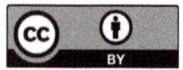

© 2020 by the authors. Licensee MDPI, Basel, Switzerland. This article is an open access article distributed under the terms and conditions of the Creative Commons Attribution (CC BY) license (http://creativecommons.org/licenses/by/4.0/).

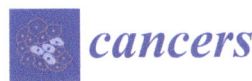

Review

Direct Oral Anticoagulants in Cancer Patients. Time for a Change in Paradigm

Marek Z. Wojtukiewicz [1,2,*], **Piotr Skalij** [1,2], **Piotr Tokajuk** [1,2], **Barbara Politynska** [3,4], **Anna M. Wojtukiewicz** [3], **Stephanie C. Tucker** [5] **and Kenneth V. Honn** [5,6,7]

1. Department of Oncology, Medical University of Białystok, 12 Ogrodowa St., 15-027 Białystok, Poland; skalij@piasta.pl (P.S.); ptokajuk@poczta.onet.pl (P.T.)
2. Department of Clinical Oncology, Comprehensive Cancer Center, 12 OgrodowaSt., 15-369 Białystok, Poland
3. Department of Philosophy and Human Psychology, Medical University of Białystok, 37 Szpitalna St., 15-295 Białystok, Poland; bpolitynska@wp.pl (B.P.); aniawojtukiewicz@gmail.com (A.M.W.)
4. Robinson College, University of Cambridge, Cambridge CB3 9AN, UK
5. Bioactive Lipids Research Program, Department of Pathology-School of Medicine, Detroit, MI 48202, USA; stucker@med.wayne.edu (S.C.T.); k.v.honn@wayne.edu (K.V.H.)
6. Department of Chemistry, Wayne State University, Detroit, MI 48202, USA
7. Department of Oncology, Karmanos Cancer Institute, Detroit, MI 48202, USA
* Correspondence: mzwojtukiewicz@gmail.com

Received: 10 April 2020; Accepted: 30 April 2020; Published: 2 May 2020

Abstract: Thrombosis is a more common occurrence in cancer patients compared to the general population and is one of the main causes of death in these patients. Low molecular weight heparin (LMWH) has been the recognized standard treatment for more than a decade, both in cancer-related thrombosis and in its prevention. Direct oral anticoagulants (DOACs) are a new option for anticoagulation therapy. Recently published results of large randomized clinical trials have confirmed that DOAC may be a reasonable alternative to LMWH in cancer patients. The following review summarizes the current evidence on the safety and efficacy of DOAC in the treatment and prevention of cancer-related thrombosis. It also draws attention to the limitations of this group of drugs, knowledge of which will facilitate the selection of optimal therapy.

Keywords: thrombosis; cancer; treatment; prophylaxis; anticoagulants; DOAC

1. Introduction

As early as the nineteenth century, Armand Trousseau observed a relationship between the occurrence of venous thromboembolism (VTE) and cancer. Around one in five of all VTE cases are found in patients with oncological disease [1]. The risk of occurrence of VTE shows a four- to six-fold increase in patients with active oncological disease compared to the general population and is found in around 5–10% of patients with malignant disease. After progression of the malignant condition itself, it is the second most common cause of death in these patients [2]. Oncological treatment itself is an additional factor in raising the risk of thromboembolism. The co-occurrence of thrombosis and cancer creates many clinical problems. Firstly, VTE in patients with cancer worsens the prognosis by reducing objective survival rates. Secondly, the risk of recurrence of VTE and that of significant bleeding during the treatment of thrombosis is significantly increased in cancer patients compared to those without cancer (by three- and two-fold, respectively) [3]. In the absence of contradictions to its use, low molecular weight heparin (LMWH) remains the standard treatment for cancer-associated thrombosis (CAT), and LMWH has been confirmed to be superior to antagonists of vitamin K (VKA) in terms of efficacy and safety in many clinical trials [4–7]. Equally, a Cochrane meta-analysis demonstrated that LMWH reduces the risk of recurrent CAT without a significant increase in the risk of major or minor bleeding. This means that until recently LMWH has formed the backbone of most evidence-based recommendations for the treatment and prevention of venous thromboembolism in cancer patients, and many of these recommendations are still in operation [8–10]. Direct oral anticoagulants (DOAC), which include thrombin inhibitors (dabigatran) and factor Xa inhibitors (rivaroxaban, apixaban, and edoxaban) present a new option in the treatment and prevention of CAT. The specific properties of DOAC are particularly attractive due to the limitations of therapies in current use, such as the need for parenteral administration of LMWH as well as the need to monitor and modify the dose, and the high risk of interaction with food and other drugs in the case of VKA [11]. In the last two years, knowledge concerning the use of DOAC in cancer patients has significantly expanded. Is the emerging evidence sufficient to refute the current paradigm of the unrivaled role of LMWH in these patients? Below, the authors attempt to provide an answer to this question.

2. The Place of Direct Oral Anticoagulants in the Treatment of VTE in Patients with Cancer

To the best of the authors' knowledge, no studies have, as yet, been specifically dedicated to directly comparing VKA and DOAC in the treatment of CAT in cancer patients. Large clinical trials carried out in members of the general population with a diagnosis of VTE have demonstrated the superiority of DOAC over VKA in terms of the effectiveness and safety of treatment, which has allowed the standards for management of patients without cancer to be modified accordingly, replacing warfarin with DOAC [12–15]. However, additional analyses of major clinical trials have also been performed. Selected sub-groups of cancer patients did not show significant differences between warfarin and DOAC with regard to the risk of VTE recurrence and major bleeding [16–18], defined as requiring transfusion or lowering hemoglobin by at least 2 g/dL [19]. However, it should be noted that the percentage of cancer patients in these studies was small. Additionally, the presence of variously-defined active cancers is likely to have been part of the exclusion criteria for the studies, and thus patients in the more advanced stages of the disease would not have been included. A meta-analysis of the results of patients meeting these exclusion criteria from six key phase III clinical studies demonstrated a statistically insignificant increase in the effectiveness and safety of DOAC as compared to VKA [20]. In turn, another meta-analysis covering the same sub-population of patients with cancer included in the studies described, showed a significant reduction in the risk of CAT recurrence among patients receiving DOAC as compared to patients in the control arm of the study receiving warfarin, while showing a similar risk of major bleeding [21].

The above data, suggesting the potential efficacy of DOAC in the treatment of CAT, prompted researchers to conduct randomized clinical trials directly comparing DOAC and LMWH in this condition. The results of four such studies have been published in the last two years. The first of them, Hokusai VTE Cancer, included 1050 cancer patients with newly diagnosed deep vein thrombosis, and symptomatic or accidental pulmonary embolism. Patients were given LMWH for five days and then continued on edoxaban (60 mg daily) or subcutaneous dalteparin (200 IU/kg/day for a month, then 150 IU/kg/day) for a period of 6–12 months. The primary efficacy endpoint was a composite factor that included recurrence of VTE or major bleeding. Edoxaban proved no worse than dalteparin (12.8% vs. 13.5%, respectively; $p = 0.006$ on noninferiority analysis). Statistically, the number of VTE recurrences was not significantly different between DOAC and LMWH treated groups (7.9% vs. 11.3%, $p = 0.09$), while major bleeding was more common in patients receiving edoxaban (6.9% vs. 4.0%, $p = 0.04$). No statistically significant differences were found in the number of clinically relevant non-major bleeding episodes (CRNMB). Of interest is the fact that attention was drawn to the high rate of CRNMB which reached 11.1% in the deltaparin arm in the Hokusai VTE Cancer clinical trial in which CRNMB was a secondary outcome. However, it is difficult to compare this result with the same parameter in other clinical trials due to the different protocol designs employed, distinct prespecified CRNMB definitions and different patient populations. Survival in both arms of the study was similar [22]. Another study (SELECT-D) compared the efficacy of rivaroxaban (given at a dose of 15 mg twice a day for three weeks, then 20 mg daily for six months) with dalteparin (200 IU/kg/day for a month, then 150 IU/kg/day for five months) in 406 patients with newly diagnosed CAT, defined as pulmonary embolism or deep vein thrombosis. The recurrence rate of VTE after six months was 4% in patients receiving rivaroxaban (95% CI 2–9%) and 11% (95% CI 7–17%) in patients receiving dalteparin. The number of major bleeds was similar in both arms of the study, 6% (95% CI 3–10%) in the rivaroxaban arm, and 4% in the dalteparin arm (95% CI 1–6%). However, there were differences in the number of CRNMBs and these were more frequent in patients receiving rivaroxaban (13% vs. 4%, HR 3.75; 95% CI, 1.63–8.69%). Survival was similar in both groups [23]. In the third study (ADAM VTE), administration of apixaban (2 × 10 mg for a week then 2 × 5 mg for six months) was compared with dalteparin (200 IU/kg/day for a month, and then 150 IU/kg/day for five months) in 300 patients with CAT. The primary efficacy endpoint for the study was the number of major bleeds that occurred, and no significant differences were found between the two trial arms (0.0% in the apixaban arm and 2.1% in the dalteparin arm; $p = 0.138$). Similarly, the total number of major bleeds and CRNMBs did not differ significantly between the two arms of the study (6.2% vs. 6.3%, respectively, $p = 0.88$). However, the number of VTE recurrences was significantly smaller in the group of patients receiving apixaban in comparison to the group treated with dalteparin (0.7% vs. 6.3%, respectively, $p = 0.02$). Mortality for both groups was similar [24]. A meta-analysis of the above studies has recently been published that confirms the reduced risk of VTE recurrence in cancer patients receiving DOAC as compared to dalteparin, although this is at the cost of an increased number of episodes of major bleeding [25]. In recent days, the results of the Caravaggio study, which is an extension of the ADAM-VTE study, were published and included 1155 cancer patients with newly diagnosed thrombosis who were randomly assigned to one of two arms identical to those found in the ADAM-VTE study. The primary endpoint of this study was the number of CAT relapses over a six-month period. No differences were found between the study drugs (5.6% for the apixaban arm and 7.9% for the dalteparin arm, $p < 0.001$ for noninferiority and $p = 0.09$ for superiority). Interestingly, in the subgroup analysis, in patients less than 65 years of age, apixaban was more effective than dalteparin in preventing the recurrence of venous thromboembolism, and its effectiveness decreased inversely in proportion to the age of the patients. As in other studies, the separation of curves describing the number of CAT relapses over time occurs after a month in keeping with a decrease in the dose of dalteparin. There were also no differences in the main safety point, which was major bleeding, observed in 3.8% of patients receiving apixaban compared to 4.0% of patients in the control group ($p = 0.6$). Importantly, this also concerned major gastrointestinal bleeding. In terms of absolute numbers, CRNMB episodes occurred more frequently after apixaban (9.0% vs. 6.0%, respectively). However, total mortality was similar in both groups [26]. The results of the studies referred to above are summarized in Table 1.

Primary or metastatic lesions of the CNS (*central nervous system*) are associated with an increased risk of thrombosis, while at the same time there is an increased risk of intracranial hemorrhage in such patients. In practice, tumor lesions in the CNS are not an absolute contraindication to anticoagulant therapy, and LMWH is used to treat thrombosis in these patients.

Patients with neoplastic lesions of the CNS were not included in the studies described above, or they constituted only a marginal percentage of subjects. One single comparative cohort study has been performed in which a retrospective analysis of patients with primary or metastatic cancer of the CNS, in whom thrombosis occurred, was carried out. Increased risk of intracranial hemorrhage among patients receiving DOAC compared to patients treated with LMWH was not found. Moreover, much less severe bleeding was observed after DOAC treatment in the subgroup of patients with primary CNS tumors [27].

Table 1. Data from prospective clinical trials comparing the safety and efficacy of direct oral anticoagulants and low molecular weight heparin in the treatment of thrombosis in cancer patients.

Study	Hokusai Cancer VTE		SELECT-D		ADAM-VTE		Caravaggio	
Patient Population	Adults with cancer and newly diagnosed symptomatic or incidental thrombosis		Adults with cancer and newly diagnosed symptomatic or incidental thrombosis		Adults with cancer and newly diagnosed symptomatic or incidental thrombosis		Adults with cancer and newly diagnosed symptomatic or incidental thrombosis	
Observation time (months)	12		6		6		6	
Anticoagulant	Edoxaban	Dalteparin	Rivaroxaban	Dalteparin	Apixaban	Dalteparin	Apixaban	Dalteparin
Treatment	LMWH for 5 days, then edoxaban 60 mg daily	200 IU/kg/day for 30 days, then 150 IU/kg/day	15 mg twice daily for 3 weeks, then 20 mg once daily	200 IU/kg/day for 1 month, then 150 IU/kg/day	10 mg twice daily for 7 days, then 5 mg twice daily	200 IU/kg/day for 1 month, then 150 IU/kg/day	10 mg twice daily for 7 days, then 5 mg twice daily	200 IU/kg/day for 1 month, then 150 IU/kg/day
Sample size	522	524	203	203	145	142	576	579
Mean age of patients (years)	64.3 (SD = 11)	63.7 (SD = 11.7)	67 (22–87)	67 (34–87)	64.4 (SD = 11.3)	64.0 (SD = 10.8)	67.2 (SD = 11.3)	67.2 (SD = 10.9)
Metastatic disease (%)	52.2	53.4	58	58	65.3	66.0	67.5	68.4
Recurrence of thrombosis (%)	7.9 HR 0.71, 95% CI 0.48–1.06 $p = 0.09$	11.3	4 HR 0.43, 95% CI 0.19–0.99 $p = NR$	11	0.7 HR 0.099, 95% CI 0.01–0.78 $p = 0.0281$	6.3	5.6 HR 0.63, 95% CI 0.37–1.07 $p = 0.09$	7.9
Major bleeding (%)	6.9 HR 1.77, 95% CI 1.03–3.04 $p = 0.04$	4	6 HR 1.83, 95% CI 0.68–4.96 $p = NR$	4	0 $p = 0.138$	2.1	3.8 HR 0.82, 95% CI 0.40–1.69 $p = 0.60$	4.0
CRNMB (%)	14.6 HR 1.38, 95% CI 0.98–1.94 $p = NR$	11.1	13 HR 3.76, 95% CI 1.63–8.69 $p = NR$	4	6.2 NR *	4.2	9.0 HR 1.42, 95% CI 0.88–2.30 $p = NR$	6.0
Mortality (%)	39.5 HR 1.12, 95% CI 0.92–1.37 $p = NR$	36.6	25 NR	30	16 HR 1.40, 95% CI 0.82–2.43 $p = 0.307$	11	23.4 HR 0.82, 95% CI 0.62–1.09 $p = NR$	26.4
Median duration of treatment	211 days	184 days	5.9 months	5.8 months	5.78 months	5.65 months	178 days	175 days

CRNMB—clinically relevant non-major bleeding, NR—not reported; * statistics for CRNMB and major bleeding were tested cumulatively. The results of the comparison were statistically insignificant.

3. The Use of DOAC in the Primary Prevention of CAT

Current guidelines recommend the primary prevention of VTE in patients with cancer during hospitalization [28]. However, it is not a standard procedure in outpatient settings, remaining an option in selected patients at high risk of CAT, which can be estimated using prognostic scales such as the well validated Khorana scale (see Table 2) [29]. The usefulness of DOAC in primary CAT prevention has been assessed in two large clinical trials. In the CASSINI study, the effectiveness of rivaroxaban used for a period of six months at a standard dose (10 mg per day) was compared to placebo for the prophylaxis of VTE in cancer patients starting systematic outpatient treatment. A total of 841 patients in whom the Khorana score was 2 or more at baseline were entered into the study, after the exclusion of patients with primary or metastatic CNS lesions due to the significantly increased risk of bleeding complications in these patients. In addition, during the process of selection for the study, patients underwent ultrasound assessment for asymptomatic deep vein thrombosis in order that those with positive results be excluded from the study (4.5% of patients originally qualified to take part). The primary efficacy endpoint for the study was the composite of symptomatic or asymptomatic proximal deep vein thrombosis of the lower limbs, symptomatic deep vein thrombosis of the upper limb or distal part of the lower limb, symptomatic or asymptomatic pulmonary embolism, or VTE-related death, which was objectively assessed by an independent clinical endpoint committee. These events occurred during six months of follow-up in 6.0% of patients receiving rivaroxaban compared to 8.8% of patients in the placebo control group (HR 0.66, 95% CI: 0.40–1.09; $p = 0.10$). There were no differences in the number of complications, both in terms of major bleeding (2.7% in the study group vs. 2.0% in the control group; HR 1.96; 95% CI, 0.59–6.49) and CRNMB (respectively: 2.7% vs. 2.0%; HR 1.34; 95% CI, 0.54–3.32) [30]. The study thus confirmed the safety of rivaroxaban in a selected population of patients with cancer, while demonstrating no effect of such prophylaxis on reducing the incidence of CAT compared to placebo in these patients. It is worth noting that 47% of patients enrolled in the study prematurely terminated participation while remaining under observation, which had a significant impact on the results obtained, as nearly 40% of events related to the primary endpoint occurred in this group of patients. Additional analysis, including observation limited to the treatment period, showed a statistically significant reduction in the number of primary endpoint events in the rivaroxaban arm of the study (6.4% vs. 2.6%; HR 0.40, 95% CI, 0.20–0.80).

Table 2. Khorana scale (with modifications by the *American Society of Clinical Oncology*) for assessing the risk of venous thromboembolism in patients receiving chemotherapy in an ambulatory setting.

Clinical Characteristics:	No. of Points:
Type of cancer: stomach, pancreas, primary brain tumors (very high risk)	2
Lungs, lymphoma, reproductive organs, bladder, kidneys (high risk)	1
Platelet count prior to chemotherapy ≥350,000/μL	1
Leukocyte count prior to chemotherapy >11,000/μL	1
Concentration of hemoglobin prior to chemotherapy <10 g/dL and/or use of erythropoietin	1
BMI ≥ 35 kg/m^2	1

Interpretation: 0 points—minimal risk, 1–2 points—medium risk, ≥3 points—high risk.

Different results were obtained in the AVERT study that included 574 patients with cancer who were initiating systemic outpatient treatment and in whom, as in the CASSINI study, the risk of VTE was assessed on the Khorana scale with a cut-off of at least 2 points. Patients with myeloproliferative neoplasms, acute leukemias, and those at increased risk of major bleeding, such as occurring in liver disease associated with coagulopathy, were excluded from the study. Patients were assigned to one of two study arms in which they received apixaban 2.5 mg twice daily for six months or a placebo in the control arm. The primary endpoint was defined as the percentage of confirmed VTE (defined as symptomatic or asymptomatic proximal deep vein thrombosis in the lower and upper extremities, pulmonary embolism, or death due to pulmonary embolism) within six months of randomization.

It is worth noting that unlike in the CASSINI study, no routinely repeated ultrasound examinations were performed. Statistically, apixaban significantly reduced the incidence of VTE (4.2% vs. 10.2%, HR 0.41; 95% CI: 0.26–0.65; $p < 0.001$) compared to placebo. At the same time, major bleeding was more frequently observed in the apixaban arm (3.5% vs. 1.8%, HR 2.00, 95% CI: 1.01–3.95) [31]. While the overall mortality in the above studies was similar in relation to the study arms, it differed significantly between the two studies. This is most likely due to differences in the types of cancer included in the two studies, in the first of which, half of the patients were being treated for pancreatic or stomach cancer, while in the second, patients with lymphomas or gynecological cancers predominated. Significant differences in the observed frequency of thrombosis and hemorrhagic complications between the two studies can be explained in terms of the design, course, and analysis (on-treatment analysis and intention-to-treat analysis) of both studies. Firstly, the initial screening test for patients with VTE in the CASSINI study likely led to a reduction in the number of events during the study, and these individuals were not included in the analysis (4.5% of the patients originally qualified to participate). Secondly, the longer average period of pharmacotherapy among patients in the AVERT trial may have contributed to the increased number of complications. The most relevant data that support use of DOAC have been extracted from both studies in Table 3.

Table 3. Data from prospective clinical trials assessing the efficacy and safety of direct oral anticoagulants in the prevention of thrombosis in cancer patients.

Study	CASSINI		AVERT	
Population	Adult patients starting chemotherapy assessed according to the Khorana scale ≥2 points		Adult patients starting chemotherapy assessed according to the Khorana scale ≥2 points	
Period of observation (months)	6		6	
Anticoagulant	rivaroxaban	placebo	apixaban	placebo
Group size	420	421	291	283
Mean age of patients (years)	63 (23–87)	62 (28–88)	61.2 (SD = 12.4)	61.7 (SD = 11.3)
Type of analysis	on-treatment analysis		intention-to-treat analysis	
Occurrence of thrombosis (%)	2.62 HR 0.40, 95% CI 0.20–0.80 $p = 0.007$	6.41	4.2 HR 0.41, 95% CI 0.26–0.65 $p < 0.001$	10.2
Major bleeding (%)	1.98 HR 1.96, 95% CI 0.59–6.49 $p = 0.265$	0.99	3.5 HR 2.00, 95% CI 1.01–3.95 $p = 0.046$	1.8
CRNMB (%)	2.72 HR 1.34, 95% CI 0.54–3.32 $p = 0.53$	1.98	7.3 HR 1.28, 95% CI 0.89–1.84 $p = $ NR	5.5
Mortality (%)	20.0 HR 0.83, 95% CI 0.62–1.11 $p = 0.213$	23.8	12.2 HR 1.29, 95% CI 0.98–1.71 $p = $ NR	9.8

CRNMB—clinically relevant non-major bleeding, NR—not reported.

4. Limitations of Direct Oral Anticoagulant Therapy

The wide therapeutic window for DOAC makes it possible to achieve the correct therapeutic plasma concentrations in people weighing 40–120 kg using the same standard dose. Due to the etiology of tumors as well as their impact on metabolism, there is an increased likelihood of weight disorders among patients with malignant tumors. It is estimated that obesity is currently one of the main causes of cancer [32], and hence obese people constitute a significant percentage of patients with malignant tumors. In these patients, however, the use of DOAC may not be sufficiently clinically effective; moreover, data on the effectiveness of DOAC in this group of patients are lacking. At the opposite end of the spectrum, over the course of cancer, some patients suffer from extreme cachexia. For people severely debilitated in this way, the use of DOAC may increase the risk of hemorrhagic complications.

Hence, LMWH would appear to be a better choice in the treatment/prevention of CAT in people with significant weight disorders.

Interactions with other drugs may be problematic during DOAC therapy. All DOACs are transported by P-glycoprotein, and in addition, rivaroxaban and apixaban are substrates for cytochrome P450 (CYP3A4) [33]. Many drugs used in systematic anticancer therapy and adjunctive therapy are inhibitors or inducers of P-glycoprotein and/or CYP3A4, which may potentially result in a change in plasma DOAC concentration, taking it outside the therapeutic window. The consequence of this may be lack of a therapeutic effect or an increase in the number of bleeding complications [34]. Despite the fact that any direct interactions between DOAC and oncological drugs have not been evaluated so far, in patients qualifying for DOAC therapy, it is necessary to take into account the systemic treatments used that include both classic cytostatics and drugs used in hormone therapy, targeted therapy, and supportive therapy. In addition, some oncological surgery and radiation therapy may affect DOAC absorption, thereby interfering with therapeutic concentrations [35]. Drugs used in the treatment of cancer patients that have known effects on CYP3A4 and/or P-glycoprotein, and consequently affect the pharmacokinetics of DOAC, are summarized in Table 4 [36,37].

Table 4. Drugs used in oncological therapy with known effects on cytochrome P450 and/or P-glycoprotein.

Type of Interaction	CYP3A4	P-Glycoprotein
Inducers (may increase DOAC plasma levels)	Cytostatics: paclitaxel, docetaxel, vincristine, vinorelbine Hormonal drugs: **enzalutamide** * Immunomodulators: **dexamethasone**, prednisone	Cytostatics: **vinblastine, doxorubicin** Tyrosine kinase inhibitors: **vandetanib, sunitinib** Immunomodulators: **dexamethasone**
Inhibitors (may reduce DOAC plasma levels)	Cytostatics: etoposide, doxorubicin, idarubicin, ifosfamide, cyclophosphamide, lomustine Tyrosine kinase inhibitors: imatinib, crizotinib, nilotinib, lapatinib, dasatinib Hormonal drugs: abiraterone, anastrozole Immunomodulators: cyclosporine, tacrolimus, temsirolimus	Tyrosine kinase inhibitors: **imatinib, crizotinib**, nilotinib, lapatinib Hormonal drugs: **abiraterone, enzalutamide, tamoxifen** Immunomodulators: cyclosporine, tacrolimus
Other substrates for CYP3A4 or/and P-glycoprotein	Cytostatics: vinblastine, irinotecan, busulfan Tyrosine kinase inhibitors: vemurafenib, vandetanib, sunitinib, erlotinib, gefitinib Monoclonal antibodies: brentuximab Hormonal drugs: bicalutamide, tamoxifen, flutamide, letrozole, fulvestrant Immunomodulators: everolimus	Cytostatics: paclitaxel, docetaxel, vincristine, vinorelbine, methotrexate, irinotecan, etoposide, daunorubicin, bendamustine

Adapted from Steffel et al., 2018 [37]; * especially strong interactions are printed in bold type.

Furthermore, renal impairment limits the use of DOAC. Most clinical trials assessing the usefulness of DOAC in VTE excluded patients with creatinine clearance below 30 mL/min (for apixaban: below 25 mL/min) and DOAC should not be used in these patients. However, no data are available on the appropriate management of patients with less severe renal dysfunction. The only available dose reduction recommendations during VTE therapy are for edoxaban, which requires a half dose reduction in patients with creatinine clearance between 30 and 50 mL/min [22]. Despite the favorable DOAC safety profile demonstrated in studies in patients without active cancer [38], bleeding complications are more common in patients with cancer. A detailed analysis of hemorrhagic complications in the HOKUSAI VTE study has provided interesting information. Major bleeding occurred mainly in the upper gastrointestinal tract (56.2% of all major bleeds in the edoxaban arm compared to 18.8% in the dalteparin arm). Bleeding was most commonly observed in patients with gastrointestinal cancer, among whom 12.7% experienced major bleeding during treatment with DOAC compared to 3.6% of patients treated with LMWH (a statistically significant difference). Significant differences in the frequency of major bleeding between these trial arms also occurred in patients with genitourinary cancers (4.3% vs. 1.4%), especially bladder cancers (12.5% vs. 0.0%) [39]. Somewhat different data are provided by the Caravaggio study in which no increase in major bleeding was observed among patients with gastrointestinal malignancies. At present, due to conflicting data, the use of DOAC for patients with gastrointestinal or urological malignancies would appear risky. Based on the findings of the Caravaggio study, it seems that apixaban is the safest of the DOAC medications; however, caution has to be exercised with regard to possible bleeding complications with apixaban probably being the safest in this group of patients.

Central vein catheters and vascular ports are increasingly implanted during systemic therapy. The presence of a catheter in cancer patients predisposes them to thrombosis in the veins of the upper extremities. Although no direct comparison has been made between the various anticoagulants in the treatment of VTE in these patients, LMWH remains the standard. A small prospective study evaluated the efficacy of rivaroxaban in 70 cancer patients with VTE associated with central venous catheter placement. The large number of bleeding complications occurring during 12 weeks of treatment (12.9%), and the occurrence of fatal pulmonary embolism call into question the safety of DOAC in patients with a diagnosis of cancer [40].

Thrombocytopenia is one of the factors affecting the individual risk of bleeding. At the same time, thrombocytopenia does not reduce the number of VTE recurrences. DOAC therapy in patients with malignant tumors can be safely carried out with a platelet count above 50 G/L. In patients with a platelet count below 50 G/L, DOAC should be discontinued in favor of LMWH. Further anticoagulation therapy during periods of severe thrombocytopenia should be carried out in accordance with LMWH guidelines.

The optimal duration of CAT anticoagulation therapy is unknown. The risk of recurrence of VTE due to active oncological disease still exists even after six months from the first VTE episode [41]. Data from studies on the use of LMWH in patients with cancer confirm the validity and safety of prolonged anticoagulant therapy, with the number of episodes of major bleeding dropping significantly after six months of treatment [42,43]. The safety of prolonged treatment with DOAC is indirectly confirmed by the HOKUSAI VTE study in which the period of active therapy included periods of up to 12 months. An ongoing study (API-CAT, NCT03692065) is currently assessing the benefits of full vs. reduced dose apixaban at the end of six months of standard CAT therapy. To sum up, despite limited evidence, prolonged DOAC therapy in CAT treatment seems justified, which is partly extrapolated from studies involving LMWH.

Bearing in mind that DOAC is absorbed in the gastrointestinal tract, concerns about the pharmacokinetics of this group of drugs in patients after oncological surgery of the gastrointestinal tract or in other disorders that reduce the absorbent surface of the gut seem justified. No data are available on the characteristics of individual DOAC medicinal products in this regard, and the available literature is limited to case reports [44]. Therefore, caution in these patients would seem justified.

The above limitations mean that the use of DOAC for the treatment of VTE in patients with cancer requires appropriate selection of patients. The following algorithm, proposed by Suryanarayan [44,45] and modified by the authors, takes into account the specificity of this group of drugs and would appear to enable the appropriate selection of patients for treatment using DOAC (Figure 1).

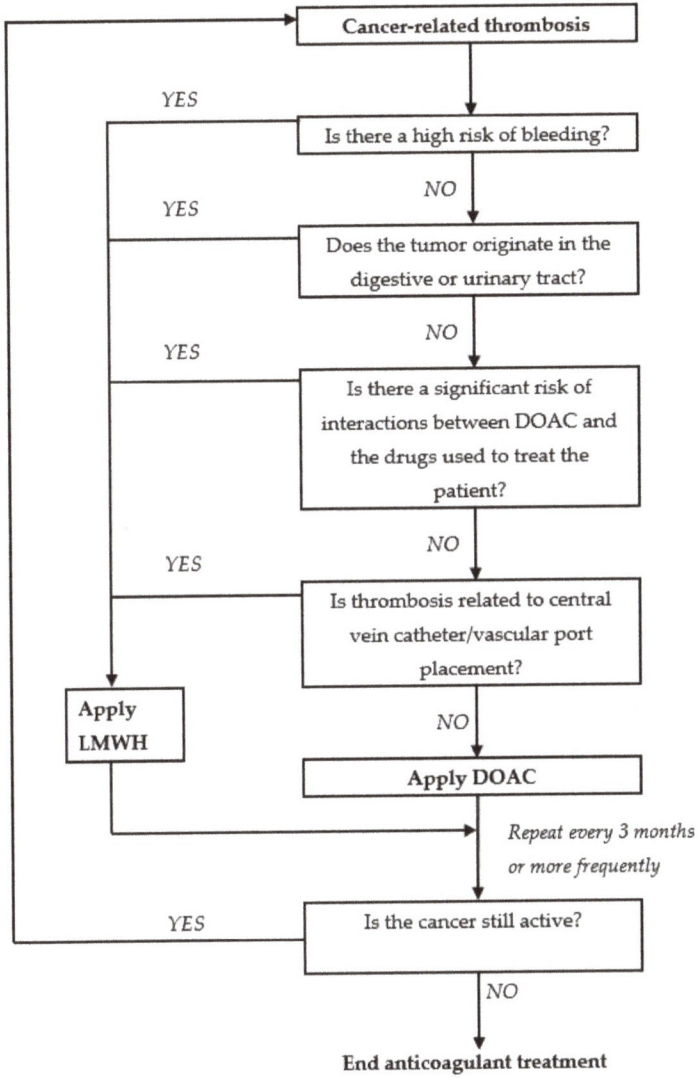

Figure 1. A proposed algorithm for facilitating a safe choice between direct oral anticoagulants and low molecular weight heparin for thrombosis treatment in patients with malignant tumors. Adapted from Suryanarayan, 2019 [43,44].

5. Patient Preferences and the Route of Administration of Anticoagulants

From the physician's perspective, patients' preferences in choosing the route of drug administration are unequivocal: oral anticoagulants are superior to LMWH in this respect. Adherence to medical recommendations has a significant impact on the effectiveness of treatment, including successful anticoagulation. Therefore, in terms of patients' preferences that take into account such factors as fear of injections, the choice of therapy may be important. However, in this respect most patients with malignant tumors express a viewpoint that is contrary to expectations. A study was conducted in which 100 oncology patients being treated for CAT were asked to assess the most important attributes of anticoagulants (LMWH or VKA), after being given specific information in this regard. The results revealed that the greatest concern to patients was that anticoagulant therapy should not interfere with cancer treatment (39%), which suggests that cancer is perceived as more important than VTE despite the inherent risk of the latter. The reduction of thrombosis recurrence (24%) was in second place, followed by low risk of bleeding (19%). The superiority of oral administration over injections (13%) was ranked in fourth place [46]. On the other hand, quality of life (QoL) analyses conducted in the ADAM study showed significantly better results among those receiving oral anticoagulants compared to those receiving them in the form of injection. The discomfort associated with daily injections may have an impact on compliance with medical recommendations, and this may have caused the difference in the median duration of treatment between the arms of the HOKUSAI study (211 days vs. 184 days; $p = 0.01$). Nevertheless, the authors believe that from the perspective of an oncological patient, the choice between the use of DOAC and LMWH would not be significantly affected by the route of drug administration.

6. Anticoagulation Therapy and the Use of DOAC in Hospice patients

After exhausting the possibilities for causal treatment in patients with advanced malignancy, symptomatic treatment is required in most cases. As the disease progresses and end-of-life care becomes a necessity, for some patients such treatment is delivered in the form of hospice care. The occurrence of CAT in this group of patients, who are frequently in a poor general condition and have additional comorbidities, is a further challenge. The incidence of VTE in patients receiving palliative care remains unknown. However, as the risk of VTE increases with the progression of oncological disease, hospitalization, dehydration, and prolonged immobilization, the increased risk for CAT is also likely to affect patients in hospice care [47,48]. Focusing hospice treatment on maintaining the highest QoL, even at the expense of prolonging it, is an additional problem in the event of symptomatic CAT, which may be manifested by limb or chest pain, shortness of breath, and mental suffering. The occurrence of these symptoms significantly worsens QoL, which should be taken into account when making therapeutic decisions [49]. Guidelines for CAT treatment recommend anticoagulant therapy without specifying its duration in patients with active cancer, and there are no guidelines to define its legitimacy in end-of-life management [50]. Analysis of a series of 214 cases of patients with CAT who died during a two-year follow-up, found that treatment was continued until death in half of the patients, while in 11% it was discontinued ≤7 days before death (patients treated with LMWH). Patients whose anticoagulant treatment was terminated did not have any recurrence of previous CAT symptoms. However, CRNMB was observed in 7% of patients in whom anticoagulant therapy was continued until death [51]. Another observational study involving nearly 1200 patients admitted to palliative care wards, 90% of whom had malignancies, demonstrated a low incidence of VTE. In nearly 10% of patients clinically significant bleeding was observed and was associated primarily with prophylactic anticoagulation [52]. On the basis of these data, LMWH anticoagulation prophylaxis in hospice patients would seem to be inadvisable. There have been no studies dedicated to the use of DOAC in patients with cancer at the end of life. Furthermore, the large randomized DOAC studies in cancer patients described previously did not include patients with a life expectancy of less than six months. It is also worth noting that organ dysfunction, polypharmacy, and cachexia are common among hospice patients, and this may affect the safety of DOAC therapy. These considerations lead to the conclusion that DOAC should not currently be used in this patient population, and in the event of deteriorating QoL symptomatic of CAT, the use of LMWH should remain the treatment of choice.

7. The Effect of DOAC on Tumor Growth and Metastatic Dissemination in Experimental Models

The two-way relationship between coagulation and cancer is well known. Preclinical studies, mainly in animal models where drugs were applied before inoculation with cancer cells, have demonstrated the influence of VKA and LMVH on reducing tumor growth and inhibiting the formation of metastases [53,54]. The increasing role of DOAC in the treatment of cancer patients has prompted researchers to conduct experimental studies that assess the effects of DOAC on cancer biology [55]. Most of the available data relate to drugs currently not in clinical use with cancer patients.

The carcinogenicity of ximelagatran was assessed by comparing mice given the drug for 18 months to a control group. Pancreatic cell hyperplasia discovered in individual mice on post-mortem examination prompted the researchers to continue the study in rats, among which, a selected group received a particularly high daily dose of ximelagatran for 24 months. In this group, the development of hyperplastic pancreatic tissue, adenomas or cancer of the pancreas were observed among male rats. There were no changes in other organs. This may indicate a dose- and time-dependent effect on carcinogenesis [56]. Another study demonstrated an increase in lung metastases in mice vaccinated with melanoma cells and treated with ximelagatran prior to inoculation. However, somewhat different results were provided by a study in which female mice were injected with breast cancer cells and administration of dabigatran was started concurrently. In the following weeks, a decrease in tumor volume was observed and there was a tendency for metastatic changes in the lungs and liver to decrease [57]. By contrast, however, in two experiments, Alexander et al. did not observe reduction of the primary tumor [58] nor any effect on metastatic changes [59] in mice during the administration of dabigatran, initiated during the development of the neoplastic changes. Thus, the effect of dabigatran on tumor reduction appears to be negligible for already established tumors. Moreover, in an experiment in which mice were vaccinated with pancreatic cancer cells and dabigatran was started after one week, an increase in tumor dissemination was observed in comparison to the control group. Researchers explained this in terms of increased bleeding within the tumor [60]. Interesting results have been provided by studies using rivaroxaban. In the first of these, fibrosarcoma cells were injected into mice, and after 14 days the animals were randomized for rivaroxaban treatment. A reduction of approximately 50% in tumor mass and a significant reduction in lung metastases was observed. In a further experiment, when randomization was carried out at a later point in time, the effect of rivaroxaban on tumor size was smaller. Similar data were obtained in additional experiments using colorectal and breast cancer models [61]. The effect of rivaroxaban on tumor growth or tumor cell proliferation, in turn, has not been confirmed in pancreatic cancer or triple-negative breast cancer experimental models in immunodeficient mice [62,63]. The above data suggest that the role of DOAC in cancer biology is uncertain and requires further research.

8. Conclusions

Direct oral anticoagulants provide an attractive alternative to LMWH in the treatment of VTE in cancer patients. Studies have confirmed both the efficacy and safety of this group of drugs in the treatment of CAT. However, the limitations of DOAC associated with an increased risk of major bleeding, interaction with other drugs, unknown or inappropriate pharmacokinetics in patients with large deviations from normal body weight, and in patients with impaired renal function means that CAT therapy using DOAC requires patients to be carefully selected for this form of treatment. Currently, DOAC in CAT treatment is an alternative to LMWH in the recommendations of some scientific societies, including the National Comprehensive Cancer Network (NCCN) and the International Society on Thrombosis and Haemostasis (ISTH) [64,65]. Direct oral anticoagulants have also been included in the recently published American Society of Clinical Oncology (ASCO) recommendations: supporting the use of rivaroxaban in initial anticoagulant therapy and in combination with edoxaban in prolonged therapy. These recommendations are based on the strength and quality of the evidence available [66]. Furthermore, data obtained from studies assessing DOAC in the primary prevention of CAT in high-risk patients are very encouraging, which prompted the inclusion of rivaroxaban and apixaban in the latest ASCO and The International Initiative on Thrombosis and Cancer (ITAC) guidelines [67]. Ongoing subsequent phase III studies, as well as data from actual clinical practice, will determine the optimal role of DOAC in cancer patients, both in the treatment and prevention of VTE. However, DOAC is a long-awaited alternative that has irrevocably ended the dominance of LMWH in oncology.

Author Contributions: Concept and design: M.Z.W., P.S., and K.V.H.; acquisition and assembly of data: P.S., P.T., B.P., and A.M.W.; data analysis and interpretation: M.Z.W., P.S., and P.T.; writing the draft of the manuscript: P.S., P.T., B.P., and A.M.W.; critical revision of the manuscript: M.Z.W., S.C.T., and K.V.H.; final proofreading: M.Z.W., S.C.T., K.V.H., and B.P.; approval of the version for publication: M.Z.W. All authors have read and agree to the published version of the manuscript.

Funding: This research received no external funding.

Conflicts of Interest: The authors declare no conflict of interest.

References

1. Lee, A.Y. Management of thrombosis in cancer: Primary prevention and secondary prophylaxis. *Br. J. Haematol.* **2005**, *128*, 291–302. [CrossRef] [PubMed]
2. Levitan, N.; Dowlati, A.; Remick, S.C.; Tahsildar, H.I.; Sivinski, L.D.; Beyth, R.; Rimm, A.A. Rates of initial and recurrent thromboembolic disease among patients with malignancy versus those without malignancy. Risk analysis using Medicare claims data. *Medicine* **1999**, *78*, 285–291. [CrossRef] [PubMed]
3. Prandoni, P.; Lensing, A.W.A.; Piccioli, A.; Bernardi, E.; Simioni, P.; Girolami, B.; Marchiori, A.; Sabbion, P.; Prins, M.H.; Noventa, F.; et al. Recurrent venous thromboembolism and bleeding complications during anticoagulant treatment in patients with cancer and venous thrombosis. *Blood* **2002**, *100*, 3484–3488. [CrossRef] [PubMed]
4. Meyer, G.; Marjanovic, Z.; Valcke, J.; Lorcerie, B.; Gruel, Y.; Solal-Celigny, P.; Le Maignan, C.; Extra, J.M.; Cottu, P.; Farge, D. Comparison of low-molecular-weight heparin and warfarin for the secondary prevention of venous thromboembolism in patients with cancer: A randomized controlled study. *Arch. Intern. Med.* **2002**, *162*, 1729–1735. [CrossRef]
5. Lee, A.Y.Y.; Levine, M.N.; Baker, R.I.; Bowden, C.; Kakkar, A.K.; Prins, M.; Rickles, F.R.; Julian, J.A.; Haley, S.; Kovacs, M.J.; et al. Low-molecular-weight heparin versus a coumarin for the prevention of recurrent venous thromboembolism in patients with cancer. *N. Engl. J. Med.* **2003**, *349*, 146–153. [CrossRef]
6. Hull, R.D.; Pineo, G.F.; Brant, R.F.; Mah, A.F.; Burke, N.; Dear, R.R.; Wong, T.; Cook, R.; Solymoss, S.; Poon, M.C.; et al. Long-term low-molecular-weight heparin versus usual care in proximal-vein thrombosis patients with cancer. *Am. J. Med.* **2006**, *119*, 1062–1072. [CrossRef]
7. Lee, A.Y.Y.; Kamphuisen, P.W.; Meyer, G.; Bauersachs, R.; Janas, M.S.; Jarner, M.F.; Khorana, A.A. Tinzaparin vs warfarin for treatment of acute venous thromboembolism in patients with active cancer: A randomized clinical trial. *JAMA* **2015**, *314*, 677–686. [CrossRef]
8. Mandalà, M.; Falanga, A.; Roila, F. ESMO Guidelines Working Group. Management of venous thromboembolism (VTE) in cancer patients: ESMO clinical practice guidelines. *Ann. Oncol.* **2011**, *22*, 85–92. [CrossRef]
9. Kearon, C.; Akl, E.A.; Ornelas, J.; Blaivas, A.; Jimenez, D.; Bounameaux, H.; Huisman, M.; King, C.S.; Morris, T.A.; Sood, N.; et al. Antithrombotic therapy for VTE disease: CHEST guideline and expert panel report. *Chest* **2016**, *149*, 315–352. [CrossRef]
10. Wojtukiewicz, M.Z.; Sierko, E.; Tomkowski, W.; Zawilska, K.; Undas, A.; Podolak-Dawidziak, M.; Wysocki, P.; Krzakowski, M.; Warzocha, K.K.; Windyga, J. Guidelines for the prevention and treatment of venous thromboembolism in non-surgically treated cancer patients. *Oncol. Clin. Pract.* **2016**, *12*, 67–91. [CrossRef]
11. Frere, C.; Benzidia, I.; Marjanovic, Z.; Farge, D. Recent advances in the management of cancer-associated thrombosis: New hopes but new challenges. *Cancers* **2019**, *11*, 71. [CrossRef]
12. Agnelli, G.; Buller, H.R.; Cohen, A.; Curto, M.; Gallus, A.S.; Johnson, M.; Masiukiewicz, U.; Pak, R.; Thompson, J.; Raskob, G.E.; et al. Oral apixaban for the treatment of acute venous thromboembolism. *N. Engl. J. Med.* **2013**, *369*, 799–808. [CrossRef]
13. Büller, H.R.; Décousus, H.; Grosso, M.A.; Mercuri, M.; Middeldorp, S.; Prins, M.H.; Raskob, G.E.; Schellong, S.M.; Schwocho, L.; Segers, A.; et al. Edoxaban versus warfarin for the treatment of symptomatic venous thromboembolism. *N. Engl. J. Med.* **2013**, *369*, 1406–1415.
14. Bauersachs, R.; Berkowitz, S.D.; Brenner, B.; Buller, H.R.; Decousus, H.; Gallus, A.S.; Lensing, A.W.; Misselwitz, F.; Prins, M.H.; Raskob, G.E.; et al. Oral rivaroxaban for symptomatic venous thromboembolism. *N. Engl. J. Med.* **2010**, *363*, 2499–2510. [PubMed]

15. Büller, H.R.; Prins, M.H.; Lensin, A.W.; Decousus, H.; Jacobson, B.F.; Minar, E.; Chlumsky, J.; Verhamme, P.; Wells, P.; Agnelli, G.; et al. Oral rivaroxaban for the treatment of symptomatic pulmonary embolism. *N. Engl. J. Med.* **2012**, *366*, 1287–1297. [PubMed]

16. Schulman, S.; Goldhaber, S.Z.; Kearon, C.; Kakkar, A.K.; Schellong, S.; Eriksson, H.; Hantel, S.; Feuring, M.; Kreuzer, J. Treatment with dabigatran or warfarin in patients with venous thromboembolism and cancer. *Thromb. Haemost.* **2015**, *114*, 150–157. [PubMed]

17. Prins, M.H.; Lensing, A.W.; Brighton, T.A.; Lyons, R.M.; Rehm, J.; Trajanovic, M.; Davidson, B.L.; Beyer-Westendorf, J.; Pap, Á.F.; Berkowitz, S.D.; et al. Oral rivaroxaban versus enoxaparin with vitamin K antagonist for the treatment of treatment of symptomaticvenous thromboembolism in patients with cancer (EINSTEIN-DVT and EINSTEIN-PE): A pooled subgroup analysis of two randomised controlled trials. *Lancet Haematol.* **2014**, *1*, e37–e46. [CrossRef]

18. Agnelli, G.; Buller, H.R.; Cohen, A.; Gallus, A.S.; Lee, T.C.; Pak, R.; Raskob, G.E.; Weitz, J.I.; Yamabe, T. Oral apixaban for the treatment of venous thromboembolism in cancer patients: Results from the AMPLIFY trial. *J. Thromb. Haemost.* **2015**, *13*, 2187–2191. [CrossRef]

19. Schulman, S.; Kearon, C. Definition of major bleeding in clinical investigations of antihemostatic medicinal products in non-surgical patients. *J. Thromb. Haemost.* **2005**, *3*, 692–694. [CrossRef]

20. Posch, F.; Königsbrügge, O.; Zielinski, C.; Pabinger, I.; Ay, C. Treatment of venous thromboembolism in patients with cancer: A network meta-analysis comparing efficacy and safety of anticoagulants. *Thromb. Res.* **2015**, *136*, 582–589. [CrossRef]

21. Van Es, N.; Coppens, M.; Schulman, S.; Middeldorp, S.; Buller, H.R. Direct oral anticoagulants compared with vitamin K antagonists for acute venous thromboembolism: Evidence from phase 3 trials. *Blood* **2014**, *124*, 1968–1975. [CrossRef]

22. Raskob, G.E.; van Es, N.; Verhamme, P.; Carrier, M.; Di Nisio, M.; Garcia, D.; Grosso, M.A.; Kakkar, A.K.; Kovacs, M.J.; Mercuri, M.F.; et al. Edoxaban for the treatment of cancer-associated venous thromboembolism. *N. Engl. J. Med.* **2018**, *378*, 615–624. [CrossRef] [PubMed]

23. Young, A.M.; Marshall, A.; Thirlwall, J.; Chapman, O.; Lokare, A.; Hill, C.; Hale, D.; Dunn, J.A.; Lyman, G.H.; Hutchinson, C.; et al. Comparison of an oral factor Xa inhibitor with low molecular weight heparin in patients with cancer with venous thromboembolism: Results of a randomized trial (SELECT-D). *J. Clin. Oncol.* **2018**, *36*, 2017–2023. [CrossRef] [PubMed]

24. McBane, R.D., II; Wysokinski, W.E.; Le-Rademacher, J.G.; Zemla, T.; Ashrani, A.; Tafur, A.; Perepu, U.; Anderson, D.; Gundabolu, K.; Kuzma, C.; et al. Apixaban and dalteparin in active malignancy associated venous thromboembolism: The ADAM VTE Trial. *J. Thromb. Haemost.* **2019**. [CrossRef] [PubMed]

25. Fuentes, H.E.; McBane, R.D.; Wysokinski, W.E.; Tafur, A.J.; Loprinzi, C.L.; Murad, M.H.; Riaz, I.B. Direct oral factor Xa inhibitors for the treatment of acute cancer-associated venous thromboembolism: A systematic review and network meta-analysis. *Mayo Clin. Proc.* **2019**, *94*, 2444–2454. [CrossRef] [PubMed]

26. Agnelli, G.; Becattini, C.; Meyer, G.; Muñoz, A.; Huisman, M.V.; Connors, J.M.; Cohen, A.; Bauersachs, R.; Brenner, B.; Torbicki, A.; et al. Apixaban for the treatment of venous thromboembolism associated with cancer. *N. Engl. J. Med.* **2020**, *382*, 1599–1607. [CrossRef]

27. Carney, B.J.; Uhlmann, E.J.; Puligandla, M.; Mantia, C.; Weber, G.M.; Neuberg, D.S.; Zwicker, J.I. Intracranial hemorrhage with direct oral anticoagulants in patients with brain tumors. *J. Thromb. Haemost.* **2019**, *17*, 72–76. [CrossRef]

28. Khorana, A.A.; Carrier, M.; Garcia, D.A.; Lee, A.Y. Guidance for the prevention and treatment of cancer-associated venous thromboembolism. *J. Thromb. Thrombolysis* **2016**, *41*, 81–91. [CrossRef]

29. Khorana, A.A.; Francis, C.W. Risk prediction of cancer-associated thrombosis: Appraising the first decade and developing the future. *Thromb. Res.* **2018**, *164*, 70–76. [CrossRef]

30. Khorana, A.A.; Soff, G.A.; Kakkar, A.K.; Vadhan-Raj, S.; Riess, H.; Wun, T.; Streiff, M.B.; Garcia, D.A.; Liebman, H.A.; Belani, C.P.; et al. Rivaroxaban for thromboprophylaxis in high-risk ambulatory patients with cancer. *N. Engl. J. Med.* **2019**, *380*, 720–728. [CrossRef]

31. Carrier, M.; Abou-Nassar, K.; Mallick, R.; Tagalakis, V.; Shivakumar, S.; Schattner, A.; Kuruvilla, P.; Hill, D.; Spadafora, S.; Marquis, K.; et al. Apixaban to prevent venous thromboembolism in patients with cancer. *N. Engl. J. Med.* **2019**, *380*, 711–719. [CrossRef] [PubMed]

32. Pischon, T.; Nimptsch, K. Obesity and risk of cancer: An introductory overview. *Recent Results Cancer Res.* **2016**, *208*, 1–15. [PubMed]

33. Galgani, A.; Palleria, C.; Iannone, L.F.; De Sarro, G.; Giorgi, F.S.; Maschio, M.; Russo, E. Pharmacokinetic interactions of clinical interest between direct oral anticoagulants and antiepileptic drugs. *Front. Neurol.* **2018**, *9*, 1067. [CrossRef] [PubMed]
34. Vazquez, S.R. Drug-drug interactions in an era of multiple anticoagulants: A focus on clinically relevant drug interactions. *Hematol. Am. Soc. Hematol. Educ. Program.* **2018**, *132*, 2230–2239. [CrossRef] [PubMed]
35. Bellesoeur, A.; Thomas-Schoemann, A.; Allard, M.; Smadja, D.; Vidal, M.; Alexandre, J.; Goldwasser, F.; Blanchet, B. Pharmacokinetic variability of anticoagulants in patients with cancer-associated thrombosis: Clinical consequences. *Crit. Rev. Oncol. Hematol.* **2018**, *129*, 102–112. [CrossRef]
36. Farge, D.; Frere, C. Recent advances in the treatment and prevention of venous thromboembolism in cancer patients: Role of the direct oral anticoagulants and their unique challenges. *F1000 Res.* **2019**, *8*, 974. [CrossRef]
37. Steffel, J.; Verhamme, P.; Potpara, T.S.; Albaladejo, P.; Antz, M.; Desteghe, L.; Haeusler, K.G.; Oldgren, J.; Reinecke, H.; Roldan-Schilling, V.; et al. The 2018 European heart rhythm association practical guide on the use of non-vitamin K antagonist oral anticoagulants in patients with atrial fibrillation. *Eur. Heart J.* **2018**, *39*, 1330–1393. [CrossRef]
38. Lip, G.Y.; Mitchell, S.A.; Liu, X.; Liu, L.Z.; Phatak, H.; Kachroo, S.; Batson, S. Relative efficacy and safety of non-vitamin K oral anticoagulants for non-valvular atrial fibrillation: Network meta-analysis comparing apixaban, dabigatran, rivaroxaban and edoxaban in three patient subgroups. *Int. J. Cardiol.* **2016**, *204*, 88–94. [CrossRef]
39. Kraaijpoel, N.; Di Nisio, M.; Mulder, F.I.; van Es, N.; Beyer-Westendorf, J.; Carrier, M.; Garcia, D.; Grosso, M.; Kakkar, A.K.; Mercuri, M.F.; et al. Clinical impact of bleeding in cancer-associated venous thromboembolism: Results from the Hokusai VTE cancer study. *Thromb. Haemost.* **2018**, *118*, 1439–1449. [CrossRef]
40. Davies, G.A.; Lazo-Langner, A.; Gandara, E.; Rodger, M.; Tagalakis, V.; Louzada, M.; Corpuz, R.; Kovacs, M.J. A prospective study of Rivaroxaban for central venous catheter associated upper extremity deep vein thrombosis in cancer patients (catheter 2). *Thromb. Res.* **2018**, *162*, 88–92. [CrossRef]
41. Chee, C.E.; Ashrani, A.A.; Marks, R.S.; Petterson, T.M.; Bailey, K.R.; Melton, L.J., III; Heit, J.A. Predictors of venous thromboembolism recurrence and bleeding among active cancer patients: A population-based cohort study. *Blood* **2014**, *123*, 3972–3978. [CrossRef] [PubMed]
42. Francis, C.W.; Kessler, C.M.; Goldhaber, S.Z.; Kovacs, M.J.; Monreal, M.; Huisman, M.V.; Bergqvist, D.; Turpie, A.G.; Ortel, T.L.; Spyropoulos, A.C.; et al. Treatment of venous thromboembolism in cancer patients with dalteparin for up to 12 months: The DALTECAN Study. *J. Thromb. Haemost.* **2015**, *13*, 1028–1035. [CrossRef] [PubMed]
43. Jara-Palomares, L.; Solier-Lopez, A.; Elias-Hernandez, T.; Asensio-Cruz, M.; Blasco-Esquivias, I.; Marin-Barrera, L.; de la Borbolla-Artacho, M.R.; Praena-Fernandez, J.M.; Montero-Romero, E.; Navarro-Herrero, S.; et al. Tinzaparin in cancer associated thrombosis beyond 6months: TiCAT study. *Thromb. Res.* **2017**, *157*, 90–96. [CrossRef] [PubMed]
44. Carrier, M.; Blais, N.; Crowther, M.; Kavan, P.; Le Gal, G.; Moodley, O.; Shivakumar, S.; Tagalakis, V.; Wu, C.; Lee, A.Y.Y. Treatment algorithm in cancer-associated thrombosis: Canadian expert consensus. *Curr. Oncol.* **2018**, *25*, 329–337. [CrossRef]
45. Suryanarayan, D.; Lee, A.Y.Y.; Wu, C. Direct oral anticoagulants in cancer patients. *Semin. Thromb. Hemost.* **2019**, *45*, 638–647. [CrossRef]
46. Noble, S.; Matzdorff, A.; Maraveyas, A.; Holm, M.V.; Pisa, G. Assessing patients' anticoagulation preferences for the treatment of cancer-associated thrombosis using conjoint methodology. *Haematologica* **2015**, *100*, 1486–1492. [CrossRef]
47. Johnson, M.J.; McMillan, B.; Fairhurst, C.; Gabe, R.; Ward, J.; Wiseman, J.; Pollington, B.; Noble, S.I. Primary thromboprophylaxis in hospices: The association between risk of venous thromboembolism and development of symptoms. *J. Pain Symptom Manag.* **2014**, *48*, 56–64. [CrossRef]
48. Noble, S.; Shelley, M.D.; Coles, B.M.; Williams, S.M.; Wilcock, A.; Johnson, M.J. Management of venous thromboembolism in patients with advanced cancer: A systematic review and meta-analysis. *Lancet Oncol.* **2008**, *9*, 577–584. [CrossRef]
49. Noble, S. Thromboembolic disease and breathlessness. *Curr. Opin. Support. Palliat. Care* **2016**, *10*, 249–255. [CrossRef]
50. Noble, S. Venous thromboembolism and palliative care. *Clin. Med.* **2019**, *19*, 315–318. [CrossRef]

51. Chin-Yeea, N.; Tanuseputroa, P.; Carriera, M.; Noble, S. Thromboembolic disease in palliative and end-of-life care: A narrative review. *Thromb. Res.* **2019**, *175*, 84–89. [CrossRef] [PubMed]
52. Tardy, B.; Picard, S.; Guirimand, F.; Chapelle, C.; Danel Delerue, M.; Celarier, T.; Ciais, J.F.; Vassal, P.; Salas, S.; Filbet, M.; et al. Bleeding risk of terminally ill patients hospitalized in palliative care units: The RHESO study. *J. Thromb. Haemost.* **2017**, *15*, 420–428. [CrossRef] [PubMed]
53. Kirane, A.; Ludwig, K.F.; Sorrelle, N.; Haaland, G.; Sandal, T.; Ranaweera, R.; Toombs, J.E.; Wang, M.; Dineen, S.P.; Micklem, D.; et al. Warfarin blocks Gas6-mediated Axl activation required for pancreatic cancer epithelial plasticity and metastasis. *Cancer Res.* **2015**, *75*, 3699–3705. [CrossRef] [PubMed]
54. Niers, T.M.; Klerk, C.P.; DiNisio, M.; Van Noorden, C.J.; Buller, H.R.; Reitsma, P.H.; Richel, D.J. Mechanisms of heparin induced anti-cancer activity in experimental cancer models. *Crit. Rev. Oncol. Hematol.* **2007**, *61*, 195–207. [CrossRef] [PubMed]
55. Najidh, S.; Versteeg, H.H.; Buijs, J.T. A systematic review on the effects of direct oral anticoagulants on cancer growth and metastasis in animal models. *Thromb. Res.* **2020**, *187*, 18–27. [CrossRef]
56. Stong, D.B.; Carlsson, S.C.; Bjurstrom, S.; Fransson-Steen, R.; Healing, G.; Skanberg, I. Two-year carcinogenicity studies with the oral direct thrombin inhibitor ximelagatran in the rat and the mouse. *Int. J. Toxicol.* **2012**, *31*, 348–357. [CrossRef]
57. DeFeo, K.; Hayes, C.; Chernick, M.; Ryn, J.V.; Gilmour, S.K. Use of dabigatran etexilate to reduce breast cancer progression. *Cancer Biol. Ther.* **2010**, *10*, 1001–1008. [CrossRef]
58. Alexander, E.T.; Minton, A.R.; Hayes, C.S.; Goss, A.; Van Ryn, J.; Gilmour, S.K. Thrombin inhibition and cyclophosphamide synergistically block tumor progression and metastasis. *Cancer Biol. Ther.* **2015**, *16*, 1802–1811. [CrossRef]
59. Alexander, E.T.; Minton, A.R.; Peters, M.C.; van Ryn, J.; Gilmour, S.K. Thrombin inhibition and cisplatin block tumor progression in ovarian cancer by alleviating the immunosuppressive microenvironment. *Oncotarget* **2016**, *7*, 85291–85305. [CrossRef]
60. Shi, K.; Damhofer, H.; Daalhuisen, J.; Ten Brink, M.; Richel, D.J.; Spek, C.A. Dabigatran potentiates gemcitabine-induced growth inhibition of pancreatic cancer in mice. *Mol. Med.* **2017**, *23*, 13–23. [CrossRef]
61. Graf, C.; Wilgenbus, P.; Pagel, S.; Pott, J.; Marini, F.; Reyda, S.; Kitano, M. Macher-Goppinger, S.; Weiler, H.; Ruf, W. Myeloid cell-synthesized coagulation factor X dampens antitumor immunity. *Sci. Immunol.* **2019**, *4*, eaaw8405. [CrossRef]
62. Rondon, A.M.R.; Kroone, C.; Kapteijn, M.Y.; Versteeg, H.H.; Buijs, J.T. Role of tissue factor in tumor progression and cancer-associated thrombosis. *Semin. Thromb. Hemost.* **2019**, *45*, 396–412. [CrossRef] [PubMed]
63. Buijs, J.T.; Laghmani, E.H.; van den Akker, R.F.P.; Tieken, C.; Vletter, E.M.; van der Molen, K.M.; Crooijmans, J.J.; Kroone, C.; Le Devedec, S.E.; van der Pluijm, G.; et al. The direct oral anticoagulants rivaroxaban and dabigatran do not inhibit orthotopic growth and metastasis of human breast cancer in mice. *J. Thromb. Haemost.* **2019**, *17*, 951–963. [CrossRef] [PubMed]
64. NCCN. *Guidelines for Venous Thromboembolic Disease*, version 1; NCCN: Plymouth Meeting, PA, USA, 2019.
65. Wang, T.; Zwicker, J.I.; Ay, C.; Pabinger, I.; Falanga, A.; Antic, D.; Noble, S.; Khorana, A.A.; Carrier, M.; Meyer, G. The use of direct oral anticoagulants for primary thromboprophylaxis in ambulatory cancer patients: Guidance from the SSC of the ISTH. *J. Thromb. Haemost.* **2019**, *17*, 1772–1778. [CrossRef] [PubMed]
66. Key, N.S.; Khorana, A.A.; Kuderer, N.M.; Bohlke, K.; Lee, A.Y.Y.; Arcelus, J.I.; Wong, S.L.; Balaban, E.P.; Flowers, C.R.; Francis, C.W.; et al. Venous thromboembolism prophylaxis and treatment in patients with cancer: ASCO clinical practice guideline update. *J. Clin. Oncol.* **2020**, *38*, 496–520. [CrossRef] [PubMed]
67. Farge, D.; Frere, C.; Connors, J.M.; Ay, C.; Khorana, A.A.; Munoz, A.; Brenner, B.; Kakkar, A.; Rafii, H.; Solymoss, S.; et al. 2019 international clinical practice guidelines for the treatment and prophylaxis of venous thromboembolism in patients with cancer. *Lancet Oncol.* **2019**, *20*, e566–e581. [CrossRef]

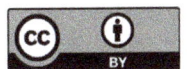

© 2020 by the authors. Licensee MDPI, Basel, Switzerland. This article is an open access article distributed under the terms and conditions of the Creative Commons Attribution (CC BY) license (http://creativecommons.org/licenses/by/4.0/).

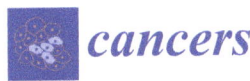

Review

Primary Thromboprophylaxis in Pancreatic Cancer Patients: Why Clinical Practice Guidelines Should Be Implemented

Dominique Farge [1,2,3,*], Barbara Bournet [4,5], Thierry Conroy [6], Eric Vicaut [7,8], Janusz Rak [9], George Zogoulous [9], Jefferey Barkun [9], Mehdi Ouaissi [10], Louis Buscail [4,5] and Corinne Frere [11,12]

1. Institut Universitaire d'Hématologie, Université de Paris, EA 3518, F-75010 Paris, France
2. Assistance Publique Hôpitaux de Paris, Saint-Louis Hospital, Internal Medicine, Autoimmune and Vascular Disease Unit, F-75010 Paris, France
3. Department of Medicine, McGill University, Montreal, Québec, QC H4A 3J1, Canada
4. University of Toulouse, F-31059 Toulouse, France; bournet.b@chu-toulouse.fr (B.B.); buscail.l@chu-toulouse.fr (L.B.)
5. CHU de Toulouse, Department of Gastroenterology and Pancreatology, F-31059 Toulouse, France
6. Institut de Cancérologie de Lorraine, Department of Medical Oncology, Université de Lorraine, APEMAC, EA4360, F-54519 Vandoeuvre-lès-Nancy, France; t.conroy@nancy.unicancer.fr
7. Department of Biostatistics, Université de Paris, F-75010 Paris, France; eric.vicaut@aphp.fr
8. Assistance Publique Hôpitaux de Paris, Department of Biostatistics, Fernand Widal Hospital, F-75010 Paris, France
9. McGill University and the Research Institute of the McGill University Health Centre, Montreal, Québec, QC H4A 3J1, Canada; janusz.rak@mcgill.ca (J.R.); george.zogoulous@mcgill.ca (G.Z.); jefferey.barkun@mcgill.ca (J.B.)
10. Department of Digestive, Oncological, Endocrine, and Hepatic Surgery, and Hepatic Transplantation, Trousseau Hospital, CHRU Trousseau, F-37170 Chambray-les-Tours, France; m.ouaissi@chu-tours.fr
11. Institute of Cardiometabolism and Nutrition, Sorbonne Université, INSERM UMRS_1166, GRC 27 GRECO, F-75013 Paris, France; corinne.frere@aphp.fr
12. Assistance Publique Hôpitaux de Paris, Department of Haematology, Pitié-Salpêtrière Hospital, F-75013 Paris, France
* Correspondence: dominique.farge-bancel@aphp.fr

Received: 12 February 2020; Accepted: 4 March 2020; Published: 6 March 2020

Abstract: Exocrine pancreatic ductal adenocarcinoma, simply referred to as pancreatic cancer (PC) has the worst prognosis of any malignancy. Despite recent advances in the use of adjuvant chemotherapy in PC, the prognosis remains poor, with fewer than 8% of patients being alive at 5 years after diagnosis. The prevalence of PC has steadily increased over the past decades, and it is projected to become the second-leading cause of cancer-related death by 2030. In this context, optimizing and integrating supportive care is important to improve quality of life and survival. Venous thromboembolism (VTE) is a common but preventable complication in PC patients. VTE occurs in one out of five PC patients and is associated with significantly reduced progression-free survival and overall survival. The appropriate use of primary thromboprophylaxis can drastically and safely reduce the rates of VTE in PC patients as shown from subgroup analysis of non-PC targeted placebo-controlled randomized trials of cancer patients and from two dedicated controlled randomized trials in locally advanced PC patients receiving chemotherapy. Therefore, primary thromboprophylaxis with a Grade 1B evidence level is recommended in locally advanced PC patients receiving chemotherapy by the International Initiative on Cancer and Thrombosis clinical practice guidelines since 2013. However, its use and potential significant clinical benefit continues to be underrecognized worldwide. This narrative review aims to summarize the main recent advances in the field including on the use of individualized risk assessment models to stratify the risk of VTE in each patient with individual available treatment options.

Keywords: pancreatic cancer; venous thromboembolism; thromboprophylaxis; low-molecular weight heparin; direct oral anticoagulant; survival

1. Introduction

Exocrine pancreatic ductal adenocarcinoma (PDAC), often referred to simply as pancreatic cancer (PC) is a malignancy with the highest mortality rate of any solid cancer and with a growing incidence, partly due to aging of the population and improvements in diagnostic techniques [1,2]. The global burden of PC as reported by the Global Burden of Disease 2017 PC collaborators showed a 2.3-fold increase in incidence between 1990 and 2017, with 441,000 documented cases in 2017 compared to 196,000 in 1990, and this rise is expected to continue [3]. The prevalence of PC is projected to increase by approximately 40% over the next decade in North America and Europe [4], and it is predicted to become the second-leading cause of cancer-related death by 2030 [5]. However, the factors contributing to the current increasing rate of incidence are not fully understood.

Only 15–20% of PC patients have a potentially resectable tumor at diagnosis, while most patients have locally advanced tumors and over 50% have metastatic disease, due to a lack of early symptoms or available biological markers, with a life expectancy of less than one year [2,6]. Patients undergoing curative resection for PC mostly develop recurrent disease; 69–75% of patients relapse within 2 years and 80–90% relapse within 5 years [7]. Palliative and adjuvant chemotherapy remains the appropriate therapeutic option in unresectable cases and the 5-year survival rate for patients with unresectable tumor is less than 8% [8–10]. FOLFIRINOX, which was demonstrated to improve clinical status and survival by Conroy et al. in 2011, is now the current treatment standard for metastatic PC [9]. More recently, Conroy et al. also showed that adjuvant therapy with a modified FOLFIRINOX regimen led to significantly longer survival than gemcitabine (GEM) monotherapy among patients with resected PC [11]. However, despite recent advancements, prognosis remains poor, with few patients surviving to 10 years [7]. In this context, there is a need for optimizing and integrating supportive care in the management of PC patients to improve survival and quality of life. The importance of taking charge of the main physical symptoms related to disease evolution, which include pain, anorexia, depression, duodenal obstruction, ascites and venous thromboembolism (VTE) is well recognized and advocated by disease specialist experts [7]. Although recommended by the International Thrombosis and Cancer Initiative (ITAC) clinical practice guidelines (CPGs) since 2013 [12–14] and more recently by the American Society of Clinical Oncology (ASCO) guidelines [15], the use of primary thromboprophylaxis, a supportive treatment with potential significant clinical benefit, continues to be underrecognized [16].

2. Pancreatic Cancer and Venous Thomboembolism

2.1. Burden of Venous Thromboembolism (VTE) in Pancreatic Cancer: the Highest Incidence of VTE Among All Cancer Types

Cancer is an independent major risk factor for VTE [17,18], the latter occurring in 4% to 20% of all cancer patients [19,20]. The extent of VTE risk is determined by the type of cancer, the stage of the disease, and the location of the tumor [17,21]. PC is the malignancy associated with the highest rate of VTE [19,22]. A strong association between VTE and PC was first reported in an autopsy study of 4258 consecutive necropsies, which documented a VTE event in 56.2% of pancreatic patients compared to 15–25% in other cancer patients [23]. The reported incidence of VTE in PC patients varies from 5% to 41% in retrospective cohorts, depending on the diagnostic methods used (Table 1) [24–42]. Deep vein thrombosis (DVT) and pulmonary embolism (PE) are the most common VTE events observed [43], but visceral vein thrombosis (VVT), including portal vein thrombosis, splenic vein thrombosis, mesenteric vein thrombosis and hepatic veins thrombosis, accounts for approximatively 30–50% of all reported VTE events [31,38,41,44]. The main risk factors for the onset of VTE in PC patients are advanced or metastatic disease, surgery, or use of chemotherapy [35,39]. The highest incidence of VTE has been reported in a retrospective cohort of PC patients receiving palliative chemotherapy, with a VTE diagnosis in 41.3% of patients [36]. In this study, symptomatic VTE (12.2%) was identified as an independent risk factor for death by multivariate analysis (hazard ratio [HR]: 2.22, 95% CI: 1.05–2.60, $p < 0.05$). We recently investigated the incidence and risk factors for VTE in the BACAP-VTE study, a large prospective multicenter cohort of patients with histologically proven PC. Diagnosis of the index VTE, including DVT, VVT, Catheter-Related Thrombosis (CRT), or PE, was established by the referring physician and based on objective standard routine clinical practice criteria, as previously detailed [41]. During a median follow-up of 19.3 months (95% CI 17.45–22.54), 152 out of 731 (20.79%) patients developed a VTE event. In competing-risk analysis, the cumulative probabilities of VTE were 8.07% (95% CI 6.31–10.29) at 3 months and 19.21% (95% CI 16.27–22.62) at 12 months. The median time from PC diagnosis to VTE was 4.49 months (range 0.8–38.26). The rates of VTE did not differ between patients treated with GEM and those treated with FOLFIRINOX. In a multivariate analysis, primary pancreatic tumor location (isthmus *versus* head, HR 2.06, 95% CI 1.09–3.91, $p = 0.027$) and tumor stage (locally advanced *versus* resectable or borderline, HR 1.66, 95% CI 1.10–2.51, $p = 0.016$ and metastatic *versus* resectable or borderline, HR 2.50, 95% CI 1.64–3.79, $p < 0.001$) were independent predictors for onset of VTE [41]. The PRODIGE 4/ACCORD 11 [9] and PRODIGE 24/ACCORD 24 [11] randomized controlled trials (RCT) reported lower rates of VTE both in metastatic patients (cumulative incidence of grade 3–4 VTE at 6 months, 6.6% in the FOLFIRINOX arm vs. 4.1% in the GEM arm) [9] and in resected pancreatic patients (cumulative incidence of any grade VTE at 6 months, 5.9% in the FOLFIRINOX arm vs. 7.9% in the GEM arm) [11]. Of note, only Common Terminology Criteria for Adverse Events (CTCAE) [45] grade 3 and 4 VTE events were reported in the PRODIGE 24/ACCORD study [11], leading to an underestimate of the overall rate of VTE. In a recent retrospective cohort of 150 PC patients receiving either GEM-based chemotherapy or FOLFIRINOX, there was a 21.4% incidence of incidental and symptomatic VTE (grade 2 or higher) in the FOLFIRINOX group vs. 29.5% in the GEM group, suggesting that patients treated with FOLFIRINOX carry the same risk for VTE as patients treated with GEM-based therapy [38].

2.2. Association of VTE with Progression Free Survival and OverAll Survival in Pancreatic Cancer

VTE is the second-leading cause of death after metastasis in cancer patients [46,47]. Patients with cancer who develop VTE have a shorter overall survival compared to those without VTE who have a similar tumor stage and anti-cancer treatment [19]. In a study of 235-149 cancer patients (with 6712 patients with PC) included in the California Cancer Registry, adjusted for age, race, and stage, VTE was a significant predictor of decreased survival during the first year for all cancer types (hazard ratios, 1.6–4.2; $p < 0.01$) and when measured in person-time, the incidence of VTE during the first year after cancer diagnosis, was the highest among patients with metastatic PC (20.0 events per 100 patient-years) [21]. Early retrospective studies assessing the association of VTE with progression-free survival (PFS) and overall survival (OS) in PC patients reported conflicting results. Two monocentric cohorts of PC patients found no difference in OS between patients who developed VTE and those who did not [29,35]. The lack of difference in survival between patients with and without VTE might be explained by patient short life expectancy, since most patients included in both studies had stage III-IV disease. In contrast, several studies have found an association between the onset of VTE and poorer prognosis. In an early monocentric retrospective cohort of 227 patients with unresectable PC, the onset of VTE during chemotherapy was associated with decreased PFS (HR 2.59, 95% CI 1.69–3.97, $p < 0.0001$) and OS (HR 1.64, 95% CI 1.04–2.58, $p = 0.032$) [25]. Similarly, VTE, including VVT, was associated with increased mortality in a small cohort of 135 PC patients. [31] Of note, anticoagulant therapy improved survival in those patients with VTE (HR 0.30, 95% CI 0.12–0.74, $p = 0.009$) [31]. Two retrospective studies focusing on the association of VVT with survival also found an association between the onset of VVT and increased mortality [44,48]. Few studies have investigated the association between early VTE (defined by a VTE at diagnosis or within 30 days after the beginning of palliative chemotherapy) and survival.

Table 1. Main studies reporting the rates of venous thromboembolism in pancreatic cancer (PC) patients.

Reference	Study Type	n	Study Period or Duration of Follow-Up	Rates of VTE	Type of VTE	Risk Factors for VTE/Survival
Blom et al. 2006 [24]	Cohort Study	202	From January 1990 to December 2000	Incidence rate of VTE: 108.3 per 1000 patient-year (95% CI 64.4–163.8) Overall cumulative incidence of VTE: 94.1 per 1000 patient-year (95% CI 90.9–97.3)	Early VTE: 15 out of 19 cases of VTE occurred in the first 6 months after cancer diagnosis	Risk factors for VTE: Tumor of the corpus (HR 1.9, 95% CI 0.5–6.7) and of the cauda (HR 2.9, 95% CI 1.0–8.5) Chemotherapy (HR 4.8, 95% CI 1.1–20.8) Postoperative period of 30 days (HR 4.5, 95% CI 0.5–40.9) Distant metastases (HR 1.9, 95% CI 0.7–5.1)
Mandala et al. 2007 [25]	Retrospective	227	From December 2001 to December 2004	VTE = 26% (n = 59)	VTE at cancer diagnosis in 28 patients (12.3%) VTE occurring during chemotherapy in 15 patients (6.6%)	
Mitry et al. 2007 [26]	Retrospective	90	-	26.7% (n = 24)	4 PE, 2 fatal PE	Risk factors for VTE: Use of thromboprophylaxis (HR 0.03, 95% CI 0.003–0.27) Biological inflammatory syndrome (HR 9.0, 95% CI 2.30–34.4) Metastatic disease (HR 4.4, 95% CI 1.1–17.9)
Oh et al. 2008 [27]	Retrospective	75	From June 2003 to December 2005	5.3% (n = 4) Incidence rate of VTE: 157 per 1000 patient-year (95% CI 59–418)		
Poruk et al. 2010 [28]	Retrospective	133	-	20% Incidence rate of VTE: 169 per 1000 patient-year (95% CI 109–263)		
Shaib et al. 2010 [29]	Retrospective	201	From July 2003 to December 2008	28.9% (n = 58)	Multiple thrombosis: 17.2% (n = 10)	
Epstein et al. 2012 [30]	Retrospective	1915	From January 2000 to December 2009	32% (n = 650)	Arterial Thrombosis in 1.5% patients (n = 30)	
Menapace et al. 2011 [31]	Retrospective	135	From 2006 to 2009	34.8% patients (n = 47)	12 PE, 28 DVT and 47 VVT Incidental events: 33.3% PE, 21.4% DVT and 100% VVT	Anticoagulants reduced the risk of death by 70% (95% CI 26–88%, p = 0.009)
Afsar et al. 2014 [33]	Retrospective	77	From 2007 to 2012	18.1% (n = 14)		
Munoz-Martin et al. 2014 [33]	Retrospective	84	From 2008 to 2011	35.7% (n = 30)	Multiple thrombosis: 7.1% (n = 68) 66 % of the events diagnosed during the first 6 months after diagnosis.	

Table 1. Cont.

Reference	Study Type	n	Study Period or Duration of Follow-Up	Rates of VTE	Type of VTE	Risk Factors for VTE/Survival
Larsen et al. 2015 [49]	Prospective	121	Duration of follow-up: 24 months	At the time of cancer diagnosis: 12.4% (n = 15) First VTE during follow-up: 20.7% (n = 25)		
Ouiassi et al. 2015 [42]	Retrospective	162	Median follow-up of 15 months after diagnosis	17.3% (n = 28)		VTE associated with shorter survival (HR 1.995, 95% CI 1.209–3.292)
Krepline et al. 2016 [34]	Retrospective	260	From 2009 to 2014	10% (n = 26)	All VTE events were incident events: 9 (35%) PE, 9 (35%) DVT, and 8 (31%) VVT	
Lee et al. 2016 [35]	Retrospective	1115	From 2005 to 2010	11.8% (n = 132) 2 years cumulative incidence rate of VTE 9.2%	72% of incidental VTE	Major risk factors associated with VTE events: advanced cancer stage, major surgery, and poor performance status
Kruger et al. 2017 [36]	Retrospective	172	From 2002 to 2017	41.3%	50.2% of asymptomatic VTE	
Van Es et al. 2017 [37]	Retrospective	178	Median of follow-up of 234 days	12.4% (n = 22) - Estimated 2 years overall VTE incidence rate: 13.9% (95% C, 8.3–19.5)	50% of incidental VTE	
Berger et al. 2017 [38]	Retrospective	150	From initiation of first-line treatment until last follow-up or death	25% (n = 37)	43.2% of incidental VTE	
Chen et al 2018 [39]	Retrospective	816	From 2010 to 2016	8.0% (n = 67)		Leukocyte count > 11,000/μL (HR 1.75, 95% CI 1.07–3.03; $p = 0.032$) Presence of liver metastases (HR 1.65, 95% CI 1.03–3.99; $p = 0.046$)
Kim et al. 2018 [40]	Retrospective	216	From 2005 to 2015	23.6% (n = 51)		Risk factors for VTE: Low serum sodium (OR 10.30; 95% CI 1.04–102.47; $p = 0.047$) High Khorana score ≥3 (OR 5.11; 95% CI 1.01–25.84; $p = 0.049$)
Frere et al. 2019 [41]	Prospective	731	From study entry until last follow-up or death Median follow-up of 19.3 months	20.79% (n = 152) Cumulative probabilities of VTE: 8.07% (95% CI 6.31–10.29) at 3 months 19.21% (95% CI 16.27–22.62) at 12 months	54% of incidental VTE Median time from PC diagnosis to VTE: 4.49 months (range 0.8–38.26).	Risk factors for VTE:PC tumor location (isthmus versus head, HR 2.06, 95% CI 1.09–3.91, $p = 0.027$) Tumor stage (locally advanced versus resectable or borderline, HR 1.66, 95% CI 1.10–2.51, $p = 0.016$ and metastatic versus resectable or borderline, HR 2.50, 95% CI 1.64–3.79, $p < 0.001$)

Abbreviations: CI, Confidence interval; DVT, deep vein thrombosis; HR, Hazard ratio; OR, odds ratio; PC, pancreatic cancer; PE, pulmonary embolism; VTE, venous thromboembolism; VVT, visceral vein thrombosis.

In 227 unresectable PC patients, Mandala et al. reported that presence of synchronous VTE at cancer diagnosis was associated with a higher probability of not responding to treatment (odds ratio [OR] 2.98, 95% CI 1.42–6.27, p = 0.004), but were not associated with PFS or OS on multivariate analysis, while the occurrence of a VTE during chemotherapy was associated with significant shorter PFS (HR 2.59, 95% CI 1.69–3.97, p< 0.0001) and OS (HR 1.64, 95%CI 1.04–2.58, p = 0.032) [25].

In another monocentric retrospective cohort of 216 metastatic PC patients receiving GEM-based palliative chemotherapy, early VTE occurred in 10.6% patients and was associated with a significantly shorter OS (3.7 months vs. 6.4 months in patients with late VTE or without VTE, p = 0.005) [40].

Only two prospective studies have investigated the impact of VTE on survival in PC patients. A small cohort of 121 PC patients reported a significant association between the onset of VTE within the study and shorter OS (median OS 4.4 months vs. 11.9 months in patients without VTE; HR 2.15, 95% CI 1.28–3.60, p = 0.004) [49]. In the BACAP-VTE study, patients developing VTE during follow-up had shorter PFS even after adjustment for cancer stage and other risk factors for decreased PFS (6.66 months vs. 9.56 months in patients without VTE; HR 1.74, 95% CI 1.19–2.54, p = 0.004). The onset of VTE was also associated with shorter OS, even after adjustment for age, cancer stage and other risk factors for decreased OS (9.13 months vs. 14.55 months in patients without VTE; HR 2.02, 95% CI 1.57–2.60, p = 0.004). PC patients who developed VTE after study entry had a higher mortality rate compared to patients who did not develop VTE: 109 out of 152 (72%) patients with VTE died vs. 343 out 531 (65%) patients without VTE (OR 2.88, 95% CI 1.96–4.21, p < 0.0001) [41]. These results deserve attention since this association between VTE and mortality suggests that preventing VTE might improve survival in PC patients.

2.3. VTE in Pancreatic Cancer: A Model of Hypercoagulability and the Effects of Heparins

Cancer leads to a hypercoagulable state which confers advantages to cancer cells. This hypercoagulable state is attributed to high expression of tissue factor (TF) and transmembrane proteins (e.g.: PSGL-1, Muc1) by cancer cells [50], leading to thrombin generation and platelet activation and aggregation [51]. Aggregation of blood platelets around cancer cells provides protection from immune responses, and also facilitates circulation of cancer cells in the blood stream and their adhesion at potential sites of metastasis [52–54]. In cancer multiple oncogenic events including activation of proto-oncogenes *KRAS* [55], *EGFR*, and inactivation of tumor suppressor genes such as *P53* and *PTEN*, promote TF expression and contribute to other procoagulant changes in the tumor microenvironment [56]. Of note is the fact that in sporadic PC/PDAC over 90% of lesions carry an activating *KRAS* mutation [57] and elevated TF expression is common in advanced stages [58]. Moreover, cancer cells spontaneously release TF-positive microvesicles (MVs) in the circulation [59–61]. TF-positive MVs bind to Factor VII (FVII), promoting the activation of the extrinsic pathway and thrombin generation. An additional mechanism of thrombin generation is related to Factor XII activation, which initiates the intrinsic coagulation pathway. Moreover, Plasminogen Activator Inhibitor 1 (PAI-1) can be released by pancreatic tumor cells, as well as by activated platelets [62]. TF initiates angiogenesis via both a) a clotting-dependent mechanism where thrombin formation and fibrin deposition support angiogenesis, and TF induces VEGF expression, and b) a clotting-independent mechanism in which TF-FVIIa complex activates pro-angiogenic protease-activated receptor 2 (PAR-2). In addition, an alternatively spliced TF (asTF, soluble variant of TF) is expressed in PDAC as opposed to normal pancreas, and stimulates angiogenesis independently of FVIIa [63,64]. Unruh et al. demonstrated that asTF binds β1-integrins on the surface of PDAC cells and also on microvascular endothelial cells [63,64], thereby promoting tumor growth, metastatic dissemination, and monocyte recruitment to the stroma through an autocrine paracrine manner [64]. Overall, TF overexpression by the PC cells which induces thrombin generation and platelet activation all directly contribute to cancer progression and dissemination [65]. Whether and how preceding intermittent inflammation and PC-associated desmoplasia contribute to these events remain of great interest [57].

Circulating extracellular MVs derived from cancer-cells contribute to hypercoagulability and to metastatic invasion. Experimental data have shown that MVs released by cultured PC cells exhibit TF-dependent procoagulant activity [66]. In a mouse model of PC, cancer cell-derived MVs expressing TF accumulate at sites of endothelial injury in a *p*-selectin-dependent manner [67].

Several publications demonstrate the presence of TF-bearing MVs in patients with cancer [68–75]. In PC patients specifically, around 50% of TF-positive MVs detected in platelet-poor plasma are also positive for MUC-1 antigen, suggesting that they are derived from the underlying malignancy. TF-positive MVs are highly procoagulant [69]. A retrospective study of 117 patients with pancreatic or biliary cancer (68% of PC) reported a 44.4% rate of VTE. In these patients, elevated TF levels were significantly associated with VTE events (p = 0.04), and with decreased overall survival (HR 1.05; p = 0.01) [70]. A first prospective study suggested that MVs-TF activity may be predictive of VTE in PC patients [71]. In a cohort study of 73 PDAC patients, elevated MVs-TF activity was present only in patients with poorly differentiated metastatic, unresectable tumors and correlated with CA 19–9 and D-dimer levels [73]. In a prospective cohort study on 79 PDAC patients, MVs-TF activity did not correlate with the intensity of TF expression in adenocarcinoma cells but to the number of TF-positive macrophages in the surrounding stroma [74]. More recently, Faille et al. showed that MVs-TF activity was predictive of VTE in 48 PDAC patients [75]. Both D-dimers and MVs-TF activity were associated with the occurrence of VTE [75].

Many studies have analyzed the effect of heparins and of low molecular weight heparin (LMWH) on tumor progression, metastasis formation, and angiogenesis [76,77]. In addition to its action on the coagulation cascade, heparin also inhibits the binding of P-selectin to its ligands [78], which is involved in hypercoagulability and metastasis process. Heparins as well as heparan sulfate (HS) belong to the glycosaminoglycan family and bind antithrombin via a pentasaccharide sequence. HS are key components of the extracellular matrix (ECM). Heparanase, which is overexpressed in PC, acts by cleaving heparan sulfate side chains from proteoglycans, contributing to ECM disruption and vascular endothelial growth factor A (VEGF-A) and fibroblast growth factor 2 (FGF-2) release [51]. In addition, heparanase has a non-enzymatic pro-coagulant activity in which removal of glycocalyces containing tissue factor pathway inhibitor (TFPI) enhances TF activity [79]. By inhibiting heparanase, heparins may potentially inhibit tumor growth [80].

LMWHs can also contribute to the inhibition of cancer progression. LMWHs were shown to inhibit P-and L-selectin as well as integrin-mediated formation of tumor thrombi, and to alter tumor neo-angiogenesis. This effect is primarily based on their ability to induce the prolonged release of TFPI from binding sites on endothelial cells [81,82]. TFPI acts by inhibiting TF-FVIIa complex, leading to activation of Factor X, inhibition of thrombin generation and PAR-2 activation, and disruption of pro-angiogenic signaling [83,84]. Thus, anticoagulants could possess both biological and antithrombotic activities in cancer albeit possibly exerted through different mechanisms.

3. Risk Assessment Models (RAM) for Prediction of VTE in Patients with PC

Risk assessment models (RAM) have been developed to help identify cancer patients at high risk of VTE who may benefit from primary thromboprophylaxis (Table 2). Nonetheless, VTE risk factors vary according to cancer type and during the course of malignancy, from diagnosis through treatment, metastasis, and end-of-life care. Therefore, repeated individual risk assessments are important.

The most widely used RAM for VTE prediction in ambulatory cancer patients is the Khorana score (KS). This score was developed in a prospective derivation cohort of 2701 cancer outpatients in the United States more than ten years ago and validated in an independent cohort of 1365 patients from the same study [85]. The KS assigns different points to five clinical and pre-chemotherapy laboratory parameters, namely: primary tumor site (+2 points for PC and gastric cancer), platelet count $\geq 350 \times 10^9 \cdot dL^{-1}$ (+1 point), hemoglobin concentration ≤ 10 g.dL^{-1} or use of erythropoiesis-stimulating agents (+1 point), leukocyte count $\geq 11 \times 10^9 \cdot L^{-1}$ (+1 point), and a BMI ≥ 35 kg/m^2 (+1 point). The KS discriminates three groups of patients according to risk of VTE: a low-risk group (score of 0), an intermediate-risk group (score of 1–2) and a high-risk group (score ≥3). Several small retrospective studies in PC patients undergoing chemotherapy found no difference in the rates of VTE between intermediate and high-risk patients, as estimated by the Khorana score (Table 3) [33,36–38,86]. In the BACAP-VTE study, the KS did not discriminate between patients with intermediate vs. high VTE risk scores [41]. However, all PC patients have a sum score ≥ 2 and being subsequently classified as at least intermediate-risk or high risk of VTE should be considered for prophylaxis. Other RAMs, such as the Vienna modification of the Khorana score (addition of biomarkers D-dimer and soluble P-selectin) [87], the PROTECHT score (addition of GEM and platinum-based chemotherapy), [88] and the CONKO score (addition of WHO performance status) [86] have been developed. However, none of these scores have been externally validated in PC patients.

The ONKOTEV score [89] was developed using a large multicenter prospective cohort of 843 cancers patients. Overall, 73 (8.6%) VTE events occurred during a median follow-up of 8.3 months. In a multivariate analysis, the presence of a metastatic disease, the compression of vascular/lymphatic structures by the tumor, a history of previous VTE, and a KS ≥2 were significantly associated with the risk of VTE. The resulting ONKOTEV score assigns one point to each of these four variables, and according to a sum score of 0, 1, 2, or ≥ 2 points patients are classified as being at "score = 0", "score = 1", "score = 2", or "score > 2", respectively. In the development cohort, patients with "score = 0" (37%) had a cumulative probability of VTE at 12 months of 3.69%, compared to 9.74% for patients with "score = 1" (43.1%), 19.39% for patients with "score = 2" (9.2%), and 33.87% for patients with "score > 2" (6.3%). As expected, the ONKOTEV score demonstrated a significantly higher predictive power than the KS in the same cohort. However, overfitting of the ONKOTEV model is likely and these results should be interpreted with caution. This model was recently externally validated in a retrospective single-center cohort of 165 PC patients [90]. Cumulative incidence of VTE was 3.3%, 12.7%, 50.9%, and 82.4% for patients with ONKOTEV scores of 0 (18.2% of the overall population), 1 (38.2% of the overall population), 2 (33.3% of the overall population), and >2 (10.3% of the overall population), respectively [90]. This study has several limitations including its retrospective and single-center design, and the inclusion of patients with VTE at cancer diagnosis and deserve further confirmation in prospective cohorts of ambulatory PC patients.

Table 2. Risk assessment models that have been evaluated in pancreatic cancer patients.

KHORANA SCORE [85]	
Very high-risk tumors (stomach, pancreas)	+2
High risk tumors (lung, gynecologic, genitourinary excluding prostate)	+1
Hemoglobin <10 g/dl or erythropoietin stimulating agents	+1
White blood cell count >11 × 10^9/L	+1
Platelet count ≥ 350 × 10^9/L	+1
BMI >35 kg/m^2	+1
A score of 0 = low-risk category A score of 1–2 = intermediate-risk category A score of >2 = very high-risk category	
ONKOTEV SCORE [89]	
Khorana score of >2	+1
Previous venous thromboembolism	+1
Metastatic disease	+1
Vascular/lymphatic macroscopic compression	+1
Total ONKOTEV score	4

Abbreviations: BMI = body mass index.

Table 3. Studies assessing the predictive values of risk assessment models in pancreatic cancer patients.

Reference	Type	RAMs	Study Population, n	VTE Screening at Study Entry	Median Follow Up (Months)	Number of Patients in Each Group	Patients with VTE During the Total Follow-Up, n (%)	Rates of VTE
Pelzer et al. 2013 [86]	Retrospective	Khorana score	144	No	12	Intermediate risk: 38% High risk: 62%	21 (14.6%)	At 6 months: Intermediate risk: 7.2% High risk: 19.1%
Munoz-Martin et al. 2014 [33]	Retrospective	Khorana score	73	No	9.5	Intermediate risk: 51% High risk: 49%	22 (30.1%)	At 6 months: Intermediate risk: 10.8% High risk: 27.8%
Van Es et al. 2017 [37]	Retrospective	Khorana score	147	No	7.7	Intermediate risk: 31% High risk: 69%	20 (13.6%)	At 6 months: Intermediate risk: 8.9% High risk: 8.7%
Kruger et al. 2017 [36]	Retrospective	Khorana score	111	No	9.2	Intermediate risk: 62% High risk: 38%	16 (14.4%)	At 6 months: Intermediate risk: 8.7% High risk: 11.9%
Berger et al. 2017 [38]	Retrospective	Khorana score	150	No	NS	Intermediate risk: 58% High risk: 42%	37 (24.7%)	NS During the total follow-up: no difference between groups ($p = 0.44$)
Godinho et al. 2019 [90]	Retrospective	Onkotev score	165	no	6.3	Score 0: 18.2% Score 1: 38.2% Score 2: 33.3% Score ≥3: 10.3%	51 (31%)	During the total follow-up: Score 0: < 10% Score 1: <10% Score 2: 41.8% Score ≥3: 70.6%
Frere et al. 2019 [41]	Prospective	Khorana score	731	Yes	19.3	Intermediate risk: 73% High risk: 27%	152 (20.1%)	NS During the total follow-up: Intermediate risk: 21% High risk: 18% Intermediate vs. high risk: HR 0.83 (95% CI 0.56–1.23), $p = 0.363$

Abbreviations: NS, not specified; RAM, risk assessment model; VTE, venous thromboembolism.

4. Studies Assessing the Benefit of Anticoagulants in Pancreatic Cancer Patients

4.1. Primary Thromboprophylaxis in Ambulatory Pancreatic Cancer Patients

4.1.1. Primary Thromboprophylaxis with LMWH in Cancer Patients

Several RCTs have assessed the efficacy and safety of LMWH for primary thromboprophylaxis in patients with different cancers treated with chemotherapy. The PROTECHT [91] and SAVE-ONCO [92] trials enrolled more than 4000 patients with non-selected solid cancers, but few data were generated from the subgroup analyses of PC patients (Table 4).

In PROTECHT [91], 1150 patients with different cancers were randomized to receive either nadroparin (3800 IU once daily) or placebo for the duration of chemotherapy, up to a maximum of 4 months. A significant reduction in the rate of VTE was observed in the nadroparin arm (2.0% vs. 3.9% in the placebo arm, $p = 0.02$) without difference in major bleeding (0.7% in the nadroparin arm vs. 0 in the placebo arm, $p = 0.18$). Only 53 out of 1150 (4.7%) patients included in PROTECHT had PC, and the rates of VTE did not differ between the placebo and nadroparin treatment arms in this subgroup of PC patients ($p = 0.755$). This lack of difference might be related to the small number of PC patients included in PROTECHT.

In SAVE-ONCO [92], 3212 patients with metastatic or locally advanced cancers beginning a course of chemotherapy were randomized to receive either semuloparin (20 mg once daily) or placebo for the duration of chemotherapy. In the overall population, a significant reduction in the rates of VTE was observed in the semuloparin arm (1.2% vs. 3.4% in the placebo arm; HR 0.36, 95% CI 0.21–0.60; $p < 0.001$), and there was no difference in major bleeding (1.2% vs. 1.1% in the placebo arm; HR 1.05, 95% CI 0.55–1.99; $p =$ ns). Two hundred fifty four out of 3212 (7.9%) patients had a PC in SAVE-ONCO. In this PC patient subgroup, a significant reduction in the rates of VTE was observed in the semuloparin arm (2.4% vs. 10.9% in the placebo arm; HR 0.22, 95 CI 0.06–0.76; $p = 0.015$). This subgroup effect was not statistically significant different, from the overall effect in the overall population.

4.1.2. Primary Thromboprophylaxis with LMWHs in Pancreatic Cancer Patients

Two dedicated RCTs evaluated the efficacy and safety of primary thromboprophylaxis with LMWH in patients with advanced PC receiving chemotherapy (Table 4) [93,94]. In total, these two studies enrolled more than 400 PC patients.

The phase 2b FRAGEM trial randomized 123 advanced PC patients to receive either GEM with weight-adjusted dalteparin (GEM-WAD, dalteparin 200 IU/kg daily during 4 weeks, then 150 IU/kg daily) for 12 weeks or GEM alone [93]. The primary end point was the occurrence of all-type VTE (symptomatic or incidentally diagnosed). Addition of weight-adjusted dalteparin reduced the rate of VTE from 23% to 3.4% during the treatment period (RR 0.145, 95% CI 0.035–0.612, $p = 0.002$) and from 28% to 12% during the entire follow-up period (RR 0.42, 95% CI 0.19–0.94, $p = 0.039$). VTE-related deaths were observed in 5 (8.3%) patients in the GEM alone arm compared to 0 patients in the GEM with weight-adjusted dalteparin arm (RR 0.092, 95% CI 0.005–1.635, $p = 0.057$). The rates of major bleeding events were low in both arms (3.4% in the GEM-WAD arm vs. 3.2% in the GEM arm), but there was a higher incidence of trivial bleeding (skin bruising, minor epistaxis) in the GEM-WAD arm (9% vs. 3% in the GEM arm) [93].

The prospective, open-label, multicenter phase 2b PROSPECT-CONKO 004 study randomized 312 advanced PC patients to receive enoxaparin during the first 12 weeks of chemotherapy (1 mg/kg daily for the first 3 months, then 40 mg daily, $n = 160$) or chemotherapy alone (i.e., single-agent GEM or an intensified regimen including fluorouracil and folinic acid, depending on performance status and renal function, $n = 152$) [94]. The primary end point was the first event rate of symptomatic VTE within 3 months. Asymptomatic VTE events found on routine imaging during the study were excluded from the analysis. Enoxaparin reduced the cumulative incidence rate of symptomatic VTE from 10.2% to 1.3% within the first 3 months (HR 0.12, 95% CI 0.03–0.52, $p = 0.001$) and from 15.1%

to 6.4% during the entire follow-up period (HR 0.40, 95% CI 0.19–0.83, $p = 0.01$), without an overall difference in major bleeding (8.3% in the enoxaparin arm vs. 6.9% in the control arm, HR 1.23, 95% CI 0.54–2.79, $p = 0.63$). Three fatal bleeding events occurred in the overall population, including one fatal bleed from esophageal varices in the enoxaparin arm and two fatal bleeds from fulminant cancer ulceration in the duodenum in the control arm. There was no significant difference in PFS (HR, 1.06; 95% CI, 0.84 to 1.32; $p = 0.64$) or OS (HR, 1.01; 95% CI, 0.87 to 1.38; $p = 0.44$).

A recent meta-analysis pooling the results from both the FRAGEM [93] and PROSPECT-CONKO 004 [94] trials reported a significant reduction in crude rates of VTE in advanced PC patients receiving LMWH compared to control (2.1% vs. 11.2%, RR 0.18, 95% CI 0.08–0.40), corresponding to a 82% relative risk reduction, without difference in the rate of bleeding events (4.1% vs. 3.3%, RR 1.25, 95% CI 0.48–3.3) [95]. While standard prophylactic doses of LMWH were used in PROTECHT [91] and SAVE-ONCO [92] trials, dalteparin was administered at therapeutic doses in the FRAGEM trial, [93] and enoxaparin was administered at supra-prophylactic doses in the PROSPECT-CONKO 004 trial, [94] suggesting that PC patients might require higher than standard prophylactic doses of anticoagulant for effective VTE prophylaxis.

4.1.3. Direct Oral Anticoagulants (DOAC) As Primary Thromboprophylaxis in Various Cancers, with PC as A Subgroup

Despite limited data on their efficacy and safety in this setting, there is growing interest in the potential role of DOACs for thromboprophylaxis in patients with cancer. Two recent randomized controlled trials evaluated the efficacy and safety of primary thromboprophylaxis with DOACs in various cancers with different inclusion criteria and primary endpoints (Table 4).

The double-blind placebo-controlled CASSINI trial randomized 841 cancer patients initiating chemotherapy at intermediate-to-high risk of VTE (as defined by a Khorana score ≥2) to receive either primary prophylaxis with rivaroxaban (10 mg once daily) or placebo for up to 6 months. [96] Four hundred eight patients (54.5%) had stage IV disease at enrollment. Screening ultrasound was performed at baseline and every 8 weeks during the follow-up period. The primary efficacy endpoint was a composite of symptomatic DVT, asymptomatic proximal DVT, any PE and VTE-related death within the first 180 days after randomization. During the entire follow-up, there was no statistically significant difference in the primary end point between the two arms: 6.0% in the rivaroxaban arm vs. 8.8% in the placebo arm (HR 0.66, 95% CI 0.40–1.09; $p = 0.10$). However, during the on-treatment period, patients treated with rivaroxaban experienced fewer VTE events compared to those receiving placebo (2.6% vs. 6.4%, HR 0.40, 95% CI 0.20–0.80). There was no difference in major bleeding between the two groups (HR 1.96, 95% CI 0.59–6.49). In a prespecified subgroup analysis of PC patients included in CASSINI ($n = 273$, 32.6%), the primary composite endpoint occurred in five out of 135 (3.7%) PC patients in the rivaroxaban arm compared to 14 out of 138 (10.1%) patients in the placebo arm (HR 0.35, 95% CI 0.13–0.97) during intervention. In PC patients, there was no difference in major bleeding between the two groups (1.5% in the rivaroxaban arm vs. 2.3% in the placebo arm) [97].

The Double-Blind Placebo-Controlled Phase 3 AVERT Trial [98] randomized 574 ambulatory cancer patients initiating chemotherapy at intermediate-to-high risk of VTE (as defined by a Khorana score ≥2) to receive either primary prophylaxis with apixaban (2.5 mg twice daily) or a placebo for up to 6 months. Five hundred and sixty-three patients were included in the modified intention-to-treat analysis. One hundred forty (24.8%) patients had metastatic disease at enrollment and 77 (13.8%) patients had PC. Screening ultrasound was not performed at baseline, nor during the follow-up period. The primary outcome was the occurrence of objectively documented major VTE (proximal DVT or PE) within the first 180 days after randomization. During the on-treatment period, patients receiving apixaban had a significant lower risk of VTE (1% vs. 7.3% in the placebo arm; HR 0.14, 95% CI 0.05–0.42, $p < 0.001$) with no difference in major bleeding (2.1% in the apixaban arm vs. 1.1% in the placebo arm; HR 1.89, 95% CI 0.39–9.24).

Table 4. Studies assessing the clinical benefit of anticoagulants for the prevention of venous thromboembolism in ambulatory pancreatic cancer (PC) patients.

Reference Study Design	Number of Patients Analyzed	Follow-Up	Population	Intervention	VTE Incidence	Safety	Survival
PROTECHT Agnelli et al. 2009 [91] Randomized, placebo-controlled, double-blind, multicenter study	Overall population Arm A: 769 patients Arm B: 381 patients PC subgroup Arm A: 36 patients Arm B: 17 patients	120 days	Ambulatory patients >18 years on chemotherapy with metastatic or locally advanced lung, gastrointestinal, breast, ovarian, or head and neck cancer	Arm A: nadroparin 3800 IU/day Arm B: placebo For duration of chemotherapy (up to 4 months maximum)	Overall population Arm A: 11/769 (1.4%) Arm B: 11/381 (2.9%) $p = 0.02$ PC subgroup Arm A: 3/36 (8.3%) Arm B: 1/17 (5.9%) $p = 0.755$	Overall population Major bleeding Arm A: 5/769 (0.7%) Arm B: 0/381 $p = 0.18$ Minor bleeding Arm A: 57/769 (7.4%) Arm B: 30/381 (7.9%) $p = ns$ PC subgroup NS	Overall population Arm A: 33/769 (4.3%) Arm B: 16/381 (4.2%) $p = ns$ PC subgroup NS
SAVE ONCO Agnelli et al. 2012 [92] Randomized, placebo-controlled, double-blind, multicenter study	Overall Population Arm A: 1608 patients Arm B: 1604 patients PC subgroup Arm A: 126 patients Arm B: 128 patients	3 months	Patients with metastatic or locally advanced lung, pancreatic, gastric, colorectal, bladder, and ovarian cancer beginning to receive a course of chemotherapy	Arm A: Semuloparin, 20 mg/day Arm B: placebo For duration of chemotherapy (median: 3.5 months)	Overall population Arm A: 20/1608 (1.2%) Arm B: 55/1064 (1.2%) HR 0.36 (95%CI 0.21–0.60) $p < 0.001$ PC subgroup Arm A: 3/126 (2.4%) Arm B: 14/128 (10.9%) HR 0.22 (95%CI 0.06–0.76) $p = 0.015$	Overall population Major bleeding Arm A: 19/1589 (1.2%) Arm B: 18/1583 (1.1%) OR 1.05 (95% CI 0.55–2.04) CRNMB Arm A: 26/1589 (2.8%) Arm B: 14/1583 (0.9%) OR 1.86 (95% CI 0.98–3.68) PC subgroup NS	NS
FRAGEM Marayevas et al. 2012 [93] Randomized, controlled Phase 2b study	Arm A: 59 patients Arm B: 62 patients	3 months	Patients aged 18 years or older Histologically/cytologically confirmed advanced or metastatic pancreatic cancer Karnofsky performance status (KPS): 60–100	Arm A: Gemcitabine + Dalteparin 200 IU/kg sc, od, for 4 weeks, followed by a step-down regimen to 150 IU/kg for a further 8 weeks) Arm B: Gemcitabine alone For up to 12 weeks	At 3 months Arm A: 2/59 (3%) Arm B: 14/62 (23%) RR 0.145 (95% CI 0.035–0.612) $p = 0.002$ Entire study Arm A: 7/59 (12%) Arm B: 17/62 (28%) RR 0.419 (95%CI 0.187–0.935) $p = 0.039$	ISTH severe Arm A: 2/59 (3%) Arm B: 2/62 (3%) ISTH non severe Arm A: 5/59 (9%) Arm B: 2/62 (3%)	Arm A: 8.7 months Arm B: 9.7 months

Table 4. *Cont.*

Reference Study Design	Number of Patients Analyzed	Follow-Up	Population	Intervention	VTE Incidence	Safety	Survival
CONKO-0004 Pelzer et al. 2015 [94] Prospective, open label, randomized, multicenter and group-sequential 2b trial	Arm A: 160 patients Arm B: 152 patients	3 months	Patients with histologically proven advanced pancreatic cancer were randomly assigned to ambulant first-line chemotherapy	Arm A: Enoxaparin 1 mg/kg/day Arm B: no enoxaparin	**At 3 months** Arm A: 2/160 (1.25%) Arm B: 15/152 (9.8%) HR 0.12 (95%CI 0.03–0.52) $p = 0.001$ **Cumulative incidence rates** Arm A: 6.4% Arm B: 15.1% HR 0.40 (95% CI 0.19–0.83) $p = 0.01$	**Cumulative incidence rates Of major bleeding** Arm A: 8.3% Arm B: 6.9% HR 1.23 (95% CI 0.54–2.79) $p = 0.63$	Arm A: 8.2 months Arm B: 8.51 months HR 1.01 (95% CI 0.87–1.38) $p = 0.44$
CASSINI Khorana et al. 2019 [96] Double-blind, randomized, placebo-controlled, parallel-group, multicenter study	Overall population Arm A: 420 patients Arm B: 404 patients PC patients Arm A: 135 patients Arm B: 138 patients	6 months	Adult ambulatory patients with various cancers initiating a new systemic regimen and at increased risk for VTE (defined as Khorana score ≥ 2).	Arm A: rivaroxaban 10 mg once daily up to day 180 Arm B: placebo up to day 180	**Overall population VTE at 6 months** Arm A: 25/420 (5.95%) Arm B: 37/421 (8.79%) HR 0.66 (95% CI 0.40–1.09) $p = 0.101$ NNT = 35 **VTE during the on-treatment period** Arm A: 11/420 (2.62%) Arm B: 27/420 (6.41%) HR 0.40 (95% CI 0.20–0.80) $p = 0.007$ NNT = 26 **PC subgroup Composite of VTE and death from VTE** Arm A: 5/135 (3.7%) Arm B: 14/138 (10.1%) HR 0.35 (95% CI 0.130–0.97) $p = 0.03$	**Overall population Major bleeding** Arm A: 8/405 (1.98%) Arm B: 4/404 (0.99%) HR 1.96 (95% CI 0.59–6.49) $p = 0.265$ NNH = 101 **Clinically relevant non-major bleeding** Arm A: 2.72% Arm B: 1.98% HR 1.96 (95% CI 0.59–6.49) $p = 0.265$ NNH = 101 **PC subgroup Major bleeding** Arm A: 2/135 (1.5%) Arm B: 3/138 (2.3%)	**Overall population All-cause mortality** Arm A: 20.0% Arm B: 23.8% HR, 0.83, 95% CI 0.62–1.11 $p = 0.213$. PC subgroup NS

Table 4. Cont.

Reference Study Design	Number of Patients Analyzed	Follow-Up	Population	Intervention	VTE Incidence	Safety	Survival
AVERT Carrier et al. 2019 [98] Double-blind, randomized, placebo-controlled, multicenter study	Overall population Arm A: 288 patients Arm B: 275 patients PC patients: 77	6 months	Ambulatory cancer patients receiving chemotherapy who are at high-risk for VTE (as defined by a Khorana score of ≥2)	Arm A: apixaban 2.5 mg twice daily up to day 180 Arm B: placebo up to day 180	Overall population VTE at 6 months Arm A: 12/288 (4.2%) Arm B: 28/275 (10.2%) HR 0.41 (95% CI 0.26–0.65) $p < 0.001$ PC subgroup NS	Overall population Major bleeding Arm A: 10/288 (3.5%) Arm B: 5/275 (1.8%) HR 2.00 (95% CI 1.01–3.95) $p = 0.046$ Clinically relevant non-major bleeding Arm A: 21/288 (7.3%) Arm B: 15/276 (5.5%) HR, 1.28; 95% CI, 0.89–1.84 PC subgroup NS	All-cause mortality Arm A: 35/288 (12.2%) Arm B: 27/275 (9.8%) HR 1.29 (95% CI 0.98–1.71) $p =$ ns PC subgroup NS
Ramathan et al. 2018 [99] Open-label multicenter phase 2	Arm A: 18 patients Arm B: 16 patients	Median of 8 weeks	Locally advanced ductal adenocarcinoma of the pancreas diagnosed ≤6 months prior to enrollment	Arm A: Gemcitabine +PCI-27483 1.2 mg/kg/bid Arm B: Gemcitabine alone	VTE (any grade) Arm A: 10/18 (56%) Arm B: 3/16 (19%)	Bleeding (any grade) Arm A: 1/18 (6%) Arm B: 2/16 (13%)	Arm A: 5.7 months Arm B: 5.6 months

Abbreviations: CI, confidence interval; CRNMB, clinically relevant non major bleeding; HR, hazard ratio; OR, odds ratio; NNH, number needed to harm; NNT, number needed to treat; NS, not specified; PC, pancreatic cancer; RR, relative risk; VTE, venous thromboembolism.

During the entire follow-up, patients receiving apixaban experienced fewer VTE events compared to those receiving placebo (4.2% vs. 10.2%; HR 0.41, 95% CI 0.26–0.65, $p < 0.001$). In the modified intention-to-treat analysis, patients receiving apixaban had a significant higher risk of major bleeding (3.5% vs. 1.8% in the placebo arm; HR 2.00, 95% CI 1.01–3.95; $p = 0.046$). Results were not reported separately for the subgroup of PC patients.

The percentage of patients who prematurely discontinued the trial regimen was relatively high in both trials (47% in CASSINI and 38% in AVERT) and there was no significant difference in overall survival between patients receiving DOAC or placebo.

In an updated meta-analysis pooling the results from FRAGEM, [93] PROSPECT-CONKO 004 [94] and from subgroups of PC patients included in PROTECHT [91], SAVE-ONCO [92] and CASSINI, [96] PC patients receiving primary thromboprophylaxis with either LMWH or a DOAC had significantly lower rates of VTE compared to controls (5.43% vs. 12.07%, RR 0.44, 95% CI 0.29–0.70), with a risk difference of −0.06 (95% CI −0.11–0.01, $p = 0.01$) with no difference in the rate of major bleeding between the two groups (4.11% vs. 3.27%) [100]. However, pooling subgroup analyses of RCTs is prone to biased results and these results should be interpreted with caution.

Compared to LMWH, DOACs have the advantage of being orally administered at fixed doses. However, there are some limitations for their use in cancer patients that should be taken in consideration. Certain patient characteristics (e.g.: weight and age) and comorbidities (e.g.: renal or hepatic impairment), as well as potential drug-drug interactions may affect anticoagulant pharmacokinetics and result in over or under-coagulating [101–103]. Vomiting and diarrhea, common side effects of cancer treatment, can also limit drug absorption in these patients. Finally, DOACs have been associated with an increased risk of GI bleeding, particularly in cancers of the upper GI tract. In each case, full consideration of the appropriate balance of benefits and harms is warranted.

4.2. Anticoagulants as Adjuvant Treatment to Improve Survival in Pancreatic Cancer Patients

Several studies evaluated the hypothesis that targeted inhibition of the coagulation cascade might improve survival in cancer patients. However, few data were obtained from PC patients due to their short life expectancy.

The FAMOUS trial [104] randomized 385 cancer patients to receive either dalteparin (5000 IU daily) or placebo for 1 year. One year after randomization, OS was 46% in patients receiving dalteparin compared to 41% in patients receiving placebo ($p = 0.19$). Thirty eight (10%) PC patients were included in the study, but results were not reported for this subgroup [104].

The MALT trial [105] assessed the effect of nadroparin compared to placebo for 6 weeks on survival in 302 patients with advanced cancer without VTE. In the intention-to-treat population, the median survival was significantly longer in the nadroparin group (8.0 months vs. 6.6 months in the placebo group; HR 0.75, 95% CI 0.59–0.96; $p = 0.021$), even after adjustment for WHO performance status, concomitant treatment, and type and histology of cancer (HR 0.76, 95% CI 0.58–0.99). In a pre-specified subgroup of patients with a life expectancy longer than 6 months at enrollment, the median survival was 15.4 months in the nadroparin group compared to 9.4 to months in the placebo group (HR 0.64, 95% CI 0.45–0.90; $p = 0.01$). These results are difficult to extrapolate to PC patients since only 18 out of 302 (6%) patients included in the MALT trial had PC [105].

In a multicenter, open-label, randomized controlled trial, 503 patients with non-small-cell lung cancer, hormone-refractory prostate cancer, or locally advanced PC received either nadroparin for 6 weeks (2 weeks at therapeutic dose, and 4 weeks at half therapeutic dose) in addition to their cancer treatment, or no nadroparin. One hundred thirty four out of 503 (27%) patients had PC. In PC patients, the mortality rate did not differ between the two study arms (79% in the nadroparin arm vs. 73.6% in the control arm; HR 1.14, 95% CI 0.77–1.68; $p = 0.53$). The median survival was 8.0 months in the nadroparin arm compared to 10.4 months in the control arm ($p = $ ns) [106].

Finally, a non-randomized trial reported that the use of nadroparin improved survival in 69 consecutive patients with advanced pancreatic ductal adenocarcinoma treated with GEM plus cisplatin every 21 days with or without nadroparin until disease progression. The overall response rate on PFS was 58.8% with nadroparin compared to 12.1% without nadroparin ($p = 0.0001$). Patients receiving nadroparin had longer median time to progression and survival compared to those without (7.3 vs. 4.0 months, $p = 0.0001$ and 13.0 vs. 5.5 months, $p = 0.0001$, respectively) [107].

Survival was a secondary efficacy end point in FRAGEM [93] and PROSPECT-CONKO 004 [94], but despite established association between VTE and mortality in PC patients, both studies failed to demonstrate a benefit of LMWH on overall survival (Table 4). This lack of difference between the LMWH and placebo arms might be related to the short life expectancy of PC patients included in these studies [108], or might suggest that the activities driving VTE and progression are not equally susceptible to LMWH. It may well be that clinical VTE per se is not the sole determinant of survival and neither could be FXa and FIIa since TF activities unrelated to those e.g., PAR2 would not be altered by LMWH.

A recent phase 2 study evaluated the safety and efficacy of PCI-27483, a reversible small-molecule inhibitor of activated factor VII. This study randomized 34 patients with metastatic or locally advanced PC to receive PCI-27483-GEM ($n = 18$) or GEM alone ($n = 16$). OS did not significantly differ between patients treated with PCI-27483- GEM and those with GEM alone but there was a nonsignificant trend toward longer PFS in patients receiving PCI-27483- GEM compared to those receiving GEM alone (PFS: 3.7 months vs. 1.9 months; HR 0.62; $p = 0.307$) [99]. There was no difference in the rates of grade ≥ 3 bleeding between the two arms and there was a trend toward lower rates of VTE in the PCI-27483-GEM arm (6% vs. 13% in the GEM arm). Overall, there is yet no evidence that points towards any survival benefit of anticoagulants as adjuvant treatment in PC patients.

5. Current Guidelines for VTE Thromboprophylaxis in PC Patients

Since 2013, the ITAC CPGs have recommended the use of thromboprophylaxis with LMWH in surgical PC patients undergoing major surgery, hospitalized patients with acute medical illness and reduced mobility [12–14], and in locally advanced or metastatic ambulatory PC patients receiving chemotherapy [12–14]. New data have now emerged on the benefit of DOACs for primary thromboprophylaxis, which provide another option in selected patients [96,98]. The ITAC working group [14], the American Society of Clinical Oncology (ASCO) [15], and the National Comprehensive Cancer Network (NCCN) [109] updated their recommendations for VTE prophylaxis in cancer patients in 2019.

5.1. Thromboprophylaxis in Surgical PC Patients

Thromboprophylaxis is recommend in PC patients undergoing major surgery by all current guidelines [12–15,109]. The 2019 ITAC CPGs [14] recommend thromboprophylaxis with the highest prophylactic dose of LMWH in PC patients undergoing major surgery, in the absence of contraindications (creatinine clearance <30 mL·min^{-1}, high bleeding risk, active bleeding) [Grade 1A]. Low dose of unfractionated heparin (UFH) three times daily can also be used [Grade 1A]. There are insufficient data to support the use of fondaparinux as an alternative to LMWH in surgical PC patients [2C] and no data to support the use of DOACs [Best clinical practice]. Extended prophylaxis for 4 weeks should be used in patients undergoing laparotomy or laparoscopic surgery with a low bleeding risk [Grade 1A]. External compression devices are not recommended as monotherapy, except when pharmacological methods are contraindicated [Grade 2B], and the use of inferior vena cava filter is not recommended for routine thromboprophylaxis [Grade 1A] [14].

5.2. Thromboprophylaxis in Hospitalized PC Patients with Acute Medical Illness or with A Reduced Mobility

All current CPGs recommend thromboprophylaxis in hospitalized PC patients with acute medical illness or reduced mobility in the absence of bleeding or other contraindications [12–15,109]. The 2019 ITAC CPGs [14] recommend to use of prophylactic dose of LMWH in hospitalized PC patients with acute medical illness or with a reduced mobility in the absence of contraindications (creatinine clearance <30 mL·min^{-1}, high bleeding risk, active bleeding) [Grade 1B]. Prophylaxis with UFH or fondaparinux can also be used [Grade 1B], but DOACs are not recommended routinely in this setting due to the lack of data [Best clinical practice] [14].

5.3. Thromboprophylaxis in Ambulatory PC Patients Receiving Chemotherapy

The KS assigns +2 points for PC patients. Therefore, according to the most recent guidelines, all ambulatory PC patients should be considered for thromboprophylaxis with either LMWH or DOACs. [14,15] In locally advanced or metastatic PC patients, the 2019 ITAC CPGs [14] recommend primary prophylaxis with LMWH for those patients having a low risk of bleeding and receiving systemic anticancer therapy [Grade 1B] [14], based on available evidence. [93–95] The 2019 ITAC CPGs [14] also recommend thromboprophylaxis with apixaban or rivaroxaban in cancer outpatients at intermediate-to-high risk (KS ≥2 prior to starting chemotherapy) with a low bleeding risk and in the absence of drug-drug interactions [Grade 1B] [14].

Similarly, the ASCO guidelines recommend that thromboprophylaxis with apixaban, rivaroxaban or LMWH may be offered in high-risk cancer outpatients (KS ≥2 or higher prior to starting a new systemic chemotherapy regimen) in the absence of significant risk factors for bleeding and drug interactions [15].

6. Conclusions

Evidence (Grade 1B) that appropriate use of primary thromboprophylaxis significantly and safely reduces the burden of VTE in PC patients has been available since 2013. Despite this fact, thromboprophylaxis remains largely underused. Increased awareness among healthcare professionals and adherence to evidence-based guidelines can decrease the burden of VTE in PC patients. Clinical tools based on the 2019 ITAC-CME international guidelines, such as a free accessible web-based mobile application with a decision-tree algorithm (downloadable at www.itaccme.com), can be used to assist clinicians in optimizing treatment in daily clinical practice. In the absence of head-to-head comparison between LMWH and DOACs, a discussion with the patient about the relative benefits and risks, drug cost, duration and tolerance of prophylaxis is warranted before prescribing thromboprophylaxis in PC ambulatory patients.

Author Contributions: D.F. and C.F. wrote the first draft of the manuscript and contributed to the concept and design, critical of intellectual content, and final approval; all other authors contributed to critical of intellectual content of the manuscript, and final approval. All authors have read and agreed to the published version of the manuscript.

Funding: This research received no external funding.

Conflicts of Interest: D.F. reports non-financial support from Leo Pharma, Aspen Pharmacare, and Pfizer, outside of the submitted work. C.F. reports personal fees and non-financial support from Leo Pharma, personal fees and non-financial support from Bayer, Aspen Pharma Care, and Pfizer, outside of the submitted work. Other authors declare no conflicts of interest.

References

1. Siegel, R.L.; Miller, K.D.; Jemal, A. Cancer statistics, 2018. *CA Cancer J. Clin.* **2018**, *68*, 7–30. [CrossRef] [PubMed]
2. Ryan, D.P.; Hong, T.S.; Bardeesy, N. Pancreatic Adenocarcinoma. *N. Engl. J. Med.* **2014**, *371*, 1039–1049. [CrossRef] [PubMed]
3. GBD 2017 Pancreatic Cancer Collaborators The global, regional, and national burden of pancreatic cancer and its attributable risk factors in 195 countries and territories, 1990–2017: A systematic analysis for the Global Burden of Disease Study 2017. *Lancet Gastroenterol. Hepatol.* **2019**, *4*, 934–947. [CrossRef]
4. Rahib, L.; Smith, B.D.; Aizenberg, R.; Rosenzweig, A.B.; Fleshman, J.M.; Matrisian, L.M. Projecting cancer incidence and deaths to 2030: the unexpected burden of thyroid, liver, and pancreas cancers in the United States. *Cancer Res.* **2014**, *74*, 2913–2921. [CrossRef]

5. American Cancer Society. Cancer Facts & Figures 2019. Available online: https://www.cancer.org/content/dam/cancer-org/research/cancer-facts-and-statistics/annual-cancer-facts-and-figures/2019/cancer-facts-and-figures-2019.pdf (accessed on 10 October 2019).
6. Azar, I.; Virk, G.; Esfandiarifard, S.; Wazir, A.; Mehdi, S. Treatment and survival rates of stage IV pancreatic cancer at VA hospitals: A nation-wide study. *J. Gastrointest. Oncol.* **2019**, *10*, 703–711. [CrossRef]
7. Lambert, A.; Schwarz, L.; Borbath, I.; Henry, A.; Van Laethem, J.-L.; Malka, D.; Ducreux, M.; Conroy, T. An update on treatment options for pancreatic adenocarcinoma. *Ther. Adv. Med. Oncol.* **2019**, *11*, 1758835919875568. [CrossRef]
8. Burris, H.A.; Moore, M.J.; Andersen, J.; Green, M.R.; Rothenberg, M.L.; Modiano, M.R.; Cripps, M.C.; Portenoy, R.K.; Storniolo, A.M.; Tarassoff, P.; et al. Improvements in survival and clinical benefit with gemcitabine as first-line therapy for patients with advanced pancreas cancer: A randomized trial. *J. Clin. Oncol.* **1997**, *15*, 2403–2413. [CrossRef]
9. Conroy, T.; Desseigne, F.; Ychou, M.; Bouché, O.; Guimbaud, R.; Bécouarn, Y.; Adenis, A.; Raoul, J.-L.; Gourgou-Bourgade, S.; de la Fouchardière, C.; et al. FOLFIRINOX versus gemcitabine for metastatic pancreatic cancer. *N. Engl. J. Med.* **2011**, *364*, 1817–1825. [CrossRef]
10. Von Hoff, D.D.; Ervin, T.; Arena, F.P.; Chiorean, E.G.; Infante, J.; Moore, M.; Seay, T.; Tjulandin, S.A.; Ma, W.W.; Saleh, M.N.; et al. Increased survival in pancreatic cancer with nab-paclitaxel plus gemcitabine. *N. Engl. J. Med.* **2013**, *369*, 1691–1703. [CrossRef]
11. Conroy, T.; Hammel, P.; Hebbar, M.; Ben Abdelghani, M.; Wei, A.C.; Raoul, J.-L.; Choné, L.; Francois, E.; Artru, P.; Biagi, J.J.; et al. FOLFIRINOX or Gemcitabine as Adjuvant Therapy for Pancreatic Cancer. *N. Engl. J. Med.* **2018**, *379*, 2395–2406. [CrossRef]
12. Farge, D.; Debourdeau, P.; Beckers, M.; Baglin, C.; Bauersachs, R.M.; Brenner, B.; Brilhante, D.; Falanga, A.; Gerotzafias, G.T.; Haim, N.; et al. International clinical practice guidelines for the treatment and prophylaxis of venous thromboembolism in patients with cancer. *J. Thromb. Haemost.* **2013**, *11*, 56–70. [CrossRef] [PubMed]
13. Farge, D.; Bounameaux, H.; Brenner, B.; Cajfinger, F.; Debourdeau, P.; Khorana, A.A.; Pabinger, I.; Solymoss, S.; Douketis, J.; Kakkar, A. International clinical practice guidelines including guidance for direct oral anticoagulants in the treatment and prophylaxis of venous thromboembolism in patients with cancer. *Lancet Oncol.* **2016**, *17*, e452–e466. [CrossRef]
14. Farge, D.; Frere, C.; Connors, J.M.; Ay, C.; Khorana, A.A.; Munoz, A.; Brenner, B.; Kakkar, A.; Rafii, H.; Solymoss, S.; et al. 2019 international clinical practice guidelines for the treatment and prophylaxis of venous thromboembolism in patients with cancer. *Lancet Oncol.* **2019**, *20*, e566–e581. [CrossRef]
15. Key, N.S.; Khorana, A.A.; Kuderer, N.M.; Bohlke, K.; Lee, A.Y.Y.; Arcelus, J.I.; Wong, S.L.; Balaban, E.P.; Flowers, C.R.; Francis, C.W.; et al. Venous Thromboembolism Prophylaxis and Treatment in Patients With Cancer: ASCO Clinical Practice Guideline Update. *J. Clin. Oncol.* **2020**, *38*, 496–520. [CrossRef] [PubMed]
16. Moffat, G.T.; Epstein, A.S.; O'Reilly, E.M. Pancreatic cancer-A disease in need: Optimizing and integrating supportive care. *Cancer* **2019**, *125*, 3927–3935. [CrossRef]
17. Levitan, N.; Dowlati, A.; Remick, S.C.; Tahsildar, H.I.; Sivinski, L.D.; Beyth, R.; Rimm, A.A. Rates of initial and recurrent thromboembolic disease among patients with malignancy versus those without malignancy. Risk analysis using Medicare claims data. *Medicine* **1999**, *78*, 285–291. [CrossRef]
18. Heit, J.A.; Silverstein, M.D.; Mohr, D.N.; Petterson, T.M.; O'Fallon, W.M.; Melton, L.J. Risk factors for deep vein thrombosis and pulmonary embolism: A population-based case-control study. *Arch. Intern. Med.* **2000**, *160*, 809–815. [CrossRef]
19. Timp, J.F.; Braekkan, S.K.; Versteeg, H.H.; Cannegieter, S.C. Epidemiology of cancer-associated venous thrombosis. *Blood* **2013**, *122*, 1712–1723. [CrossRef]
20. Blom, J.W.; Vanderschoot, J.P.M.; Oostindiër, M.J.; Osanto, S.; van der Meer, F.J.M.; Rosendaal, F.R. Incidence of venous thrombosis in a large cohort of 66,329 cancer patients: Results of a record linkage study. *J. Thromb. Haemost.* **2006**, *4*, 529–535. [CrossRef]
21. Chew, H.K.; Wun, T.; Harvey, D.; Zhou, H.; White, R.H. Incidence of venous thromboembolism and its effect on survival among patients with common cancers. *Arch. Intern. Med.* **2006**, *166*, 458–464. [CrossRef]
22. Horsted, F.; West, J.; Grainge, M.J. Risk of venous thromboembolism in patients with cancer: A systematic review and meta-analysis. *PLoS Med.* **2012**, *9*, e1001275. [CrossRef] [PubMed]

23. Sproul, E.E. Carcinoma and Venous Thrombosis: The Frequency of Association of Carcinoma in the Body or Tail of the Pancreas with Multiple Venous Thrombosis. *Am. J. Cancer* **1938**, *34*, 566–585.
24. Blom, J.W.; Osanto, S.; Rosendaal, F.R. High risk of venous thrombosis in patients with pancreatic cancer: A cohort study of 202 patients. *Eur. J. Cancer* **2006**, *42*, 410–414. [CrossRef] [PubMed]
25. Mandalà, M.; Reni, M.; Cascinu, S.; Barni, S.; Floriani, I.; Cereda, S.; Berardi, R.; Mosconi, S.; Torri, V.; Labianca, R. Venous thromboembolism predicts poor prognosis in irresectable pancreatic cancer patients. *Ann. Oncol.* **2007**, *18*, 1660–1665. [CrossRef] [PubMed]
26. Mitry, E.; Taleb-Fayad, R.; Deschamps, A.; Mansencal, N.; Lepère, C.; Declety, G.; Lièvre, A.; Vaillant, J.-N.; Lesur, G.; Cramer, E.; et al. Risk of venous thrombosis in patients with pancreatic adenocarcinoma. *Gastroenterol. Clin. Biol.* **2007**, *31*, 1139–1142. [CrossRef]
27. Oh, S.Y.; Kim, J.H.; Lee, K.-W.; Bang, S.-M.; Hwang, J.-H.; Oh, D.; Lee, J.S. Venous thromboembolism in patients with pancreatic adenocarcinoma: Lower incidence in Asian ethnicity. *Thromb. Res.* **2008**, *122*, 485–490. [CrossRef]
28. Poruk, K.E.; Firpo, M.A.; Huerter, L.M.; Scaife, C.L.; Emerson, L.L.; Boucher, K.M.; Jones, K.A.; Mulvihill, S.J. Serum platelet factor 4 is an independent predictor of survival and venous thromboembolism in patients with pancreatic adenocarcinoma. *Cancer Epidemiol. Biomark. Prev.* **2010**, *19*, 2605–2610. [CrossRef]
29. Shaib, W.; Deng, Y.; Zilterman, D.; Lundberg, B.; Saif, M.W. Assessing risk and mortality of venous thromboembolism in pancreatic cancer patients. *Anticancer Res.* **2010**, *30*, 4261–4264.
30. Epstein, A.S.; Soff, G.A.; Capanu, M.; Crosbie, C.; Shah, M.A.; Kelsen, D.P.; Denton, B.; Gardos, S.; O'Reilly, E.M. Analysis of incidence and clinical outcomes in patients with thromboembolic events and invasive exocrine pancreatic cancer. *Cancer* **2012**, *118*, 3053–3061. [CrossRef]
31. Menapace, L.A.; Peterson, D.R.; Berry, A.; Sousou, T.; Khorana, A.A. Symptomatic and incidental thromboembolism are both associated with mortality in pancreatic cancer. *Thromb. Haemost.* **2011**, *106*, 371–378. [CrossRef]
32. Afsar, C.U.; Gunaldi, M.; Kum, P.; Sahin, B.; Erkisi, M.; Kara, I.O.; Paydas, S.; Duman, B.B.; Ercolak, V.; Karaca, F.; et al. Pancreatic carcinoma, thrombosis and mean platelet volume: Single center experience from the southeast region of Turkey. *Asian Pac. J. Cancer Prev.* **2014**, *15*, 9143–9146. [CrossRef] [PubMed]
33. Muñoz Martín, A.J.; García Alfonso, P.; Rupérez Blanco, A.B.; Pérez Ramírez, S.; Blanco Codesido, M.; Martín Jiménez, M. Incidence of venous thromboembolism (VTE) in ambulatory pancreatic cancer patients receiving chemotherapy and analysis of Khorana's predictive model. *Clin. Transl. Oncol.* **2014**, *16*, 927–930. [CrossRef] [PubMed]
34. Krepline, A.N.; Christians, K.K.; George, B.; Ritch, P.S.; Erickson, B.A.; Tolat, P.; Evans, D.B.; Tsai, S. Venous thromboembolism prophylaxis during neoadjuvant therapy for resectable and borderline resectable pancreatic cancer-Is it indicated? *J. Surg. Oncol.* **2016**, *114*, 581–586. [CrossRef] [PubMed]
35. Lee, J.-C.; Ro, Y.S.; Cho, J.; Park, Y.; Lee, J.H.; Hwang, J.-H.; Choi, H.J.; Lee, S. Characteristics of Venous Thromboembolism in Pancreatic Adenocarcinoma in East Asian Ethnics: A Large Population-Based Observational Study. *Medicine* **2016**, *95*, e3472. [CrossRef]
36. Kruger, S.; Haas, M.; Burkl, C.; Goehring, P.; Kleespies, A.; Roeder, F.; Gallmeier, E.; Ormanns, S.; Westphalen, C.B.; Heinemann, V.; et al. Incidence, outcome and risk stratification tools for venous thromboembolism in advanced pancreatic cancer—A retrospective cohort study. *Thromb. Res.* **2017**, *157*, 9–15. [CrossRef] [PubMed]
37. van Es, N.; Franke, V.F.; Middeldorp, S.; Wilmink, J.W.; Büller, H.R. The Khorana score for the prediction of venous thromboembolism in patients with pancreatic cancer. *Thromb. Res.* **2017**, *150*, 30–32. [CrossRef]
38. Berger, A.K.; Singh, H.M.; Werft, W.; Muckenhuber, A.; Sprick, M.R.; Trumpp, A.; Weichert, W.; Jäger, D.; Springfeld, C. High prevalence of incidental and symptomatic venous thromboembolic events in patients with advanced pancreatic cancer under palliative chemotherapy: A retrospective cohort study. *Pancreatology* **2017**, *17*, 629–634. [CrossRef]
39. Chen, J.-S.; Hung, C.-Y.; Chang, H.; Liu, C.-T.; Chen, Y.-Y.; Lu, C.-H.; Chang, P.-H.; Hung, Y.-S.; Chou, W.-C. Venous Thromboembolism in Asian Patients with Pancreatic Cancer Following Palliative Chemotherapy: Low Incidence but a Negative Prognosticator for Those with Early Onset. *Cancers* **2018**, *10*, 501. [CrossRef]
40. Kim, J.S.; Kang, E.J.; Kim, D.S.; Choi, Y.J.; Lee, S.Y.; Kim, H.J.; Seo, H.Y.; Kim, J.S. Early venous thromboembolism at the beginning of palliative chemotherapy is a poor prognostic factor in patients with metastatic pancreatic cancer: A retrospective study. *BMC Cancer* **2018**, *18*, 1260. [CrossRef]

41. Frere, C.; Bournet, B.; Gourgou, S.; Fraisse, J.; Canivet, C.; Connors, J.M.; Buscail, L.; Farge, D. Incidence of Venous Thromboembolism in Patients with Newly Diagnosed Pancreatic Cancer and Factors Associated With Outcomes. *Gastroenterology* **2019**. [CrossRef]
42. Ouaissi, M.; Frasconi, C.; Mege, D.; Panicot-Dubois, L.; Boiron, L.; Dahan, L.; Debourdeau, P.; Dubois, C.; Farge, D.; Sieleznef, I. Impact of venous thromboembolism on the natural history of pancreatic adenocarcinoma. *HBPD INT* **2015**, *14*, 436–442. [CrossRef]
43. Khorana, A.A.; Fine, R.L. Pancreatic cancer and thromboembolic disease. *Lancet Oncol.* **2004**, *5*, 655–663. [CrossRef]
44. Mier-Hicks, A.; Raj, M.; Do, R.K.; Yu, K.H.; Lowery, M.A.; Varghese, A.; O'Reilly, E.M. Incidence, Management, and Implications of Visceral Thrombosis in Pancreatic Ductal Adenocarcinoma. *Clin. Colorectal Cancer* **2018**, *17*, 121–128. [CrossRef] [PubMed]
45. Common Terminology Criteria for Adverse Events (CTCAE) Version 4.0. Cancer Therapy Evaluation Program: Bethesda, MD, USA, 2009.
46. Khorana, A.A.; Francis, C.W.; Culakova, E.; Kuderer, N.M.; Lyman, G.H. Frequency, risk factors, and trends for venous thromboembolism among hospitalized cancer patients. *Cancer* **2007**, *110*, 2339–2346. [CrossRef] [PubMed]
47. Khorana, A.A.; Francis, C.W.; Culakova, E.; Kuderer, N.M.; Lyman, G.H. Thromboembolism is a leading cause of death in cancer patients receiving outpatient chemotherapy. *J. Thromb. Haemost.* **2007**, *5*, 632–634. [CrossRef] [PubMed]
48. Afzal, A.; Suhong, L.; Gage, B.F.; Schoen, M.W.; Carson, K.; Thomas, T.; Sanfilippo, K. Splanchnic vein thrombosis predicts worse survival in patients with advanced pancreatic cancer. *Thromb. Res.* **2019**, *185*, 125–131. [CrossRef] [PubMed]
49. Larsen, A.C.; Brøndum Frøkjaer, J.; Wishwanath Iyer, V.; Vincents Fisker, R.; Sall, M.; Yilmaz, M.K.; Kuno Møller, B.; Kristensen, S.R.; Thorlacius-Ussing, O. Venous thrombosis in pancreaticobiliary tract cancer: outcome and prognostic factors. *J. Thromb. Haemost.* **2015**, *13*, 555–562. [CrossRef]
50. Kaur, S.; Kumar, S.; Momi, N.; Sasson, A.R.; Batra, S.K. Mucins in pancreatic cancer and its microenvironment. *Nat. Rev. Gastroenterol. Hepatol.* **2013**, *10*, 607–620. [CrossRef]
51. Campello, E.; Ilich, A.; Simioni, P.; Key, N.S. The relationship between pancreatic cancer and hypercoagulability: A comprehensive review on epidemiological and biological issues. *Br. J. Cancer* **2019**, *121*, 359–371. [CrossRef]
52. Gasic, G.J.; Koch, P.A.; Hsu, B.; Gasic, T.B.; Niewiarowski, S. Thrombogenic activity of mouse and human tumors: Effects on platelets, coagulation, and fibrinolysis, and possible significance for metastases. *Z. Krebsforsch. Klin. Onkol. Cancer Res. Clin. Oncol.* **1976**, *86*, 263–277. [CrossRef]
53. Labelle, M.; Begum, S.; Hynes, R.O. Direct signaling between platelets and cancer cells induces an epithelial-mesenchymal-like transition and promotes metastasis. *Cancer Cell* **2011**, *20*, 576–590. [CrossRef]
54. Lucotti, S.; Cerutti, C.; Soyer, M.; Gil-Bernabé, A.M.; Gomes, A.L.; Allen, P.D.; Smart, S.; Markelc, B.; Watson, K.; Armstrong, P.C.; et al. Aspirin blocks formation of metastatic intravascular niches by inhibiting platelet-derived COX-1/thromboxane A2. *J. Clin. Investig.* **2019**, *129*, 1845–1862. [CrossRef] [PubMed]
55. Buscail, L.; Bournet, B.; Cordelier, P. Role of oncogenic KRAS in the diagnosis, prognosis and treatment of pancreatic cancer. *Nat. Rev. Gastroenterol. Hepatol.* **2020**, *7*, 153–168. [CrossRef] [PubMed]
56. Yu, J.L.; May, L.; Lhotak, V.; Shahrzad, S.; Shirasawa, S.; Weitz, J.I.; Coomber, B.L.; Mackman, N.; Rak, J.W. Oncogenic events regulate tissue factor expression in colorectal cancer cells: Implications for tumor progression and angiogenesis. *Blood* **2005**, *105*, 1734–1741. [CrossRef] [PubMed]
57. Garrido-Laguna, I.; Hidalgo, M. Pancreatic cancer: From state-of-the-art treatments to promising novel therapies. *Nat. Rev. Clin. Oncol.* **2015**, *12*, 319–334. [CrossRef]
58. Kakkar, A.K.; Lemoine, N.R.; Scully, M.F.; Tebbutt, S.; Williamson, R.C. Tissue factor expression correlates with histological grade in human pancreatic cancer. *Br. J. Surg.* **1995**, *82*, 1101–1104. [CrossRef]
59. Yu, J.L.; Rak, J.W. Shedding of tissue factor (TF)-containing microparticles rather than alternatively spliced TF is the main source of TF activity released from human cancer cells. *J. Thromb. Haemost.* **2004**, *2*, 2065–2067. [CrossRef]
60. Rak, J.; Yu, J.L.; Luyendyk, J.; Mackman, N. Oncogenes, trousseau syndrome, and cancer-related changes in the coagulome of mice and humans. *Cancer Res.* **2006**, *66*, 10643–10646. [CrossRef]
61. Rak, J. Cancer: Organ-seeking vesicles. *Nature* **2015**, *527*, 312–314. [CrossRef]

62. Sawai, H.; Liu, J.; Reber, H.A.; Hines, O.J.; Eibl, G. Activation of peroxisome proliferator-activated receptor-gamma decreases pancreatic cancer cell invasion through modulation of the plasminogen activator system. *Mol. Cancer Res.* **2006**, *4*, 159–167. [CrossRef]

63. Unruh, D.; Turner, K.; Srinivasan, R.; Kocatürk, B.; Qi, X.; Chu, Z.; Aronow, B.J.; Plas, D.R.; Gallo, C.A.; Kalthoff, H.; et al. Alternatively spliced tissue factor contributes to tumor spread and activation of coagulation in pancreatic ductal adenocarcinoma. *Int. J. Cancer* **2014**, *134*, 9–20. [CrossRef]

64. Unruh, D.; Ünlü, B.; Lewis, C.S.; Qi, X.; Chu, Z.; Sturm, R.; Keil, R.; Ahmad, S.A.; Sovershaev, T.; Adam, M.; et al. Antibody-based targeting of alternatively spliced tissue factor: A new approach to impede the primary growth and spread of pancreatic ductal adenocarcinoma. *Oncotarget* **2016**, *7*, 25264–25275. [CrossRef] [PubMed]

65. Winter, P.C. The pathogenesis of venous thromboembolism in cancer: Emerging links with tumour biology. *Hematol. Oncol.* **2006**, *24*, 126–133. [CrossRef] [PubMed]

66. Davila, M.; Amirkhosravi, A.; Coll, E.; Desai, H.; Robles, L.; Colon, J.; Baker, C.H.; Francis, J.L. Tissue factor-bearing microparticles derived from tumor cells: Impact on coagulation activation. *J. Thromb. Haemost.* **2008**, *6*, 1517–1524. [CrossRef] [PubMed]

67. Thomas, G.M.; Panicot-Dubois, L.; Lacroix, R.; Dignat-George, F.; Lombardo, D.; Dubois, C. Cancer cell-derived microparticles bearing P-selectin glycoprotein ligand 1 accelerate thrombus formation in vivo. *J. Exp. Med.* **2009**, *206*, 1913–1927. [CrossRef]

68. Zwicker, J.I.; Liebman, H.A.; Neuberg, D.; Lacroix, R.; Bauer, K.A.; Furie, B.C.; Furie, B. Tumor-derived tissue factor-bearing microparticles are associated with venous thromboembolic events in malignancy. *Clin. Cancer Res.* **2009**, *15*, 6830–6840. [CrossRef]

69. Manly, D.A.; Wang, J.; Glover, S.L.; Kasthuri, R.; Liebman, H.A.; Key, N.S.; Mackman, N. Increased microparticle tissue factor activity in cancer patients with Venous Thromboembolism. *Thromb. Res.* **2010**, *125*, 511–512. [CrossRef]

70. Bharthuar, A.; Khorana, K.A.; Hutson, A.; Wang, J.; Mackman, N.; Iyer, R. Association of elevated tissue factor (TF) with survival and thromboembolism (TE) in pancreaticobiliary cancers (PBC). *J. Clin. Oncol.* **2010**, *28* (Suppl. 15), 4126. [CrossRef]

71. Khorana, A.A.; Francis, C.W.; Menzies, K.E.; Wang, J.-G.; Hyrien, O.; Hathcock, J.; Mackman, N.; Taubman, M.B. Plasma tissue factor may be predictive of venous thromboembolism in pancreatic cancer. *J. Thromb. Haemost.* **2008**, *6*, 1983–1985. [CrossRef]

72. Thaler, J.; Ay, C.; Mackman, N.; Bertina, R.M.; Kaider, A.; Marosi, C.; Key, N.S.; Barcel, D.A.; Scheithauer, W.; Kornek, G.; et al. Microparticle-associated tissue factor activity, venous thromboembolism and mortality in pancreatic, gastric, colorectal and brain cancer patients. *J. Thromb. Haemost.* **2012**, *10*, 1363–1370. [CrossRef]

73. Thaler, J.; Ay, C.; Mackman, N.; Metz-Schimmerl, S.; Stift, J.; Kaider, A.; Müllauer, L.; Gnant, M.; Scheithauer, W.; Pabinger, I. Microparticle-associated tissue factor activity in patients with pancreatic cancer: Correlation with clinicopathological features. *Eur. J. Clin. Investig.* **2013**, *43*, 277–285. [CrossRef]

74. Woei-A-Jin, F.J.S.H.; Romijn, F.P.H.T.M.; Tesselaar, M.E.T.; Rodriguez, P.G.; Bertina, R.M.; Osanto, S. Tissue factor-bearing microparticles and CA19.9: Two players in pancreatic cancer-associated thrombosis? *Br. J. Cancer* **2016**, *115*, 332. [CrossRef] [PubMed]

75. Faille, D.; Bourrienne, M.-C.; de Raucourt, E.; de Chaisemartin, L.; Granger, V.; Lacroix, R.; Panicot-Dubois, L.; Hammel, P.; Lévy, P.; Ruszniewski, P.; et al. Biomarkers for the risk of thrombosis in pancreatic adenocarcinoma are related to cancer process. *Oncotarget* **2018**, *9*, 26453–26465. [CrossRef] [PubMed]

76. Bobek, V.; Kovarík, J. Antitumor and antimetastatic effect of warfarin and heparins. *Biomed. Pharmacother.* **2004**, *58*, 213–219. [CrossRef] [PubMed]

77. Borsig, L. Heparin as an inhibitor of cancer progression. *Prog. Mol. Biol. Transl. Sci.* **2010**, *93*, 335–349.

78. Wei, M.; Tai, G.; Gao, Y.; Li, N.; Huang, B.; Zhou, Y.; Hao, S.; Zeng, X. Modified heparin inhibits P-selectin-mediated cell adhesion of human colon carcinoma cells to immobilized platelets under dynamic flow conditions. *J. Biol. Chem.* **2004**, *279*, 29202–29210. [CrossRef]

79. Mast, A.E.; Stadanlick, J.E.; Lockett, J.M.; Dietzen, D.J.; Hasty, K.A.; Hall, C.L. Tissue factor pathway inhibitor binds to platelet thrombospondin-1. *J. Biol. Chem.* **2000**, *275*, 31715–31721. [CrossRef]

80. Nadir, Y.; Brenner, B. Heparanase procoagulant activity in cancer progression. *Thromb. Res.* **2016**, *140* (Suppl. 1), S44–S48. [CrossRef]

81. Mousa, S.A.; Bozarth, J.; Barrett, J.S. Pharmacodynamic properties of the low molecular weight heparin, tinzaparin: Effect of molecular weight distribution on plasma tissue factor pathway inhibitor in healthy human subjects. *J. Clin. Pharmacol.* **2003**, *43*, 727–734. [CrossRef]
82. Sandset, P.M.; Abildgaard, U.; Larsen, M.L. Heparin induces release of extrinsic coagulation pathway inhibitor (EPI). *Thromb. Res.* **1988**, *50*, 803–813. [CrossRef]
83. Mousa, S.A.; Mohamed, S. Inhibition of endothelial cell tube formation by the low molecular weight heparin, tinzaparin, is mediated by tissue factor pathway inhibitor. *Thromb. Haemost.* **2004**, *92*, 627–633.
84. Mousa, S.A.; Mohamed, S. Anti-angiogenic mechanisms and efficacy of the low molecular weight heparin, tinzaparin: Anti-cancer efficacy. *Oncol. Rep.* **2004**, *12*, 683–688. [CrossRef]
85. Khorana, A.A.; Kuderer, N.M.; Culakova, E.; Lyman, G.H.; Francis, C.W. Development and validation of a predictive model for chemotherapy-associated thrombosis. *Blood* **2008**, *111*, 4902–4907. [CrossRef]
86. Pelzer, U.; Sinn, M.; Stieler, J.; Riess, H. Primary pharmacological prevention of thromboembolic events in ambulatory patients with advanced pancreatic cancer treated with chemotherapy? *Dtsch. Med. Wochenschr.* **2013**, *138*, 2084–2088.
87. Ay, C.; Dunkler, D.; Marosi, C.; Chiriac, A.-L.; Vormittag, R.; Simanek, R.; Quehenberger, P.; Zielinski, C.; Pabinger, I. Prediction of venous thromboembolism in cancer patients. *Blood* **2010**, *116*, 5377–5382. [CrossRef]
88. Verso, M.; Agnelli, G.; Barni, S.; Gasparini, G.; LaBianca, R. A modified Khorana risk assessment score for venous thromboembolism in cancer patients receiving chemotherapy: The Protecht score. *Intern. Emerg. Med.* **2012**, *7*, 291–292. [CrossRef]
89. Cella, C.A.; Di Minno, G.; Carlomagno, C.; Arcopinto, M.; Cerbone, A.M.; Matano, E.; Tufano, A.; Lordick, F.; De Simone, B.; Muehlberg, K.S.; et al. Preventing Venous Thromboembolism in Ambulatory Cancer Patients: The ONKOTEV Study. *Oncologist* **2017**, *22*, 601–608. [CrossRef]
90. Godinho, J.; Casa-Nova, M.; Moreira-Pinto, J.; Simões, P.; Paralta Branco, F.; Leal-Costa, L.; Faria, A.; Lopes, F.; Teixeira, J.A.; Passos-Coelho, J.L. ONKOTEV Score as a Predictive Tool for Thromboembolic Events in Pancreatic Cancer-A Retrospective Analysis. *Oncologist* **2020**, *25*, e284–e290. [CrossRef] [PubMed]
91. Agnelli, G.; Gussoni, G.; Bianchini, C.; Verso, M.; Mandalà, M.; Cavanna, L.; Barni, S.; Labianca, R.; Buzzi, F.; Scambia, G.; et al. Nadroparin for the prevention of thromboembolic events in ambulatory patients with metastatic or locally advanced solid cancer receiving chemotherapy: A randomised, placebo-controlled, double-blind study. *Lancet Oncol.* **2009**, *10*, 943–949. [CrossRef]
92. Agnelli, G.; George, D.J.; Kakkar, A.K.; Fisher, W.; Lassen, M.R.; Mismetti, P.; Mouret, P.; Chaudhari, U.; Lawson, F.; Turpie, A.G.G.; et al. Semuloparin for thromboprophylaxis in patients receiving chemotherapy for cancer. *N. Engl. J. Med.* **2012**, *366*, 601–609. [CrossRef] [PubMed]
93. Maraveyas, A.; Waters, J.; Roy, R.; Fyfe, D.; Propper, D.; Lofts, F.; Sgouros, J.; Gardiner, E.; Wedgwood, K.; Ettelaie, C.; et al. Gemcitabine versus gemcitabine plus dalteparin thromboprophylaxis in pancreatic cancer. *Eur. J. Cancer* **2012**, *48*, 1283–1292. [CrossRef] [PubMed]
94. Pelzer, U.; Opitz, B.; Deutschinoff, G.; Stauch, M.; Reitzig, P.C.; Hahnfeld, S.; Müller, L.; Grunewald, M.; Stieler, J.M.; Sinn, M.; et al. Efficacy of Prophylactic Low-Molecular Weight Heparin for Ambulatory Patients With Advanced Pancreatic Cancer: Outcomes From the CONKO-004 Trial. *J. Clin. Oncol.* **2015**, *33*, 2028–2034. [CrossRef] [PubMed]
95. Tun, N.M.; Guevara, E.; Oo, T.H. Benefit and risk of primary thromboprophylaxis in ambulatory patients with advanced pancreatic cancer receiving chemotherapy: A systematic review and meta-analysis of randomized controlled trials. *Blood Coagul. Fibrinolysis* **2016**, *27*, 270–274. [CrossRef] [PubMed]
96. Khorana, A.A.; Soff, G.A.; Kakkar, A.K.; Vadhan-Raj, S.; Riess, H.; Wun, T.; Streiff, M.B.; Garcia, D.A.; Liebman, H.A.; Belani, C.P.; et al. Rivaroxaban for Thromboprophylaxis in High-Risk Ambulatory Patients with Cancer. *N. Engl. J. Med.* **2019**, *380*, 720–728. [CrossRef] [PubMed]
97. Vadhan-Raj, S.; McNamara, M.G.; Venerito, M.; Riess, H.; O'Reilly, E.M.; Overman, M.J.; Zhou, X.; Vijapurkar, U.; Kaul, S.; Wildgoose, P.; et al. Rivaroxaban thromboprohylaxis in ambulatory patients with pancreatic cancer: Results from a prespecified subgroup analysis of the CASSINI study. *J. Clin. Oncol. Off. J. Am. Soc. Clin. Oncol.* **2019**, *37*, 4016. [CrossRef]
98. Carrier, M.; Abou-Nassar, K.; Mallick, R.; Tagalakis, V.; Shivakumar, S.; Schattner, A.; Kuruvilla, P.; Hill, D.; Spadafora, S.; Marquis, K.; et al. Apixaban to Prevent Venous Thromboembolism in Patients with Cancer. *N. Engl. J. Med.* **2019**, *380*, 711–719. [CrossRef]

99. Ramanathan, R.K.; Thomas, G.W.; Khorana, A.A.; Shah, S.; Zhou, C.; Wong, S.; Cole, G.; James, D.; Gabrail, N.Y. A Phase 2 Study of PCI-27483, a Factor VIIa Inhibitor in Combination with Gemcitabine for Advanced Pancreatic Cancer. *Oncology* **2019**, *96*, 217–222. [CrossRef]
100. Thein, K.Z.; Quick, D.P.; Oo, T.H. Updated Meta-Analysis of Randomized Controlled Trials on Primary Ambulatory Thromboprophylaxis (PATP) in Patients with Advanced Pancreatic Cancer (APC) Receiving Chemotherapy. *Blood* **2019**, *134* (Suppl. 1), 3469. [CrossRef]
101. Short, N.J.; Connors, J.M. New oral anticoagulants and the cancer patient. *Oncologist* **2014**, *19*, 82–93. [CrossRef]
102. Bellesoeur, A.; Thomas-Schoemann, A.; Allard, M.; Smadja, D.; Vidal, M.; Alexandre, J.; Goldwasser, F.; Blanchet, B. Pharmacokinetic variability of anticoagulants in patients with cancer-associated thrombosis: Clinical consequences. *Crit. Rev. Oncol. Hematol.* **2018**, *129*, 102–112. [CrossRef]
103. Mosarla, R.C.; Vaduganathan, M.; Qamar, A.; Moslehi, J.; Piazza, G.; Giugliano, R.P. Anticoagulation Strategies in Patients With Cancer: JACC Review Topic of the Week. *J. Am. Coll. Cardiol.* **2019**, *73*, 1336–1349. [CrossRef]
104. Kakkar, A.K.; Levine, M.N.; Kadziola, Z.; Lemoine, N.R.; Low, V.; Patel, H.K.; Rustin, G.; Thomas, M.; Quigley, M.; Williamson, R.C.N. Low molecular weight heparin, therapy with dalteparin, and survival in advanced cancer: The fragmin advanced malignancy outcome study (FAMOUS). *J. Clin. Oncol.* **2004**, *22*, 1944–1948. [CrossRef] [PubMed]
105. Klerk, C.P.W.; Smorenburg, S.M.; Otten, H.-M.; Lensing, A.W.A.; Prins, M.H.; Piovella, F.; Prandoni, P.; Bos, M.M.E.M.; Richel, D.J.; van Tienhoven, G.; et al. The effect of low molecular weight heparin on survival in patients with advanced malignancy. *J. Clin. Oncol.* **2005**, *23*, 2130–2135. [CrossRef] [PubMed]
106. van Doormaal, F.F.; Di Nisio, M.; Otten, H.-M.; Richel, D.J.; Prins, M.; Buller, H.R. Randomized trial of the effect of the low molecular weight heparin nadroparin on survival in patients with cancer. *J. Clin. Oncol.* **2011**, *29*, 2071–2076. [CrossRef] [PubMed]
107. Icli, F.; Akbulut, H.; Utkan, G.; Yalcin, B.; Dincol, D.; Isikdogan, A.; Demirkazik, A.; Onur, H.; Cay, F.; Büyükcelik, A. Low molecular weight heparin (LMWH) increases the efficacy of cisplatinum plus gemcitabine combination in advanced pancreatic cancer. *J. Surg. Oncol.* **2007**, *95*, 507–512. [CrossRef] [PubMed]
108. Parpia, S.; Julian, J.A.; Thabane, L.; Lee, A.Y.Y.; Rickles, F.R.; Levine, M.N. Competing events in patients with malignant disease who are at risk for recurrent venous thromboembolism. *Contemp. Clin. Trials* **2011**, *32*, 829–833. [CrossRef] [PubMed]
109. NCCN. *Cancer-Associated Venous Thromboembolic Disease (Version 1.2019)*; NCCN: Plymouth Meeting, PA, USA, 2019; p. 98.

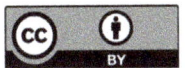

© 2020 by the authors. Licensee MDPI, Basel, Switzerland. This article is an open access article distributed under the terms and conditions of the Creative Commons Attribution (CC BY) license (http://creativecommons.org/licenses/by/4.0/).

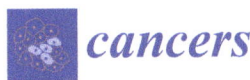

Review

Multiple Myeloma and Thrombosis: Prophylaxis and Risk Prediction Tools

Despina Fotiou, Maria Gavriatopoulou and Evangelos Terpos *

Department of Clinical Therapeutics, National and Kapodistrian University of Athens, School of Medicine, 11528 Athens, Greece; desfotiou@med.uoa.gr (D.F.); mariagabria@gmail.com (M.G.)
* Correspondence: eterpos@med.uoa.gr

Received: 26 December 2019; Accepted: 10 January 2020; Published: 13 January 2020

Abstract: Thromboembolism in multiple myeloma (MM) patients remains a common complication that renders the optimization of our thromboprophylaxis practice necessary. This review aims to make clear the need for the development of more accurate risk assessment tools and means of thrombosis prevention. Current clinical practice is guided by available guidelines published by the IMWG in 2014, but the extent to which these are implemented is unclear. Recently, several groups developed clinical scores for thrombosis risk in MM in an attempt to improve risk stratification, but these have not been validated or used in clinical practice so far. Research in this field is increasingly focusing on understanding the unique coagulation profile of the MM patient, and data on potential biomarkers that accurately reflect hypercoagulability is emerging. Finally, promising evidence on the effectiveness of direct oral anticoagulants (DOACs) in the context of thrombosis prevention in MM patients is increasingly becoming available. The critical appraisal of the above research areas will establish the necessity of combining disease-specific clinical risk factors with coagulation biomarkers to allow more effective risk stratification that will eventually lead to the reduction of this significant complication. Results from ongoing clinical trials on the role of DOACs are much anticipated.

Keywords: multiple myeloma; venous thromboembolism; risk assessment models; thromboprophylaxis; direct oral anticoagulants

1. Introduction

The extraordinary advances in the therapeutic armamentarium available for patients with a new diagnosis of multiple myeloma or relapsed/recurrent disease has led to significant increases in overall survival (OS) but has also drawn attention to the management of treatment-related complications for these patients. Among the commonest complications seen in this population is venous thromboembolism (VTE), as more than 10% will develop VTE during the course of their disease [1–4].

Data from studies that link VTE and inferior overall survival (OS) in MM patients are conflicting, and a clear association has not been established [3,5–7]. However, thrombotic events do have an adverse impact, as they may lead to treatment interruption, increased morbidity, and add to the economic burden of the disease in the population [8,9]. There is a lack of studies that have attempted to specifically assess the economic burden associated with VTE occurrence in MM patients. Data from other cancer patients demonstrate as expected increased costs associated with the long-term use of pharmaceutical agents for the treatment of thrombosis, the need for hospitalization, and increased risk of complications as well as adverse effects on patient's quality of life [8]. Given the significant improvement in the OS of MM in the era of novel agents, the conversation regarding the price and affordability of current treatments is becoming increasingly available. Formal pharmacoeconomic analyses are required to assess the cost-effectiveness of treatment options and the financial burden of managing the complications and adverse effects of these therapeutic agents, including the management of VTE [10].

Thrombogenicity in MM is multifactorial, and risk factors are traditionally distinguished in three groups [11,12]: patient-related clinical risk factors, disease-related risk factors, and treatment-related risk factors. It has become evident from clinical trial data during the last decade that immunomodulatory agents among anti-myeloma treatments stand out as having a considerable prothrombotic effect. Recognizing the significant risk associated with the use of immunomodulatory agents (IMiDs), the International Myeloma Working Group (IMWG) 2014 statement [13], and the European Myeloma Network Guidelines in 2015 [14] both included guidance on the prevention of VTE in MM patients who receive IMiDs. The risk stratification algorithm proposed is based mostly on expert opinion and the available data from clinical trials [15–20]. The National Comprehensive Cancer Network (NCCN) guidelines use a similar framework and include patients that receive non-IMiD-based regimens [21] (Table 1).

Table 1. International Myeloma Working Group, European Myeloma Network, and National Comprehensive Cancer Network risk stratification algorithm and choice of thromboprophylaxis in patients with multiple myeloma. IMiD: immunomodulatory agent, MM: multiple myeloma, VTE: venous thromboembolism.

Algorithm for MM Patient Risk Stratification		
Patient-Related Risk Factors *ASSIGN 1 Point for Each of the below:*	**Disease-Related Risk Factors:** *Assign 1 Point for Each of the below:*	**Treatment-Related Risk Factors:** *Assign Points as Seen below:*
Body mass index >25, Age >75, Personal or family history of VTE, Central venous catheter, Acute infection or Hospitalization, Blood clotting disorders or Thrombophilia, Immobility with performance status of >1, Comorbidities (liver, renal impairment, chronic obstructive pulmonary disorder, diabetes mellitus, chronic inflammatory bowel disease), Race (Caucasian is a risk factor)	• Diagnosis of multiple myeloma • Evidence of hyperviscosity	• IMiD in combination with low-dose dexamethasone (<480 mg/month) *(1 point)* • IMiD plus high-dose dexamethasone (>480 mg/month) or doxorubicin or multiagent chemotherapy *(2 points)* • IMiD alone *(1 point)* • Erythropoietin use *(1 point)*
Risk stratification and recommended thromboprophylaxis: 0 points: Low risk *None* 1 point: Intermediate risk *Aspirin at 100 mg* >1 points: High risk *Low molecular weight heparin at prophylactic dose or therapeutic dose of warfarin*		

These guidelines have been available since 2014; however, data from clinical trials demonstrate that the rates of residual VTE remain high [22–24]. Therefore, it is safe to conclude that the current risk stratification is suboptimal and fails to fully capture and distinguish between low, intermediate, and high-risk MM patients for VTE. At the same time, the extent to which the guidelines are implemented in everyday clinical practice can be questioned, increasing the complex task of assessing its effectiveness. Recent publications seem to support that most physicians tend to apply thromboprophylaxis based mostly on clinical experience. In a recent report, the rate of compliance with guidelines was only 66% in a cohort of patients who received lenalidomide-based regimens.

This review aims to highlight the multifaceted nature, the complexity, and heterogeneity that characterizes the prothrombotic environment that exists in the MM patient. It aims to demonstrate that optimum risk stratification and effective thromboprophylaxis can only be achieved through the development of a myeloma specific risk assessment models (RAM) for VTE. A RAM that includes clinical and treatment-specific risk factors in combination with disease-specific coagulation biomarkers can potentially successfully capture all aspects of the heterogenous prothrombotic environment that exists in MM patients. Research efforts need to further focus on the exploration and understanding of the interplay between markers of plasma and cellular coagulation and the MM microenvironment [25]. Following effective risk stratification, the most effective and safe tool for thromboprophylaxis needs to be established: the right agent for the right patient and for a sufficient amount of time. Increasingly, direct oral anticoagulants (DOACs) are gaining ground in the field of thrombosis treatment and venous thromboembolism prophylaxis. Randomized controlled trials are required that can provide robust data that support their use in the context of VTE prophylaxis in MM.

2. Understanding the Complex Procoagulant Profile of the MM Patient

To date, the understanding of the underlying processes that lead to enhanced coagulation in the MM patient has not been delineated. Table 2 summarizes the available data linking patient-related, disease-related, and treatment related risk factors with VTE occurrence.

Table 2. Risk factors associated with venous thromboembolism in multiple myeloma and studies that have reported the relevant association. CVC: central venous catheter, IMiD: immunomodulatory agent, CABG: coronary artery bypass graft, COPD: chronic obstructive pulmonary disease, NDMM: newly diagnosed multiple myeloma patients, DVT: deep vein thrombosis, NFκB1: nuclear factor kappa B subunit 1.

	Patient Related Risk Factors				
Age	Brown et al., 2016 [26] hazard of thrombosis for the 35–64 and 65–74 age groups compared to the 18–34 reference group, HR 2.8 for the 75 + age group (1.6–4.8 95% CI)	Baker et al. 2018 [22] Age not identified as risk factor for VTE ($p = 0.56$)	Bagratuni et al. 2013 [27] n = 200, VTEs were more frequent in patients >65 years (8.1% vs. 1.6%)		
Body mass index ≥30 kg/m^2 Family history Race	No specific studies in MM for these risk factors				
Personal history	Anaissie et al. 2012 [28] history of VTE was a strong predictor of VTE on univariate analysis ($p < 0.000005$) n = 604				
Cardiac disease (e.g., symptomatic coronary artery disease, congestive heart failure, or history of stent placement/CABG)	Brown et al. [26] congestive cardiac failure associated with hazard HR = 1.7 (95% CI, 1.4–2.1), hypertension associated with hazard (HR = 1.2 (95% CI, 1.0–1.3))				
Other comorbidity:	Diabetes mellitus, renal impairment, liver impairment, chronic inflammatory disease, COPD, immobilization, autoimmune disease, recent trauma or surgery, hospitalization, immobility, inherited thrombophilia, use of hormone replacement, acute infection *No specific data on these risk factors in patients with MM available*				
Use of erythropoietin (EPO)	Anaissie et al. 2012 [28] n = 604 prophylactic EPO ($p = 0.002$; OR, 2.488; 95% CI, 1.432–4.324)	Chalayer et al. 2018 [29] OR 0.49 (95% CI 0.18–3.83)	Knight et al. 2015 [30] n plus lenalidomide: OR 3.21 (1.72–6.01 95% CI, $p < 0.001$)	Galli et al. 2004 [31] n = 199, 8.1% prevalence with EPO vs. 9.3% without, $p > 0.5$)	Leleu et al. 2013 [5] Relative RIsk of VTE 3.46 (0.45–3.7 95% CI, $p = 0.04$)
Central venous catheter or pacemaker	Cortelezzi et al. 2005 [32] 12% VTE events in 416 patients with hematologic malignancies and CVC insertion (MM diagnosis seen in 18.8% of pts)				
	Disease-specific risk factors				
New diagnosis of MM	Zangari et al. 2003 [33] (n = 535) newly diagnosed disease (OR, 2.5; $p = 0.001$)				
Chromosome 11 abnormalities	Zangari et al. 2003 [33] (n = 535) (OR, 1.8; $p = 0.048$)				
Microparticle (MP)-associated tissue factor and tissue factor (TF)	Auwerda et al. 2011 [34]: (n = 122) NDMM; MP-TF levels prior to treatment initiation did not predict VTE, but MP-TF remained elevated in patients who developed VTE 15.1 [10.3–25.2], in contrast to patients not developing VTE (11.4 [7.0–25.2], $p < 0.001$				
Thrombin lag phase(s)	Undas et al. 2015 [35] 60 [52–60.5] vs. 50 [36–45], $p = 0.01$ in patients with VTE				
Thrombin peak concentration (nmol/L)	Undas et al. 2015 [35] higher peak concentration associated with VTE; 503.5 (418–550) vs. 344.8 (269–411) in patients without VTE, $p < 0.001$	Leiba et al. 2017 [45] higher peak height values (620 vs. 400 nM, $p < 0.001$) associated with higher VTE risk	Chalayer et al. 2018 [29] 186 nmol/L for patient with VTE vs. 149 nmol/L for not VTE, $p = 0.22$ in univariate analysis	Ay et al. 2011 [25] associated with VTE risk	
Thrombin peak time (min)	Chalayer et al. 2018 [29] at baseline; 10.8 min for patients with VTE vs. 9 min for no VTE, $p = 0.82$ in univariate analysis, no significant association with VTE		Ay et al. 2011 [25] associated with VTE risk		

Table 2. Cont.

Endogenous thrombin potential (ETP) (Mxmin)	Dargaud et al. 2019; ETP higher in MM patients versus controls [46]	Ay et al. 2011 [25] not associated with VTE risk	Leiba et al. 2017 [45] higher EPT (2896 vs. 2028 nMxmin, $p < 0.001$) associated with higher VTE risk	Chalayer et al. 2018 [29] increase in ETP between baseline and cycle 4—no association with VTE
Thrombin-activatable fibrinolysis inhibitor (TAFI) (mg/mL)	Undas et al. 2015 [35] higher levels associated with VTE 45.3 (44.6–47.4) vs. 38.9 (33.5–42.3) <0.001			
Plasminogen activator inhibitory (PAI-1) (IU/mL)	Undas et al. 2015; [35] higher PAI-1 levels associated with VTE risk 11 (9.9–12.8) vs. 8.3 (6.4–10.5), $p = 0.004$			
Lower clot permeability and clot lysis	Undas et al. 2015; [35] in patients with lower clot permeability Ks (10^{-9} cm^2) and lower D-D$_{rate}$, (maximum rate of increase in D-dimer levels in the lysis assay) associated with higher VTE risk			
Acquired activated protein C resistance (aAPC-R)	Zangari et al. 2002 [47] higher proportion of patients with APC resistance developed DVT (5/14 versus 7/38; $p = 0.04$)–41.7% prevalence of APC-R in the group of NDMM who developed VTE	Cini et al. 2010 [48] no difference in VTE occurrence between patients with APCR (6.7% vs. 10.3%, $p = 1.0$)		Elice et al. 2006 [49] higher incidence of VTE with aAPC-R; 1178 patients; 31% versus 12%; $p < 0.001$)
NFκB1 gene single nucleotide polymorphism	Bagratuni et al. 2013 [27] NFκB1 and VTE risk: OR 3.76, 95%CI 1–16, $p = 0.051$			
Factor v. Leiden (R506Q) or G20210A prothrombin mutation	Cini et al. [48] patients with polymorphisms had not increased VTE rate (10% vs. 9.4%, $p = 0.27$)		Bagratuni et al. 2013 [27] FVLeiden and FIIG20210A not associated with higher VTE rates	
P-selectin (ng/mL)	Ay et al. 2008 [50] Elevated P-selectin (>53.1 ng/mL) risk factor for VTE (HR = 2.6, 95% CI, 1.4–4.9, $p = 003$)			
vonWillenbrand (VWF) increased levels	Minnema et al. 2003 [51] N = 19 patients on thalidomide VWF-Ag in patients with VTE was 375 ± 121% vs. 235 ± 116% in patients without VTE ($p = 0.03$)		Van Marion et al. 2008 [52] higher levels of VWF not associated with VTE OR 2.69 95% CI 0.71–10.26, $p = 0.147$	
FVIII (factor VIII)	Minnema et al. 2003 [51] N = 19 patients on thalidomide FVIII:C was 352 ± 67% vs. 283 ± 114% in patients without VTE ($p = 0.17$)	Cini et al. 2010: [48] elevated FVIII activity not associated with higher VTE rate (10% vs. 7.4% $p = 0.76$)		Van Marion et al. 2008 [52] higher levels of FVIII not associated with VTE occurrence
Other biomarkers	Increased D-dimer levels, prothrombin 1 and 2 increased levels, hyperviscosity, antiphospholipid antibodies, lupus anticoagulant—resistance to protein C pathway. No data on these biomarkers and VTE risk			
Myeloma Therapy Related [53]				

- IMiD in combination with:

  High-dose dexamethasone (>480 mg/month)
  Multi-agent chemotherapy
  Doxorubicin

- IMiD alone

2.1. Patient-Related Risk Factors

Standard VTE risk factors that are specific to the patient's characteristics, past medical and surgical history, and current medications are included in the risk assessment. Age, renal impairment, immobility, and frequent hospitalizations due to immunoparesis and immunosuppression are all very relevant to the MM patient [32]. Studies have shown that the incidence of common thrombophilic polymorphisms in MM (factor V Leiden and PTG20210A polymorphism) is similar to that of the general population [27,48].

These are all well-recognized VTE risk factors, and there are no studies specific to MM that demonstrate their association with an increased risk of venous thromboembolism.

2.2. Disease-Specific Risk Factors and the Search for a Biomarker

The mechanisms underlying the prothrombotic environment observed in MM are not understood up to date. A number of plasma and cellular biomarkers of coagulation have been studied by several groups at various timepoints prior to, during, and post-treatment initiation. No group has yet identified a biomarker that accurately reflects prothrombotic risk in these patients and can be combined with clinical factors to enhance risk stratification.

The diagnosis of MM itself is a risk factor, as a newly diagnosed MM patient is at higher risk of VTE compared to a patient with relapsed or recurrent disease. A hypercoagulable environment in MM is sustained by increased levels of inflammatory cytokines and other factors of coagulation. Fibrinolysis and fibrin polymerization is also disrupted due to interference by the monoclonal component [3,12,36–39,54]. Platelet dysfunction and increased adhesion have been reported in patients with MM, which may also explain the demonstrated efficacy of aspirin as an agent for thromboprophylaxis in MM patients [38,40,41]. Some reports have also shown Lupus Antibody Coagulant (LAC)-like activity by the monoclonal component and the presence of antibodies against antithrombin and protein C and S or resistance to the activated protein C pathway [35,39,42–44]. Microparticles (MP), either tissue factor or platelet derived (TF-MP or PDMP), also seem to contribute to the procoagulant environment and are perhaps linked to VTE occurrence [34,55].

Thrombin generation (TG) is being increasingly studied by many groups who perform measurements at baseline and during treatment as well as explore the association with VTE occurrence. Most groups have reported abnormal TG in multiple parameters of the assay compared to healthy controls [56,57]. Data is variable and difficult to compare across studies as different TG assays have been used as well as different TG trigger concentrations and phospholipid reagents. Crowley et al. compared TG in MM patients, patients with Monoclonal gammopathy of undetermined significance (MGUS), and healthy controls, and found endogenous thrombin potential (ETP) to be lower, the lag time shorter, the peak shorter, and the velocity index higher in MM patients [58]. Legendre et al. in 2018 also found TG to be attenuated compared to healthy controls with prolonged lag time and time to peak with decreased peak and ETP [59]. Ay et al. demonstrated a significant association between thrombin peak concentration and time to Peak concentration (ttPeak) and VTE risk [25], and Leiba et al. found significantly higher ETP and peak thrombin concentration in patients who developed VTE compared to those who did not [45]. Another group recently published data on 71 patients with MM and performed a serial analysis of thrombin generation parameters during the first four cycles of treatment. TG parameters remained unchanged throughout treatment irrespective of treatment regimen, but they were significantly higher before cycles 2 and 3 for patients who received IMiDs. No association was determined between baseline levels of ETP, thrombin peak concentration, or time to peak and VTE [29]. In another study of 106 MM patients, the TG capacity was higher in MM patients both in platelet-poor plasma (PPP) and platelet-rich plasma (PRP). In PRP, TG was significantly higher in patients treated with lenalidomide compared to MM patients who did not receive IMiDs [46]. In a recent publication by our group as part of the ongoing ROADMAP-MM-CAT (PROspective Risk Assessment anD bioMArkers of hypercoagulability for the identification of patients with Multiple Myeloma at risk for Cancer-Associated Thrombosis) study, VTE risk was shown to be associated with longer procoagulant phospholipid-dependent clotting time (PPL-ct)® and lower endogenous thrombin potential (ETP) in patients with newly diagnosed multiple myeloma (NDMM). In this cohort of 144 patients, thrombin generation was unexpectedly attenuated compared to healthy controls [60].

The search for a useful biomarker continues through the exploration of the complex coagulation of MM patients.

2.3. Treatment-Related Risk Factors

The effects and the contribution of different anti-myeloma agents on VTE risk are the best understood among different risk factors. The use of IMiDs in the era of novel agents (thalidomide and its derivatives lenalidomide and pomalidomide) has been associated with a rise in VTE occurrence in the MM population. Thalidomide or lenalidomide (Len) monotherapy does not contribute significantly to the baseline VTE risk. It is reported to be around 3%–4% but can increase up to 26% with the addition of high dose dexamethasone or multi-agent chemotherapy or anthracyclines [39,40,48,61–64]. The rates are also low with Len maintenance post-autologous stem cell transplant (ASCT) without thromboprophylaxis, and one group reported a 6% VTE rate during a median follow up of 45 months [65]. The associated VTE risk persists over time and does not decrease as the duration of exposure increases [66,67]. Data on lenalidomide-associated VTE risk are presented more extensively in Table 3. Fewer data exist on thrombotic risk linked to pomalidomide, which is lower compared to lenalidomide but may reflect the current mandatory use of thromboprophylaxis [68]. Reported VTE rates vary depending on the dose of pomalidomide and range from 3–7% with 4 mg pomalidomide combined with dexamethasone to 0%–6% with 2 mg plus dexamethasone [69–71]. Among proteasome inhibitors, the use of bortezomib is associated with very low VTE rates and might even have a protective effect when combined with thrombogenic agents [72]. The data on the potential thrombogenic or thromboprotective effects of the second-generation protasome inhibitor, carfilzomib, is not as clear yet, and more studies are required [73]. Increased VTE risk does not seem to be one of the adverse events linked to elotozumab, daratumumab, or ixazomib among the available approved drugs for MM patients [74–79].

The exact mechanisms underlying the IMiD-induced thrombogenic effect are not known. Association studies so far have hypothesized a role for increased vonWillenbrand factor (VWF), factor VIII, and tissue factor (TF), which mediate procoagulant effects on endothelial cells. There is also enhanced platelet activation and aggregation and reports for activated protein C resistance mediated by cytokines [80]. Individual immune response and modulation might affect the effect of thalidomide on platelet activation, as immune modulation may lead to an early clearance of activated platelets [81]. High-dose dexamethasone increases the P-selectin, VWF, and FVIII levels [82], and doxorubicin seems to induce a procoagulant phenotype on endothelial cells and to increase the levels of plasma thrombin that is generated [83]. There is some data to support that lenalidomide use upregulated cathepsin G and increases the levels of endothelial stress markers sch as intercellular adhesion molecule 1 (ICAM), plasminogen activator inhibitor -1 (PAI-1), and vascular endothelial growth factor (VEGF). Higher levels of P-selectin, fibrinogen, and homocysteine following lenalidomide treatment have also been reported. The transient thrombocytopenia observed with the administration of bortezomib, and its anti-thrombotic effect is likely to be exerted via the inhibitory effects on the 26 S proteasome [80,84].

Table 3. Clinical risk assessment models for VTE prediction in MM patients. RAM: risk assessment model; VTE: venous thromboembolism; MM: multiple myeloma; BMI: body mass index; CVC: central venous catheter; LMWH: low molecular weight heparin.

CLINICAL RAMs for VTE in MM	
IMPEDE VTE Score	SAVED Score*

Immunomodulatory drug (+4)
 BMI ≥ 25 kg/m^2 (+1)
 Pathologic fracture pelvis/femur (+4)
 Erythropoiesis-stimulating agent (+1)
 Dexamethasone (High-dose) (+4)
 Dexamethasone Low-Dose (+2)
 Doxorubicin (+3)
 Ethnicity/Race = Asian (−3)
 VTE history (+5)
 Tunneled line/CVC (+2)
 Existing use of therapeutic warfarin or low molecular weight heparin (LMWH) (−5)
 Existing use of prophylactic LMWH or aspirin (−3)
	Surgery (within last 90 days) (+2)
	 Asian Race (−3)
	 VTE history (+3)
	 Eight (age >=80 years) (+1)
	 Dexamethasone dose
	     Standard (+1)
	     High (+2)
	 * for patients on IMiD-based regimens only

Stratified risk groups based on weighted scoring system	
Low risk (score ≤3) Intermediate-risk (score of 4–7) High risk (≥8 score)	High risk (score ≥2) Low risk (≤1)
Missing: recommendation on thromboprophylaxis based on risk groups	

3. Risk Assessment Tools

3.1. Guidelines and Clinical Practice

Table 1 summarizes the risk factors included in the algorithm proposed by IWMG, European myeloma network (EMN), and (National comprehensive cancer network (NCCN) guidelines. As discussed previously, the value of these guidelines is questioned given the residual rate of

VTE observed in recent trials, despite the use of thromboprophylaxis. In addition, clinicians tend to rely more on their own clinical experience rather than trust and apply the algorithm. In the Myeloma XI study, despite using thromboprophylaxis according to the IMWG guidelines for a minimum of 3 months with low molecular weight heparin (LMWH) for high-risk patients and aspirin for low-risk patients, the VTE rate was 11.8% and was highest during the first six months following diagnosis. In addition, the mode of thromboprophylaxis patients used was often inconsistent with the initial risk stratification [13,15]. Therefore, the proposed algorithm seems to fail to minimize events and optimally identify patients at high risk for VTE. A retrospective data analysis of the implementation and effectiveness of the IMWG guidelines demonstrated that among the patients that experienced a VTE event, 18% had been stratified as low risk prior to treatment initiation at baseline and 82% had been stratified as high risk. There was no association between the initial risk stratification and the mode of thromboprophylaxis of use. Therefore, it was demonstrated that guideline concordance in terms of either aspirin (ASA) or LMWH was lower than expected [22].

3.2. Risk Assessment Models

All clinical trials that currently involve the use of IMiDs either in newly diagnosed or recurrent/relapsed disease recommend thromboprophylaxis based on the IMWG guidelines. However, residual VTE rates clearly point out the suboptimal nature of the current tools. In addition, outside clinical trials, the rates of compliance and consistent use of the algorithms are low. More sensitive risk stratification tools are required that can capture all aspects of the prothrombotic profile observed in the MM patient.

The importance and the clinical benefit of using risk assessment models (RAM) for thrombosis in cancer patients have become established in recent years since the development of the Khorana risk score in 2008 [85]. The Khorana score cannot be extended to MM patients, as it does not accurately predict VTE in the MM population [86]. A RAM specific for MM that includes treatment-related parameters to adequate reflect thrombotic risk is required. The value of incorporating biomarkers into clinical RAMs has been shown previously as the incorporation of P-selectin and D-dimers into the Vienna prediction score improved the sensitivity and specificity of the original Khorana score for chemotherapy-related VTE risk in patients with solid tumors [87].

Two clinical RAMs were published in 2019 using retrospective data from databases. Sanfilippo et al. published in 2019 the IMPEDE VTE risk clinical score for MM patients based on retrospective data from the Veterans Administration Central Cancer Registry in 4446 MM patients (for a definition of IMPEDE, see Table 3). Weighting was applied to various patient-specific risk factors for patients with MM (Table 3). Three risk groups were identified, and the respective six-month cumulative incidence of VTE following treatment initiation was 3.3% for the low-risk group (scores ≤3), 8.3% for intermediate-risk group (score of 4–7), and 15.2% for the high-risk group (≥8 score). The score was externally validated using the Surveillance, Epidemiology, End Results (SEER)–Medicare database and 4256 MM patients [88]. A second group also developed a clinical RAM for MM patients who receive IMiD-based regimens using the same database to extract data retrospectively; 2397 patients with MM were selected initially using the SEER database, and the data were subsequently validated using the Veterans registry. Five variables were included in the SAVED Score RAM (Surgery, Asian race, VTE history, Eighty years old, Dexamethasone) (see Table 3) [89]. Patients were grouped into either low or high risk using this RAM, and the hazard ratios were reported for high versus low VTE risk were 1.85 ($p < 0.01$) and 1.98 ($p < 0.01$), respectively. The authors argue in favor of the higher discriminative power of the SAVED score compared to the algorithm proposed by the NCCN guidelines. Despite the fact that the two scores were developed and validated in similar settings, there are significant differences. One reason could be linked to the fact that the SAVED score was developed selecting only MM patients receiving IMiDs. The methodological approach followed is also not identical. Finally, each score possibly captures VTE risk in a unique manner; however it has significant overlap with the other score, given the particularly multifaceted nature of thrombosis in MM patients.

4. Thromboprophylaxis: To DOAC or Not To DOAC?

Robust clinical data to support the use of one pharmacological agent over the other in MM patients as thromboprophylaxis are missing. Factors to consider are effectiveness and safety as well as convenience. Essential issues in the MM patient also include renal dosing, cut-offs for use in the context of thrombocytopenias, and frailty associated with the elderly.

The rationale underlying the use of aspirin as thromboprophylaxis in low-risk MM patients who receive IMiDs lies with the evidence that supports enhanced platelet activation induced by IMiDs and altered platelet function in patients with MM [36,40,62,81]. Most clinicians chose the 100 mg dose, despite the lack of robust data to support it. One of the few RCTs ever designed to address the question of thromboprophylaxis in MM did not demonstrate a significant difference in VTE occurrence when the use of aspirin was compared to enoxaparin in a group of MM patients who received IMiD-based regimens [19]. Another RCT that compared ASA and fixed low-dose warfarin (1.25 mg/day) to LMWH (enoxaparin 40 mg/day) as agents of VTE prevention in 667 NDMM patients who received thalidomide also did not demonstrate a significant difference between the three agents; the rate of VTE was 6.3% in the ASA group, 8.2% in the warfarin group, and 5% in LMWH group [18]. The Myeloma XI study included protocol-based thrombosis risk assessment. Among patients who experienced a VTE, 9.2% were on therapeutic dose of warfarin, 44.1% were on LMWH (prophylactic dose), and 31% were on aspirin. However, given the baseline risk stratification, a direct comparison is not possible [24]. The VTE rate of 10.7% versus 1.4% for patients who received aspirin versus LMWH respectively in a recent retrospective review of over 1126 patients demonstrates the suboptimal protective effect of aspirin as thromboprophylaxis even in low-risk patients and adds controversy to its role [90]. Its use is discouraged during the initial months of treatment initiation when the VTE risk is highest for NDMM patients. It remains an option for later timepoints during disease remission [91,92].

Prophylactic LMWH is currently the standard of care based on guidelines by the IMWG, EMN, and NCCN and based on approve indications for use of this drug group. Most clinicians favor LMWH compared to warfarin particularly for patients with cyclical cytopenias, who are at higher bleeding risk. Patient compliance given the parenteral method of administration remains an issue. Two other important disadvantages of LMWH compared to warfarin include cost and the need for renal adjustment.

Currently, the most favored class of drugs are DOACs. They are inhibitors of clotting factors Xa or IIa, they are administered orally, and they do not require blood monitoring at standard doses. DOACs have been licensed for the treatment of cancer-associated thrombosis, but their role is thromboprophylaxis for these patients remains unclear up to date, as there is not enough robust data yet to support this use [93]. In a retrospective review that assessed the safety and efficacy of DOACs (dabigatran, rivaroxaban, or apixaban) versus warfarin in patients on IMiD-based regimens, there were four non-major bleeds in the DOAC group versus six in the warfarin group [94]. One group compared the VTE event rate prior and post 2014 and the introduction of a policy change in their center to use apixaban 2.5 mg twice daily as routine thromboprophylaxis for patients on IMiDs. Before 2014, the VTE rate was 20.7% in patients on aspirin and 7.4% in patients on LMWH compared to no VTE events after 2014 within six months of treatment initiation [95]. There is an ongoing single-arm phase IV study (NCT02958969) that aims to evaluate prospectively the safety and efficacy of apixaban for primary VTE prevention in MM patients. The primary objective is to assess VTE occurrence within six months in patients who receive IMiD-based therapy [96]. At interim analysis at three months, no VTE events and no major hemorrhage was reported [96]. Pergourie et al. also recently presented data from the use of apixaban as prophylaxis in MM patients on IMiDs. Two events were reported among 140 patients receiving apixaban 2.5 mg twice daily over six months [97]. DOACs are substrates of P-glycoprotein and P450; therefore an important issue to note with their use compared to the other classes of drugs is the potential drug–drug interactions. Fortunately, no anti-myeloma agent (excluding dexamethasone) is known to be a potent inhibitor or inducer of these pathways [98–100]. However, an additional issue associated with the oral route of administration is polypharmacy, which is very relevant in these patients.

Important issues to consider when deciding upon the most suitable mode of pharmacological thromboprophylaxis for the MM patients include age and associated frailty, cyclical platelet counts due to bone marrow infiltration, and the cytotoxic effects of chemotherapy in addition to renal clearance. For patients with GFR <30 mL/min, most clinicians opt for unfractionated heparin and warfarin or LMWH adjusted to anti-Xa levels. Both DOACs and LMWHs are contraindicated in patients with a glomerular filtration (GFR) rate <30 mL/min. Patients with end-stage disease are usually excluded from clinical trials; therefore, there is a paucity of data for this subgroup of patients [101]. The summary of product characteristics of each class of DOAC provides information on renal dosing adjustments [101]. Currently, using unfractionated heparin or LMWH adjusted to anti-Xa levels is considered the most legitimate option for patients with end-stage renal disease. As more safety and efficacy becomes available, DOACs are increasingly being opted for on a case-by-case basis, even for these patients [102]. The patient with thrombocytopenia is another challenge, as clear-cut instructions and thresholds for the use of different agents are absent. Most clinicians would use the empirical cut off of 50,000/mm^3 for the administration of full LMWH administration and would half the dose for platelet counts between 49,000 and 30,000 mm^3 [103–105]. Based again on clinical experience, DOAC administration is considered safe at platelet counts of >50,000/mm^3 when the indication is treatment of VTE and at >75–80.000/μL when the indication is prophylaxis [106].

Data from ongoing RCTs are much anticipated. Robust evidence that will demonstrate the effectiveness and safety of DOACs and will guide their use among different MM patient populations in the newly diagnosed and relapsed/refractory setting is required. To establish their use in this field, there is also a need for RCTs specifically designed to compared different modes of thromboprophylaxis in MM patients.

5. Conclusions and Recommendations

Existing 2014 IMWG guidelines (and 2016 EMN guidelines) propose baseline risk stratification for MM patients on IMiDs and the use of aspirin for low-risk patients and prophylactic dose LMWH for higher-risk patients. The rate of residual VTE rate reported from recent RCTs remains high, signifying the limited power of this risk stratification tool in accurately reflecting all aspects of the diverse procoagulant environment that exists in MM patients [24,60]. In addition, the extent to which the available algorithm is being applied in every day clinical practice is questionable. There is also a lack of formal recommendations for patients on non-IMiD-containing regimens [13,22,24]. There is the need for optimization of the current tool utilizing a risk assessment model (RAM) that combines disease-specific, patient-specific, and treatment specific risk factors to accurately stratify VTE risk and guide thromboprophylaxis.

The IMPEDE and the SAVED scores for VTE risk are clinical scores that have been developed retrospectively and therefore retain the advantage of a very large dataset. Weighting of the risk factors included is expected to improve their performance comparative to the current IMWG/NCCN guidelines. They both include only patient-specific risk factors and treatment-related parameters. MM-specific parameters are missing from the RAM, although there is currently no evidence to support a direct link between ISS stage, disease burden, cytogenetics, or any other disease characteristic to VTE occurrence. It should be noted that none of the groups make recommendations for thromboprophylaxis based on the proposed risk stratification. They are both simple and easy to calculate, but prospective validation will be required prior to their incorporation into clinical practice. Currently, no risk assessment tool makes a distinction between NDMM and relapsed and/or refractory MM patients (RRMM) patients. A new MM should perhaps in the future be included in RAMs as an additional risk factor. The question of whether the performance of these RAMs can be improved by the incorporation of a biomarker remains to be answered, but they could both serve as a backbone for the incorporation of additional parameters.

Given the complexities and heterogeneity of the VTE risk in the MM population, some groups have turned their research efforts toward the identification of a generic coagulation biomarker that can accurately reflect VTE risk and can be incorporated into a clinical RAM to increase its sensitivity. Such a task is demanding, given the complex and heterogeneous coagulation profile of the myeloma patient. Thrombin generation, P-selectin, platelet-derived microparticles, and procoagulant phospholipid clotting time are some of the biomarkers that have been studied. To date, no such biomarker has been identified [45,59,60]. Low-cost and simple assessment tools that do not require high-level expertise are prerequisites for the selection of a suitable biomarker. The prospective ongoing ROADMAP-MM-CAT is exploring the coagulation profile of the MM patient in the attempt to identify a marker of coagulation that can be incorporated into a clinical and disease-specific RAM.

Exploration of the complex interactions between the MM microenvironment and cellular and plasma coagulability should continue, as the understanding of the underlying mechanisms and interactions will eventually allow risk assessment optimization. At the same time, the effect of current and emerging treatments on the underlying pathways should be studied and understood. The inability to identify so far a generic biomarker to accurately reflect the above processes is perhaps a reflection of the complex and heterogeneous coagulation profile of MM patients, which results from the interaction of multiple factors.

Current recommendations propose the use of aspirin and LMWH. However, DOACs are becoming increasingly popular. Their profile is favorable, as secondary to safety and efficacy, they are administered orally and do not require routine monitoring. They are currently licensed for use in the treatment of cancer-associated thrombosis [93,107,108]. Ongoing trials will most likely establish their use in VTE prophylaxis in ambulatory cancer patients as well, and the results are much anticipated [107]. More prospective data on their use will of course be required to establish their role in the field of thromboprophylaxis. In addition, the disadvantages of using an oral administration route (diarrhea, vomiting, drug-to-drug interactions) should be taken into account. Recently, updated NCCN guidelines for cancer-associated thrombosis and thromboprophylaxis have included DOACs for the first time. Randomized controlled trials (RCTs) are required and designed to provide head-to-head comparisons of different methods of pharmacological thromboprophylaxis. These should use clear-cut risk stratification criteria to allow the generation of robust data on safety and efficacy. In addition, trials that include MM patients with renal impairment and thrombocytopenia are required to address the unanswered question of which mode of thromboprophylaxis to use for these patients. An update of the IMWG and EMN guidelines regarding MM VTE risk assessment and thromboprophylaxis is very much needed and eagerly anticipated.

Potential Algorithm for Risk Stratification of Patients

Figure 1 summarizes an ideal/future algorithm for VTE risk prediction. It uses information from current IMWG and EMN guidelines, data from RCTs, emerging data on DOACs, retrospective MM VTE risk prediction clinical scores, clinical experience, and anticipated future advances in the field. The weighting of clinical and disease-specific risk factors should be made based on the IMPEDE risk score, which should be incorporated in the RAM following prospective validation. A biomarker of coagulation that accurately reflects the prothrombotic environment of the MM patient and can be easily assessed using point-of-care tests should be incorporated into the RAM to increase its sensitivity and optimize its performance. DOACs are expected to replace LMWH, warfarin, and aspirin use. Given the heterogeneity of the MM patient profile and the complex interplay between different factors, we propose that four different levels of VTE risk should be included: no risk, low VTE risk, high risk, and very high risk.

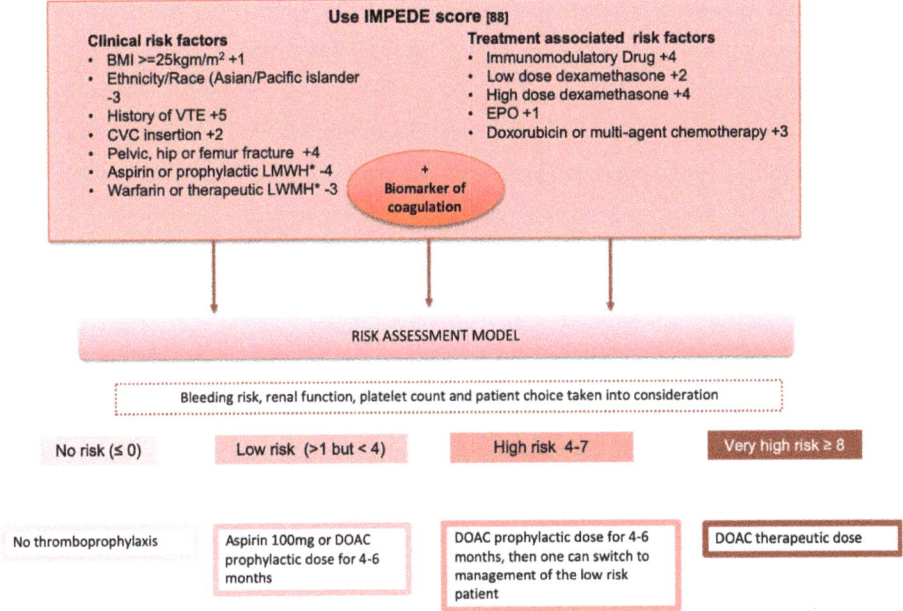

Figure 1. Algorithm for VTE risk assessment and thromboprophylaxis based on Table 1 risk factors; BMI: body mass index, CVC: central venous catheter, LMWH: low molecular weight heparin, EPO: erythropoietin, DOAC: direct oral anticoagulants. * Aspirin, LMWH, or warfarin for other clinical indication prior to treatment initiation for MM.

Funding: This research received no external funding.

Conflicts of Interest: The authors declare no conflict of interest.

References

1. Cesarman-Maus, G.; Braggio, E.; Fonseca, R. Thrombosis in multiple myeloma (MM). *Hematology* **2012**, *17* (Suppl. 1), S177–S180. [CrossRef] [PubMed]
2. Falanga, A.; Marchetti, M. Venous thromboembolism in the hematologic malignancies. *J. Clin. Oncol.* **2009**, *27*, 4848–4857. [CrossRef] [PubMed]
3. De Stefano, V.; Za, T.; Rossi, E. Venous thromboembolism in multiple myeloma. *Semin. Thromb. Hemost.* **2014**, *40*, 338–347. [CrossRef] [PubMed]
4. Kristinsson, S.Y. Thrombosis in multiple myeloma. *Hematol. Am. Soc. Hematol. Educ. Program* **2010**, *2010*, 437–444. [CrossRef] [PubMed]
5. Leleu, X.; Rodon, P.; Hulin, C.; Daley, L.; Dauriac, C.; Hacini, M.; Decaux, O.; Eisemann, J.C.; Fitoussi, O.; Lioure, B.; et al. MELISSE, a large multicentric observational study to determine risk factors of venous thromboembolism in patients with multiple myeloma treated with immunomodulatory drugs. *Thromb. Haemost.* **2013**, *110*, 844–851. [CrossRef] [PubMed]
6. Kristinsson, S.Y.; Pfeiffer, R.M.; Bjorkholm, M.; Schulman, S.; Landgren, O. Thrombosis is associated with inferior survival in multiple myeloma. *Haematologica* **2012**, *97*, 1603–1607. [CrossRef] [PubMed]
7. Schoen, M.W.; Luo, S.; Gage, B.; Carson, K.R.; Sanfilippo, K.M. Association of venous thromboembolism with increased mortality in patients with multiple myeloma. *J. Clin. Oncol.* **2018**. [CrossRef]
8. Khorana, A.A.; Dalal, M.R.; Lin, J.; Connolly, G.C. Health care costs associated with venous thromboembolism in selected high-risk ambulatory patients with solid tumors undergoing chemotherapy in the United States. *Clin. Outcomes Res.* **2013**, *5*, 101–108. [CrossRef]

9. Lee, A.Y. Anticoagulation in the treatment of established venous thromboembolism in patients with cancer. *J. Clin. Oncol.* **2009**, *27*, 4895–4901. [CrossRef]
10. Rajkumar, S.V. Value and Cost of Myeloma Therapy. *Am. Soc. Clin. Oncol. Educ. Book* **2018**, *38*, 662–666. [CrossRef]
11. Huang, H.; Li, H.; Li, D. Effect of serum monoclonal protein concentration on haemostasis in patients with multiple myeloma. *Blood Coagul. Fibrinolysis* **2015**, *26*, 555–559. [CrossRef] [PubMed]
12. Kwaan, H.C. Hyperviscosity in plasma cell dyscrasias. *Clin. Hemorheol. Microcirc.* **2013**, *55*, 75–83. [CrossRef] [PubMed]
13. Palumbo, A.; Rajkumar, S.V.; San Miguel, J.F.; Larocca, A.; Niesvizky, R.; Morgan, G.; Landgren, O.; Hajek, R.; Einsele, H.; Anderson, K.C.; et al. International Myeloma Working Group consensus statement for the management, treatment, and supportive care of patients with myeloma not eligible for standard autologous stem-cell transplantation. *J. Clin. Oncol.* **2014**, *32*, 587–600. [CrossRef] [PubMed]
14. Terpos, E.; Kleber, M.; Engelhardt, M.; Zweegman, S.; Gay, F.; Kastritis, E.; van de Donk, N.W.; Bruno, B.; Sezer, O.; Broijl, A.; et al. European Myeloma Network guidelines for the management of multiple myeloma-related complications. *Haematologica* **2015**, *100*, 1254–1266. [CrossRef]
15. Palumbo, A.; Rajkumar, S.V.; Dimopoulos, M.A.; Richardson, P.G.; San Miguel, J.; Barlogie, B.; Harousseau, J.; Zonder, J.A.; Cavo, M.; Zangari, M.; et al. Prevention of thalidomide- and lenalidomide-associated thrombosis in myeloma. *Leukemia* **2008**, *22*, 414–423. [CrossRef]
16. Dimopoulos, M.A.; Leleu, X.; Palumbo, A.; Moreau, P.; Delforge, M.; Cavo, M.; Ludwig, H.; Morgan, G.J.; Davies, F.E.; Sonneveld, P.; et al. Expert panel consensus statement on the optimal use of pomalidomide in relapsed and refractory multiple myeloma. *Leukemia* **2014**, *28*, 1573–1585. [CrossRef]
17. Dimopoulos, M.A.; Palumbo, A.; Attal, M.; Beksac, M.; Davies, F.E.; Delforge, M.; Einsele, H.; Hajek, R.; Harousseau, J.L.; da Costa, F.L.; et al. Optimizing the use of lenalidomide in relapsed or refractory multiple myeloma: Consensus statement. *Leukemia* **2011**, *25*, 749–760. [CrossRef]
18. Palumbo, A.; Cavo, M.; Bringhen, S.; Zamagni, E.; Romano, A.; Patriarca, F.; Rossi, D.; Gentilini, F.; Crippa, C.; Galli, M.; et al. Aspirin, warfarin, or enoxaparin thromboprophylaxis in patients with multiple myeloma treated with thalidomide: A phase III, open-label, randomized trial. *J. Clin. Oncol.* **2011**, *29*, 986–993. [CrossRef]
19. Larocca, A.; Cavallo, F.; Bringhen, S.; Di Raimondo, F.; Falanga, A.; Evangelista, A.; Cavalli, M.; Stanevsky, A.; Corradini, P.; Pezzatti, S.; et al. Aspirin or enoxaparin thromboprophylaxis for patients with newly diagnosed multiple myeloma treated with lenalidomide. *Blood* **2012**, *119*, 933–939. [CrossRef]
20. Fotiou, D.; Gerotziafas, G.; Kastritis, E.; Dimopoulos, M.A.; Terpos, E. A review of the venous thrombotic issues associated with multiple myeloma. *Expert Rev. Hematol.* **2016**, *9*, 695–706. [CrossRef]
21. NCCN Clinical Practice Guidelines in Oncology (NCCN Guidelines): Cancer-Associated Venous Thromboembolic Disease. Available online: www.nccn.org/professionals/physician_gls/pdf/vte.pdf (accessed on 12 December 2019).
22. Baker, H.A.; Brown, A.R.; Mahnken, J.D.; Shireman, T.I.; Webb, C.E.; Lipe, B.C. Application of risk factors for venous thromboembolism in patients with multiple myeloma starting chemotherapy, a real-world evaluation. *Cancer Med.* **2018**. [CrossRef] [PubMed]
23. Paludo, J.; Mikhael, J.R.; LaPlant, B.R.; Halvorson, A.E.; Kumar, S.; Gertz, M.A.; Hayman, S.R.; Buadi, F.K.; Dispenzieri, A.; Lust, J.A.; et al. Pomalidomide, bortezomib, and dexamethasone for patients with relapsed lenalidomide-refractory multiple myeloma. *Blood* **2017**, *130*, 1198–1204. [CrossRef] [PubMed]
24. Bradbury, C. Thrombotic Events in Patients with Myeloma Treated with Immunomodulatory Drugs; Results of the Myeloma XI Study. *Blood* **2017**, *130*, 553.
25. Ay, C.; Dunkler, D.; Simanek, R.; Thaler, J.; Koder, S.; Marosi, C.; Zielinski, C.; Pabinger, I. Prediction of venous thromboembolism in patients with cancer by measuring thrombin generation: Results from the Vienna Cancer and Thrombosis Study. *J. Clin. Oncol.* **2011**, *29*, 2099–2103. [CrossRef] [PubMed]
26. Brown, J.D.; Adams, V.R. Incidence and Risk Factors of Thromboembolism with Multiple Myeloma in the Presence of Death as a Competing Risk: An Empirical Comparison of Statistical Methodologies. *Healthcare* **2016**, *4*, 16. [CrossRef] [PubMed]
27. Bagratuni, T.; Kastritis, E.; Politou, M.; Roussou, M.; Kostouros, E.; Gavriatopoulou, M.; Eleutherakis-Papaiakovou, E.; Kanelias, N.; Terpos, E.; Dimopoulos, M.A. Clinical and genetic factors associated with venous thromboembolism in myeloma patients treated with lenalidomide-based regimens. *Am. J. Hematol.* **2013**, *88*, 765–770. [CrossRef]

28. Anaissie, E.J.; Coleman, E.A.; Goodwin, J.A.; Kennedy, R.L.; Lockhart, K.D.; Stewart, C.B.; Coon, S.K.; Bailey, C.; Barlogie, B. Prophylactic recombinant erythropoietin therapy and thalidomide are predictors of venous thromboembolism in patients with multiple myeloma: Limited effectiveness of thromboprophylaxis. *Cancer* **2012**, *118*, 549–557. [CrossRef]
29. Chalayer, E.; Tardy-Poncet, B.; Karlin, L.; Chapelle, C.; Montmartin, A.; Piot, M.; Guyotat, D.; Collet, P.; Lecompte, T.; Tardy, B. Thrombin generation in newly diagnosed multiple myeloma during the first three cycles of treatment: An observational cohort study. *Res. Pract. Thromb. Haemost.* **2019**, *3*, 89–98. [CrossRef]
30. Knight, R.; DeLap, R.J.; Zeldis, J.B. Lenalidomide and venous thrombosis in multiple myeloma. *N. Engl. J. Med.* **2006**, *354*, 2079–2080. [CrossRef]
31. Galli, M.; Elice, F.; Crippa, C.; Comotti, B.; Rodeghiero, F.; Barbui, T. Recombinant human erythropoietin and the risk of thrombosis in patients receiving thalidomide for multiple myeloma. *Haematologica* **2004**, *89*, 1141–1142.
32. Cortelezzi, A.; Moia, M.; Falanga, A.; Pogliani, E.M.; Agnelli, G.; Bonizzoni, E.; Gussoni, G.; Barbui, T.; Mannucci, P.M.; Group, C.S. Incidence of thrombotic complications in patients with haematological malignancies with central venous catheters: A prospective multicentre study. *Br. J. Haematol.* **2005**, *129*, 811–817. [CrossRef] [PubMed]
33. Zangari, M.; Barlogie, B.; Thertulien, R.; Jacobson, J.; Eddleman, P.; Fink, L.; Fassas, A.; Van Rhee, F.; Talamo, G.; Lee, C.K.; et al. Thalidomide and deep vein thrombosis in multiple myeloma: Risk factors and effect on survival. *Clin. Lymphoma* **2003**, *4*, 32–35. [CrossRef] [PubMed]
34. Auwerda, J.J.; Yuana, Y.; Osanto, S.; de Maat, M.P.; Sonneveld, P.; Bertina, R.M.; Leebeek, F.W. Microparticle-associated tissue factor activity and venous thrombosis in multiple myeloma. *Thromb. Haemost.* **2011**, *105*, 14–20. [CrossRef] [PubMed]
35. Undas, A.; Zubkiewicz-Usnarska, L.; Helbig, G.; Woszczyk, D.; Kozinska, J.; Dmoszynska, A.; Debski, J.; Podolak-Dawidziak, M.; Kuliczkowski, K. Induction therapy alters plasma fibrin clot properties in multiple myeloma patients: Association with thromboembolic complications. *Blood Coagul. Fibrinolysis* **2015**, *26*, 621–627. [CrossRef]
36. Robak, M.; Trelinski, J.; Chojnowski, K. Hemostatic changes after 1 month of thalidomide and dexamethasone therapy in patients with multiple myeloma. *Med. Oncol.* **2012**, *29*, 3574–3580. [CrossRef]
37. Carr, M.E., Jr.; Dent, R.M.; Carr, S.L. Abnormal fibrin structure and inhibition of fibrinolysis in patients with multiple myeloma. *J. Lab. Clin. Med.* **1996**, *128*, 83–88. [CrossRef]
38. Carr, M.E., Jr.; Zekert, S.L. Abnormal clot retraction, altered fibrin structure, and normal platelet function in multiple myeloma. *Am. J. Physiol.* **1994**, *266*, H1195–H1201. [CrossRef]
39. Zamagni, E.; Brioli, A.; Tacchetti, P.; Zannetti, B.; Pantani, L.; Cavo, M. Multiple myeloma, venous thromboembolism, and treatment-related risk of thrombosis. *Semin. Thromb. Hemost.* **2011**, *37*, 209–219. [CrossRef]
40. Palumbo, A.; Palladino, C. Venous and arterial thrombotic risks with thalidomide: Evidence and practical guidance. *Adv. Drug Saf.* **2012**, *3*, 255–266. [CrossRef]
41. Baz, R.; Li, L.; Kottke-Marchant, K.; Srkalovic, G.; McGowan, B.; Yiannaki, E.; Karam, M.A.; Faiman, B.; Jawde, R.A.; Andresen, S.; et al. The role of aspirin in the prevention of thrombotic complications of thalidomide and anthracycline-based chemotherapy for multiple myeloma. *Mayo Clin. Proc.* **2005**, *80*, 1568–1574. [CrossRef]
42. Deitcher, S.R.; Erban, J.K.; Limentani, S.A. Acquired free protein S deficiency associated with multiple myeloma: A case report. *Am. J. Hematol.* **1996**, *51*, 319–323. [CrossRef]
43. Gruber, A.; Blasko, G.; Sas, G. Functional deficiency of protein C and skin necrosis in multiple myeloma. *Thromb. Res.* **1986**, *42*, 579–581. [CrossRef]
44. Yasin, Z.; Quick, D.; Thiagarajan, P.; Spoor, D.; Caraveo, J.; Palascak, J. Light-chain paraproteins with lupus anticoagulant activity. *Am. J. Hematol.* **1999**, *62*, 99–102. [CrossRef]
45. Leiba, M.; Malkiel, S.; Budnik, I.; Rozic, G.; Avigdor, A.; Duek, A.; Nagler, A.; Kenet, G.; Livnat, T. Thrombin generation as a predictor of thromboembolic events in multiple myeloma patients. *Blood Cells Mol. Dis.* **2017**, *65*, 1–7. [CrossRef]

46. Dargaud, Y.; Fouassier, M.; Bordet, J.C.; Ducastelle-Lepretre, S.; Dumontet, C.; Moreau, P.; Michallet, M. The challenge of myeloma-related thromboembolic disease: Can thrombin generation assay help physicians to better predict the thromboembolic risk and personalize anti-thrombotic prophylaxis? *Leuk. Lymphoma* **2019**, 1–4. [CrossRef]
47. Zangari, M.; Saghafifar, F.; Anaissie, E.; Badros, A.; Desikan, R.; Fassas, A.; Mehta, P.; Morris, C.; Toor, A.; Whitfield, D.; et al. Activated protein C resistance in the absence of factor V Leiden mutation is a common finding in multiple myeloma and is associated with an increased risk of thrombotic complications. *Blood Coagul. Fibrinolysis* **2002**, *13*, 187–192. [CrossRef]
48. Cini, M.; Zamagni, E.; Valdre, L.; Palareti, G.; Patriarca, F.; Tacchetti, P.; Legnani, C.; Catalano, L.; Masini, L.; Tosi, P.; et al. Thalidomide-dexamethasone as up-front therapy for patients with newly diagnosed multiple myeloma: Thrombophilic alterations, thrombotic complications, and thromboprophylaxis with low-dose warfarin. *Eur. J. Haematol.* **2010**, *84*, 484–492. [CrossRef]
49. Elice, F.; Fink, L.; Tricot, G.; Barlogie, B.; Zangari, M. Acquired resistance to activated protein C (aAPCR) in multiple myeloma is a transitory abnormality associated with an increased risk of venous thromboembolism. *Br. J. Haematol.* **2006**, *134*, 399–405. [CrossRef]
50. Ay, C.; Simanek, R.; Vormittag, R.; Dunkler, D.; Alguel, G.; Koder, S.; Kornek, G.; Marosi, C.; Wagner, O.; Zielinski, C.; et al. High plasma levels of soluble P-selectin are predictive of venous thromboembolism in cancer patients: Results from the Vienna Cancer and Thrombosis Study (CATS). *Blood* **2008**, *112*, 2703–2708. [CrossRef]
51. Minnema, M.C.; Fijnheer, R.; De Groot, P.G.; Lokhorst, H.M. Extremely high levels of von Willebrand factor antigen and of procoagulant factor VIII found in multiple myeloma patients are associated with activity status but not with thalidomide treatment. *J. Thromb. Haemost.* **2003**, *1*, 445–449. [CrossRef]
52. van Marion, A.M.; Auwerda, J.J.; Lisman, T.; Sonneveld, P.; de Maat, M.P.; Lokhorst, H.M.; Leebeek, F.W. Prospective evaluation of coagulopathy in multiple myeloma patients before, during and after various chemotherapeutic regimens. *Leuk. Res.* **2008**, *32*, 1078–1084. [CrossRef] [PubMed]
53. Fotiou, D.; Gavriatopoulou, M.; Ntanasis-Stathopoulos, I.; Migkou, M.; Dimopoulos, M.A.; Terpos, E. Updates on thrombotic events associated with multiple myeloma. *Expert Rev. Hematol.* **2019**, *12*, 355–365. [CrossRef] [PubMed]
54. Joseph, L.; Fink, L.M.; Hauer-Jensen, M. Cytokines in coagulation and thrombosis: A preclinical and clinical review. *Blood Coagul. Fibrinolysis* **2002**, *13*, 105–116. [CrossRef] [PubMed]
55. Nomura, S.; Ito, T.; Yoshimura, H.; Hotta, M.; Nakanishi, T.; Fujita, S.; Nakaya, A.; Satake, A.; Ishii, K. Evaluation of thrombosis-related biomarkers before and after therapy in patients with multiple myeloma. *J. Blood Med.* **2018**, *9*, 1–7. [CrossRef]
56. Petropoulou, A.D.; Gerotziafas, G.T.; Samama, M.M.; Hatmi, M.; Rendu, F.; Elalamy, I. In vitro study of the hypercoagulable state in multiple myeloma patients treated or not with thalidomide. *Thromb. Res.* **2008**, *121*, 493–497. [CrossRef]
57. Crowley, M.P.; Kevane, B.; O'Shea, S.I.; Quinn, S.; Egan, K.; Gilligan, O.M.; Ni Ainle, F. Plasma Thrombin Generation and Sensitivity to Activated Protein C Among Patients With Myeloma and Monoclonal Gammopathy of Undetermined Significance. *Clin. Appl. Thromb. Hemost* **2016**, *22*, 554–562. [CrossRef]
58. Tiong, I.S.; Rodgers, S.E.; Lee, C.H.; McRae, S.J. Baseline and treatment-related changes in thrombin generation in patients with multiple myeloma. *Leuk. Lymphoma* **2017**, *58*, 941–949. [CrossRef]
59. Legendre, P.; Verstraete, E.; Martin, M.; Poinsard, A.; Perrot, A.; Hulin, C.; Faure, G.; Latger-Cannard, V.; Perrin, J. Hypocoagulability as assessed by thrombin generation test in newly-diagnosed patients with multiple myeloma. *Blood Cells Mol. Dis.* **2017**, *66*, 47–49. [CrossRef]
60. Fotiou, D.; Sergentanis, T.N.; Papageorgiou, L.; Stamatelopoulos, K.; Gavriatopoulou, M.; Kastritis, E.; Psaltopoulou, T.; Salta, S.; Van Dreden, P.; Sangare, R.; et al. Longer procoagulant phospholipid-dependent clotting time, lower endogenous thrombin potential and higher tissue factor pathway inhibitor concentrations are associated with increased VTE occurrence in patients with newly diagnosed multiple myeloma: Results of the prospective ROADMAP-MM-CAT study. *Blood Cancer J.* **2018**, *8*, 102. [CrossRef]
61. Fouquet, G.; Tardy, S.; Demarquette, H.; Bonnet, S.; Gay, J.; Debarri, H.; Herbaux, C.; Guidez, S.; Michel, J.; Perrot, A.; et al. Efficacy and safety profile of long-term exposure to lenalidomide in patients with recurrent multiple myeloma. *Cancer* **2013**, *119*, 3680–3686. [CrossRef]

62. Rajkumar, S.V.; Jacobus, S.; Callander, N.S.; Fonseca, R.; Vesole, D.H.; Williams, M.E.; Abonour, R.; Siegel, D.S.; Katz, M.; Greipp, P.R.; et al. Lenalidomide plus high-dose dexamethasone versus lenalidomide plus low-dose dexamethasone as initial therapy for newly diagnosed multiple myeloma: An open-label randomised controlled trial. *Lancet Oncol.* **2010**, *11*, 29–37. [CrossRef]
63. Rosovsky, R.; Hong, F.; Tocco, D.; Connell, B.; Mitsiades, C.; Schlossman, R.; Ghobrial, I.; Lockridge, L.; Warren, D.; Bradwin, G.; et al. Endothelial stress products and coagulation markers in patients with multiple myeloma treated with lenalidomide plus dexamethasone: An observational study. *Br. J. Haematol.* **2013**, *160*, 351–358. [CrossRef]
64. Zonder, J.A.; Crowley, J.; Hussein, M.A.; Bolejack, V.; Moore, D.F., Sr.; Whittenberger, B.F.; Abidi, M.H.; Durie, B.G.; Barlogie, B. Lenalidomide and high-dose dexamethasone compared with dexamethasone as initial therapy for multiple myeloma: A randomized Southwest Oncology Group trial (S0232). *Blood* **2010**, *116*, 5838–5841. [CrossRef]
65. Attal, M.; Lauwers-Cances, V.; Marit, G.; Caillot, D.; Moreau, P.; Facon, T.; Stoppa, A.M.; Hulin, C.; Benboubker, L.; Garderet, L.; et al. Lenalidomide maintenance after stem-cell transplantation for multiple myeloma. *N. Engl. J. Med.* **2012**, *366*, 1782–1791. [CrossRef]
66. Palumbo, A.; Hajek, R.; Delforge, M.; Kropff, M.; Petrucci, M.T.; Catalano, J.; Gisslinger, H.; Wiktor-Jedrzejczak, W.; Zodelava, M.; Weisel, K.; et al. Continuous lenalidomide treatment for newly diagnosed multiple myeloma. *N. Engl. J. Med.* **2012**, *366*, 1759–1769. [CrossRef]
67. Dimopoulos, M.A.; Swern, A.S.; Li, J.S.; Hussein, M.; Weiss, L.; Nagarwala, Y.; Baz, R. Efficacy and safety of long-term treatment with lenalidomide and dexamethasone in patients with relapsed/refractory multiple myeloma. *Blood Cancer J.* **2014**, *4*, e257. [CrossRef]
68. Scott, L.J. Pomalidomide: A review of its use in patients with recurrent multiple myeloma. *Drugs* **2014**, *74*, 549–562. [CrossRef]
69. Richardson, P.G.; Siegel, D.S.; Vij, R.; Hofmeister, C.C.; Baz, R.; Jagannath, S.; Chen, C.; Lonial, S.; Jakubowiak, A.; Bahlis, N.; et al. Pomalidomide alone or in combination with low-dose dexamethasone in relapsed and refractory multiple myeloma: A randomized phase 2 study. *Blood* **2014**, *123*, 1826–1832. [CrossRef]
70. Miguel, J.S.; Weisel, K.; Moreau, P.; Lacy, M.; Song, K.; Delforge, M.; Karlin, L.; Goldschmidt, H.; Banos, A.; Oriol, A.; et al. Pomalidomide plus low-dose dexamethasone versus high-dose dexamethasone alone for patients with relapsed and refractory multiple myeloma (MM-003): A randomised, open-label, phase 3 trial. *Lancet Oncol.* **2013**, *14*, 1055–1066. [CrossRef]
71. Leleu, X.; Attal, M.; Arnulf, B.; Moreau, P.; Traulle, C.; Marit, G.; Mathiot, C.; Petillon, M.O.; Macro, M.; Roussel, M.; et al. Pomalidomide plus low-dose dexamethasone is active and well tolerated in bortezomib and lenalidomide-refractory multiple myeloma: Intergroupe Francophone du Myelome 2009-02. *Blood* **2013**, *121*, 1968–1975. [CrossRef]
72. Zangari, M.; Fink, L.; Zhan, F.; Tricot, G. Low venous thromboembolic risk with bortezomib in multiple myeloma and potential protective effect with thalidomide/lenalidomide-based therapy: Review of data from phase 3 trials and studies of novel combination regimens. *Clin. Lymphoma Myeloma Leuk.* **2011**, *11*, 228–236. [CrossRef]
73. Dimopoulos, M.; Wang, M.; Maisnar, V.; Minarik, J.; Bensinger, W.; Mateos, M.V.; Obreja, M.; Blaedel, J.; Moreau, P. Response and progression-free survival according to planned treatment duration in patients with relapsed multiple myeloma treated with carfilzomib, lenalidomide, and dexamethasone (KRd) versus lenalidomide and dexamethasone (Rd) in the phase III ASPIRE study. *J. Hematol. Oncol.* **2018**, *11*, 49. [CrossRef]
74. Lonial, S.; Dimopoulos, M.; Palumbo, A.; White, D.; Grosicki, S.; Spicka, I.; Walter-Croneck, A.; Moreau, P.; Mateos, M.V.; Magen, H.; et al. Elotuzumab Therapy for Relapsed or Refractory Multiple Myeloma. *N. Engl. J. Med.* **2015**, *373*, 621–631. [CrossRef]
75. Liu, Y.C.; Szmania, S.; van Rhee, F. Profile of elotuzumab and its potential in the treatment of multiple myeloma. *Blood Lymphat. Cancer* **2014**, *2014*, 15–27. [CrossRef]
76. Kumar, S.K.; Bensinger, W.I.; Zimmerman, T.M.; Reeder, C.B.; Berenson, J.R.; Berg, D.; Hui, A.M.; Gupta, N.; Di Bacco, A.; Yu, J.; et al. Phase 1 study of weekly dosing with the investigational oral proteasome inhibitor ixazomib in relapsed/refractory multiple myeloma. *Blood* **2014**, *124*, 1047–1055. [CrossRef]

77. Kumar, S.K.; Berdeja, J.G.; Niesvizky, R.; Lonial, S.; Laubach, J.P.; Hamadani, M.; Stewart, A.K.; Hari, P.; Roy, V.; Vescio, R.; et al. Safety and tolerability of ixazomib, an oral proteasome inhibitor, in combination with lenalidomide and dexamethasone in patients with previously untreated multiple myeloma: An open-label phase 1/2 study. *Lancet Oncol.* **2014**, *15*, 1503–1512. [CrossRef]
78. Mateos, M.V.; Dimopoulos, M.A.; Cavo, M.; Suzuki, K.; Jakubowiak, A.; Knop, S.; Doyen, C.; Lucio, P.; Nagy, Z.; Kaplan, P.; et al. Daratumumab plus Bortezomib, Melphalan, and Prednisone for Untreated Myeloma. *N. Engl. J. Med.* **2018**, *378*, 518–528. [CrossRef]
79. Spencer, A.; Lentzsch, S.; Weisel, K.; Avet-Loiseau, H.; Mark, T.M.; Spicka, I.; Masszi, T.; Lauri, B.; Levin, M.D.; Bosi, A.; et al. Daratumumab plus bortezomib and dexamethasone versus bortezomib and dexamethasone in relapsed or refractory multiple myeloma: Updated analysis of CASTOR. *Haematologica* **2018**, *103*, 2079–2087. [CrossRef]
80. Rupa-Matysek, J.; Gil, L.; Wojtasinska, E.; Nowicki, A.; Dytfeld, D.; Kazmierczak, M.; Komarnicki, M. Inhibitory effects of bortezomib on platelet aggregation in patients with multiple myeloma. *Thromb. Res.* **2014**, *134*, 404–411. [CrossRef]
81. Abdullah, W.Z.; Roshan, T.M.; Hussin, A.; Zain, W.S.; Abdullah, D. Increased PAC-1 expression among patients with multiple myeloma on concurrent thalidomide and warfarin. *Blood Coagul. Fibrinolysis* **2013**, *24*, 893–895. [CrossRef]
82. Jilma, B.; Cvitko, T.; Winter-Fabry, A.; Petroczi, K.; Quehenberger, P.; Blann, A.D. High dose dexamethasone increases circulating P-selectin and von Willebrand factor levels in healthy men. *Thromb. Haemost.* **2005**, *94*, 797–801. [CrossRef]
83. Swystun, L.L.; Shin, L.Y.; Beaudin, S.; Liaw, P.C. Chemotherapeutic agents doxorubicin and epirubicin induce a procoagulant phenotype on endothelial cells and blood monocytes. *J. Thromb. Haemost.* **2009**, *7*, 619–626. [CrossRef]
84. Avcu, F.; Ural, A.U.; Cetin, T.; Nevruz, O. Effects of bortezomib on platelet aggregation and ATP release in human platelets, in vitro. *Thromb. Res.* **2008**, *121*, 567–571. [CrossRef]
85. Khorana, A.A.; Kuderer, N.M.; Culakova, E.; Lyman, G.H.; Francis, C.W. Development and validation of a predictive model for chemotherapy-associated thrombosis. *Blood* **2008**, *111*, 4902–4907. [CrossRef]
86. Sanfilippo, K.M.; Wang, T.F.; Luo, S.; Thomas, T.S.; Carson, K.R.; Keller, J.W.; Kuderer, N.M.; Calverley, D.; Gage, B. Predictive ability of the khorana score for venous thromboembolism (VTE) in multiple myeloma (MM). *J. Clin. Oncol.* **2018**, *36*. [CrossRef]
87. Syrigos, K.; Grapsa, D.; Sangare, R.; Evmorfiadis, I.; Larsen, A.K.; Van Dreden, P.; Boura, P.; Charpidou, A.; Kotteas, E.; Sergentanis, T.N.; et al. Prospective Assessment of Clinical Risk Factors and Biomarkers of Hypercoagulability for the Identification of Patients with Lung Adenocarcinoma at Risk for Cancer-associated Thrombosis. The Observational ROADMAP-CAT Study. *Oncol. Press.* **2018**, *23*, 1372–1381. [CrossRef]
88. Sanfilippo, K.M.; Luo, S.; Wang, T.F.; Fiala, M.; Schoen, M.; Wildes, T.M.; Mikhael, J.; Kuderer, N.M.; Calverley, D.C.; Keller, J.; et al. Predicting venous thromboembolism in multiple myeloma: Development and validation of the IMPEDE VTE score. *Am. J. Hematol.* **2019**. [CrossRef]
89. Li, A.; Wu, Q.; Luo, S.; Warnick, G.S.; Zakai, N.A.; Libby, E.N.; Gage, B.F.; Garcia, D.A.; Lyman, G.H.; Sanfilippo, K.M. Derivation and Validation of a Risk Assessment Model for Immunomodulatory Drug-Associated Thrombosis Among Patients With Multiple Myeloma. *J. Natl. Compr. Cancer Netw.* **2019**, *17*, 840–847. [CrossRef]
90. Al-Ani, F.; Bermejo, J.M.; Mateos, M.V.; Louzada, M. Thromboprophylaxis in multiple myeloma patients treated with lenalidomide—A systematic review. *Thromb. Res.* **2016**, *141*, 84–90. [CrossRef]
91. Swan, D.; Rocci, A.; Bradbury, C.; Thachil, J. Venous thromboembolism in multiple myeloma—Choice of prophylaxis, role of direct oral anticoagulants and special considerations. *Br. J. Haematol.* **2018**, *183*, 538–556. [CrossRef]
92. Sanfilipo, K.; Carson, K.; BF, C. Aspirin May be Inadequate Thromboprophylaxis in Multiple Myeloma. *Blood* **2017**, *130*, 3419.
93. Raskob, G.E.; van Es, N.; Verhamme, P.; Carrier, M.; Di Nisio, M.; Garcia, D.; Grosso, M.A.; Kakkar, A.K.; Kovacs, M.J.; Mercuri, M.F.; et al. Edoxaban for the Treatment of Cancer-Associated Venous Thromboembolism. *N. Engl. J. Med.* **2018**, *378*, 615–624. [CrossRef]
94. Man, L.; Morris, A.; Brown, J.; Palkimas, S.; Davidson, K. Use of direct oral anticoagulants in patients on immunomodulatory agents. *J. Thromb. Thrombolysis* **2017**, *44*, 298–302. [CrossRef]

95. Storrar, N.P.F.; Mathur, A.; Johnson, P.R.E.; Roddie, P.H. Safety and efficacy of apixaban for routine thromboprophylaxis in myeloma patients treated with thalidomide- and lenalidomide-containing regimens. *Br. J. Haematol.* **2018**. [CrossRef]
96. Cornell, R.F.; Goldhaber, S.Z.; Engelhardt, B.G.; Moslehi, J.; Jagasia, M.; Patton, D.; Harrell, S.; Hall, R.; Wyatt, H.; Piazza, G. Apixaban for Primary Prevention of Venous Thromboembolism in Patients With Multiple Myeloma Receiving Immunomodulatory Therapy. *Front. Oncol.* **2019**, *9*, 45. [CrossRef]
97. Pegourie, B.; Karlin, L.; Benboubker, L.; Orsini-Piocelle, F.; Tiab, M.; Auger-Quittet, S.; Rodon, P.; Royer, B.; Leleu, X.; Bareau, B.; et al. Apixaban for the prevention of thromboembolism in immunomodulatory-treated myeloma patients: Myelaxat, a phase 2 pilot study. *Am. J. Hematol.* **2019**, *94*, 635–640. [CrossRef]
98. Riess, H.; Prandoni, P.; Harder, S.; Kreher, S.; Bauersachs, R. Direct oral anticoagulants for the treatment of venous thromboembolism in cancer patients: Potential for drug-drug interactions. *Crit. Rev. Oncol. Hematol.* **2018**, *132*, 169–179. [CrossRef]
99. Short, N.J.; Connors, J.M. New oral anticoagulants and the cancer patient. *Oncologist* **2014**, *19*, 82–93. [CrossRef]
100. Bellesoeur, A.; Thomas-Schoemann, A.; Allard, M.; Smadja, D.; Vidal, M.; Alexandre, J.; Goldwasser, F.; Blanchet, B. Pharmacokinetic variability of anticoagulants in patients with cancer-associated thrombosis: Clinical consequences. *Crit. Rev. Oncol. Hematol.* **2018**, *129*, 102–112. [CrossRef]
101. Farge, D.; Bounameaux, H.; Brenner, B.; Cajfinger, F.; Debourdeau, P.; Khorana, A.A.; Pabinger, I.; Solymoss, S.; Douketis, J.; Kakkar, A. International clinical practice guidelines including guidance for direct oral anticoagulants in the treatment and prophylaxis of venous thromboembolism in patients with cancer. *Lancet Oncol.* **2016**, *17*, e452–e466. [CrossRef]
102. Frere, C.; Benzidia, I.; Marjanovic, Z.; Farge, D. Recent Advances in the Management of Cancer-Associated Thrombosis: New Hopes but New Challenges. *Cancers* **2019**, *11*, 71. [CrossRef]
103. Vedovati, M.C.; Giustozzi, M.; Becattini, C. Venous thromboembolism and cancer: Current and future role of direct-acting oral anticoagulants. *Thromb. Res.* **2019**, *177*, 33–41. [CrossRef]
104. Lim, M.S.; Enjeti, A.K. Safety of anticoagulation in the treatment of venous thromboembolism in patients with haematological malignancies and thrombocytopenia: Report of 5 cases and literature review. *Crit. Rev. Oncol. Hematol.* **2016**, *105*, 92–99. [CrossRef]
105. Khanal, N.; Bociek, R.G.; Chen, B.; Vose, J.M.; Armitage, J.O.; Bierman, P.J.; Maness, L.J.; Lunning, M.A.; Gundabolu, K.; Bhatt, V.R. Venous thromboembolism in patients with hematologic malignancy and thrombocytopenia. *Am. J. Hematol.* **2016**, *91*, E468–E472. [CrossRef]
106. Napolitano, M.; Saccullo, G.; Marietta, M.; Carpenedo, M.; Castaman, G.; Cerchiara, E.; Chistolini, A.; Contino, L.; De Stefano, V.; Falanga, A.; et al. Platelet cut-off for anticoagulant therapy in thrombocytopenic patients with blood cancer and venous thromboembolism: An expert consensus. *Blood Transfus.* **2018**, *17*, 171. [CrossRef]
107. Carrier, M.; Abou-Nassar, K.; Mallick, R.; Tagalakis, V.; Shivakumar, S.; Schattner, A.; Kuruvilla, P.; Hill, D.; Spadafora, S.; Marquis, K.; et al. Apixaban to Prevent Venous Thromboembolism in Patients with Cancer. *N. Engl. J. Med.* **2018**. [CrossRef]
108. Park, D.Y.; Poudel, S.K.; Jia, X.; Wilks, M.L.; Pinkava, V.; O'Brien, M.; Tripp, B.; Song, J.-M.; McCrae, K.R.; Angelini, D.E.; et al. Clinical Outcomes with Direct Oral Anticoagulants Compared to Low Molecular Weight Heparins in the Treatment of Cancer-Associated Venous Thromboembolism. *Blood* **2018**, *132*, 1237. [CrossRef]

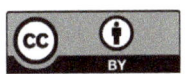

© 2020 by the authors. Licensee MDPI, Basel, Switzerland. This article is an open access article distributed under the terms and conditions of the Creative Commons Attribution (CC BY) license (http://creativecommons.org/licenses/by/4.0/).

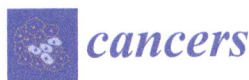

Review

Venous Thromboembolism in Lymphoma: Risk Stratification and Antithrombotic Prophylaxis

Stefan Hohaus [1,2,*], Francesca Bartolomei [2], Annarosa Cuccaro [2], Elena Maiolo [2], Eleonora Alma [2], Francesco D'Alò [1,2], Silvia Bellesi [2], Elena Rossi [1,2] and Valerio De Stefano [1,2]

1. Dipartimento di Scienze Radiologiche ed Ematologiche, Università Cattolica del Sacro Cuore, 00168 Rome, Italy; francesco.dalo@unicatt.it (F.D.); elena.rossi@unicatt.it (E.R.); valerio.destefano@unicatt.it (V.D.S.)
2. Dipartimento di Diagnostica per Immagini, Radioterapia Oncologica ed Ematologia, Fondazione Policlinico Universitario A. Gemelli, IRCCS, L.go A. Gemelli, 8, 00168 Rome, Italy; francescabarto@hotmail.it (F.B.); annarosa.cuccaro@gmail.com (A.C.); elenam86@hotmail.it (E.M.); eleonora.alma@gmail.com (E.A.); silvia.bellesi@policlinicogemelli.it (S.B.)
* Correspondence: stefan.hohaus@unicatt.it; Tel.: +39-06-30154180; Fax: +39-06-35503777

Received: 24 April 2020; Accepted: 14 May 2020; Published: 20 May 2020

Abstract: Lymphoma is listed among the neoplasias with a high risk of venous thromboembolism (VTE). Risk factors for VTE appear to differ from risk factors in solid tumors. We review the literature of the last 20 years for reports identifying these risk factors in cohorts consisting exclusively of lymphoma patients. We selected 25 publications. The most frequent studies were analyses of retrospective single-center cohorts. We also included two reports of pooled analyses of clinical trials, two meta-analyses, two analyses of patient registries, and three analyses of population-based databases. The VTE risk is the highest upfront during the first two months after lymphoma diagnosis and decreases over time. This upfront risk may be related to tumor burden and the start of chemotherapy as contributing factors. Factors consistently reported as VTE risk factors are aggressive histology, a performance status ECOG ≥ 2 leading to increased immobility, more extensive disease, and localization to particular sites, such as central nervous system (CNS) and mediastinal mass. Association between laboratory values that are part of risk assessment models in solid tumors and VTE risk in lymphomas are very inconsistent. Recently, VTE risk scores for lymphoma were developed that need further validation, before they can be used for risk stratification and primary prophylaxis. Knowledge of VTE risk factors in lymphomas may help in the evaluation of the individual risk-benefit ratio of prophylaxis and help to design prospective studies on primary prophylaxis in lymphoma.

Keywords: venous thromboembolism; lymphoma; Non-Hodgkin lymphoma; Hodgkin lymphoma; risk factors; prophylaxis

1. Introduction

Venous thromboembolism is associated with increased morbidity and mortality among patients with neoplastic diseases [1]. Diagnosis and management of thrombotic events interrupt essential anti-neoplastic treatment. VTE occurring during anti-neoplastic treatment represents a preventable complication causing a high economic burden [2]. Lymphomas are among the malignant diseases at high risk for VTE [3]. Routine assessment of VTE risk is recommended for all patients with newly-diagnosed neoplastic diseases, using validated VTE risk models [4,5]. Khorana et al. developed a risk model for predicting chemotherapy-associated VTE based on baseline clinical and laboratory variables [3]. Only a minority of patients (12.6%) in this study had lymphoma. Several studies indicate that risk factors for VTE in patients with lymphoma are different from risk factors in patients with solid tumors [6–9]. To provide more information on the VTE risk in patients with lymphoma, we conducted a systematic review of the literature to determine the incidence of VTE in patients with lymphoproliferative disease and to identify disease and patient characteristics associated with the greatest risk for VTE. VTE risk factors in lymphoma differ from VTE risk factors in solid tumors that have been used to build pan-cancer VTE risk scores, which do not capture the disease-specific VTE risk in lymphomas. As physicians increasingly specialize in the treatment of a few or single cancer type, knowledge of disease-specific risk factors will become more and more important to help treating physicians with their decisions on VTE prophylaxis. More research is needed to assess, validate, and improve VTE risk scores in patients with lymphoma.

2. Methodology

To review VTE risk factors in patients with lymphoma, we screened the Pubmed database for reports published between 1 January 2000 to 31 December 2019, using the MeSH terms "lymphoma" and "thromboembolism" and "venous". We reviewed 246 references. Publications addressing VTE risk in cohorts of adult patients with lymphoma were included for this review, and 21 studies were eligible (Figure 1).

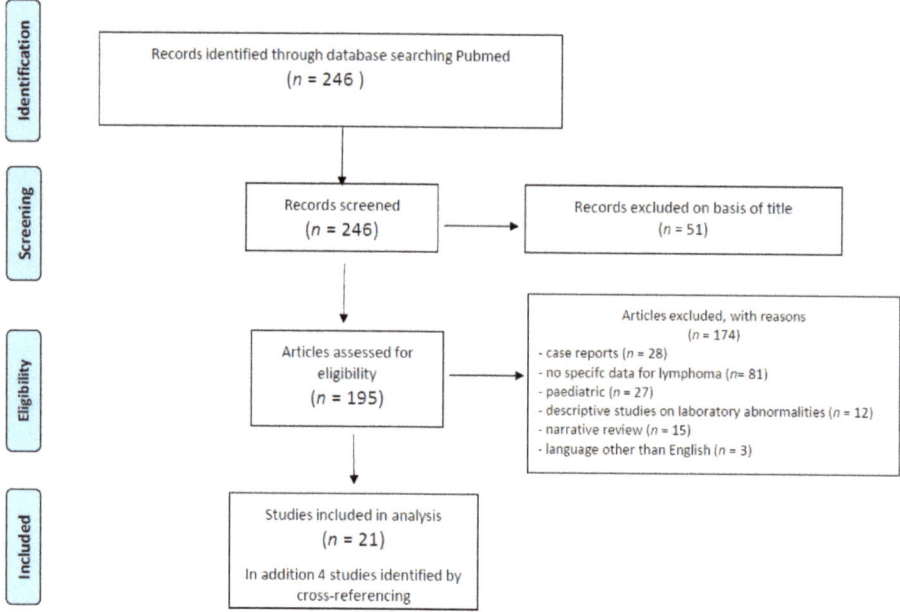

Figure 1. Flow-chart of screening process.

Four additional studies were identified by cross-referencing in the 21 published reports. The articles were divided among all the authors for a first classification and summary and then reviewed by the two senior authors (S.H. and V.D.S.). Of the 25 studies included, 12 studies were retrospective single-center studies [7,8,10–19], two studies were retrospective multicenter trials [20,21], two pooled analysis of clinical trials [9,22], two meta-analyses [23,24], two analyses of patients [25,26] and three analyses of population-based registries [27–29], and two prospective single-center studies [6,30] (Table 1).

Table 1. Characteristics and Incidence Rates of VTE in 25 studies published between 2000 and 2019.

First Author	Year	Country	Ref. No.	Type of Study	No. Pts	Histologies	Median Age	Identification of Events	Median Time	No. VTE	Cumulative Incidence
Sanfilippo	2016	USA	25	registry	2730	DLBCL, FL	64	ICD codes	28.4 mo.	246	DLBCL 10% at 6 mo.
Santi	2017	Italy	22	clinical trials	1717	NHL	57	pharmacovigilance	6 mo.	53	2.9% at 6 mo.
Antic	2016	Serbia	7	retrospective single center	1820	NHL, HL, CLL	53	records review	9 mo.	73	5.3% during therapy
Rupa-Matysek	2018	Polonia	12	retrospective single center	428	DLBCL, HL	50	records review	37 mo.	64	15%
Rupa-Matysek	2018	Polonia	13	retrospective single center	428	DLBCL, HL	50	records review	37 mo.	64	15%
Hohaus	2018	Italy	8	retrospective single center	857	NHL, HL	51	records review	15 mo.	95	11.1% at 9 mo.
Park	2012	Korea	30	prospective single center	686	NHL, HL, CLL	51	records review	21.8 mo.	54	7.9% at 1 yr
Mohren	2005	Germany	14	retrospective single center	1038	NHL, HL,	59	records review	n.a.	80	7.7%
Zhou	2010	USA	15	retrospective single center	422	NHL, HL	57	records review	2 yrs	80	17.1% at 2 yrs
Mahajan	2014	USA	27	population-based databases	16755	NHL	n.a.	ICD codes	2 yrs	670	4% at 2 yrs
Lund	2015	Denmark	28	population-based databases	10375	NHL, HL	n.a.	ICD codes	2 yrs	355	3.9% at 2 yrs
Caruso	2010	International	23	meta-analysis	18018	NHL, HL	n.a.	published studies	n.a.	1149	6.4% during therapy
Lim	2016	Korea	6	prospective single center	322	DLBCL	56	not specified	41.9 mo.	34	10.6% at 1 yr
Komrokji	2006	USA	16	retrospective single center	211	DLBCL	57	records review	n.a.	27	12.7% during therapy
Borg	2016	Denmark	6	retrospective single center	289	DLBCL	67	ICD codes	16 mo.	32	11.1% at 2 yrs
Yokoyama	2012	Japan	19	retrospective single center	142	DLBCL	63	records review	n.a.	15	11% during therapy
Goldschmidt	2003	Israel	18	retrospective single center	42	PCNSL	61	records review	n.a.	25	59.5% at 3 mo.
Byun	2019	Korea	20	retrospective multicenter	235	PCNSL	63	records review	21 mo.	33	11.7% at 1 yr
Lekovic	2010	Serbia	10	retrospective single center	42	PMBCL	34	records review	47 mo.	15	35.7% at 6 mo.
Borchmann	2019	Germany	9	clinical trials	573	HL	36	trial data	12 mo.	173	3.3%
Gebhart	2014	Austria	21	retrospective multicenter	70	SMZL	n.a.	records review	n.a.	9	13%
Hultcrantz	2014	Sweden	29	population-based databases	2190	WM/LPL	74	ICD codes	10 yrs	92	2.1% at 1 y
Gangaraju	2019	USA	26	registry	734	NHL	49	patient questionnaire	8.1 yrs	58	8.1% at 10 yrs
Yamshon	2018	International	24	meta-analysis	1433	NHL	66	published studies	n.a.	77	4.5% at 6 mo.
Zhang	2016	China	11	retrospective single center	565	lymphoma	n.a.	not specified	n.a.	40	7.1% PICC-related

Abbreviations: No., number; pts, patients; VTE, venous thromboembolism; mo, months; yrs, years; DBCL, diffuse large B cell lymphoma; FL, follicular lymphoma; NHL, Non-Hoddgkin lymphoma; HL, Hodgkin lymphoma; CLL, chronic lymphocytic leukemia; SMZL, splenic marginal zone lymphoma; PCNSL, primary central nervous system lymphoma; PMBCL, primary mediastinal B cell lymphoma; WM, Waldenstroems macroglobulinemia; LPL, lymphoplasmocytic lymphoma; ICD, international classification of diseases; IR, incidence rate; CI cumulative incidence; PICC, peripherally-inserted central catheter.

Patients included into these studies were identified by institutional databases in 14 studies [7,8,10–16,18–21,30], by the local hospital discharge registry in one study [17], by cancer registries in four studies (California Cancer Registry [27], VA Cancer registry [25], Swedish cancer registry [29], Danish lymphoma database [28]), by clinical trial registries in five studies [6,9,22,24,26], and by published patient data in one study [23]. The composition of patient cohorts varied widely both in terms of numbers, ranging from 42 to 16,755 patients, and in types of histologies included (Table 1). Ten studies analyzed the VTE risk in patient cohorts with a single histology [6,9,10,16–21,29]. Other cohort restrictions were, for example, the use of almost only male patients in the VA Cancer registry [25], only patients receiving at least one chemotherapy cycle [15], patients who had at least one hospital admission [8], or patients who had at least one serum sample available [6]. The method to identify VTE differed: record review was the most frequent tool for event identification. ICD codes were used to identify VTE in patient registries [17,25,27,28]. Other methods used included pharmacovigilance reports in a clinical trial [22] and a survey of participants of long-term survivors after bone marrow transplantation with a questionnaire [26]. The validity of coded discharge diagnoses for VTE identification was assessed in a study from Denmark [17]. The positive predictive value of the VTE discharge diagnosis was 85%, while the sensitivity of the VTE discharge diagnosis was only 53% [17].

Borg et al. note that patients may have long admissions, and therefore, an episode of VTE may get lost in other problems, and therefore not be registered [17]. Another cause of underreporting could be the exclusion of events, for example, upper extremity thrombosis, either for diagnostic uncertainty or as the presence of central venous catheters (CVC) could be the major contributing factor [27,28].

3. Epidemiology

Caruso et al. have analyzed the risk of VTE in a meta-analysis of 18 published studies, including 18,018 patients, the largest lymphoma population that has been analyzed and published so far [23]. The incidence rate (IR) of VTE for patients with NHL was 6.5% (95% CI, 6.1–6.9%), significantly greater than that observed for HL patients with an IR of 4.7% (95% CI, 3.9–5.6%). In patients with aggressive lymphomas, the IR of events increased to 8.3% (95% CI, 7.0–9.9%) [23]. Data on the second-largest population of lymphoma patients analyzed for VTE risk was published by Mahajan [27]. VTE was diagnosed within two years in 670 patients (4.0%). The rate of development of VTE was highest in the first year (47 events/1000 patient-years) and fell sharply over time (7 events/1000 patient-years in the second follow-up year) [27]. These IR are similar to another population-based study from Denmark (Lund) [28] or from pooled analyses of clinical trials [9,22]. IR reported from single-center studies tended to be higher, ranging from 10–15% (Table 1) [6,8,12,13,15–17,19–21]. Some of these studies included only patients with aggressive histology, like diffuse large B cell lymphomas (DLBCL) [6,16,17,19,20]. The highest IR ever reported for VTE in patients with lymphoma was 59.5% in patients with primary CNS lymphoma (PCNSL) [18]. Differences in reporting could be one possible explanation for these differences. Heterogeneity in risk factors for VTE present in the study population may be another reason for these differences. Risk factors for VTE in lymphoma will now be explored in the next paragraphs.

4. Risk-Modifying Factors

In a simplified model, risk factors could be classified as modifying the VTE risk by their interplay with factors pertaining to Virchow's triad [31–33]: hemostasis results from bed rest and vascular compression by the tumor mass; vessel injury is caused by intravasation of cancer cells, intravascular devices, and systemic therapies; and hypercoagulability results from the production of procoagulants and interaction of neoplastic cells with host cells, including platelets and leukocytes, mediated by direct cellular interactions and inflammatory cytokines. We will now review clinical and laboratory risk factors that are either related to the patient or the disease (Table 2). Thromboprophylaxis with low molecular heparin (LMWH) might modify VTE risk. However, the studies on VTE risk factors do not report sufficient data to evaluate the role of thromboprophylaxis.

Table 2. VTE risk factors in lymphomas.

First Author	Ref. No.	Histology	Age	Gender	BMI	PriorVTE	Cmorb.	Stage	ECOG	LDH	Hb	WBC	Plt	KS	Other
Sanfilippo	25	DLBCL	No	n.d.	Yes	Yes	No	stage	n.d.	No	Yes	n.d	n.d.	No	
Santi	22	DLBCL	Yes	Female			n.d.	No	n.d.	n.d.	n.d.	n.d.	n.d.	Yes	
Antic	7	aggressive	No	No	Yes	Yes	n.d.	E, Med	Yes	n.d.	Yes	Yes *	No	n.d.	
Rupa-Matysek	12	DLBCL	No	No	n.d.	Yes	n.d.	Med	Yes	n.d.	Yes	Yes	No	n.d.	
Rupa-Matysek	13	DLBCL	No	No	n.d.	n.d.	n.d.	Bulk	n.d.	n.d.	Yes	Yes	No	No	IPI score
Hohaus	8	aggressive	Yes	No	n.d.	No	n.d.	bulk, CNS	Yes	Yes	No	No	No	No	albumin < 4
Park	30	aggressive	Yes	No	n.d.	n.d.	Yes	stage, E, Med, CNS	Yes	Yes	n.d.	n.d.	n.d.	n.d.	
Mohren	14	aggressive	No	No	n.d.	n.d.	n.d.	No	n.d.	n.d.	n.d.	n.d.	n.d.	n.d.	
Zhou	15	n.d.	No	Female	No	n.d.	No	No	n.d.	No	Yes	No	No	n.d.	creatinine
Mahajan	27	aggressive	Yes	No	n.d.	n.d.	Yes	stage	n.d.	Yes	n.d.	No	n.d.	n.d.	Asian
Lund	28	aggressive	No	No	n.d.	n.d.	No	CNS	Yes	Yes	No	No	No	n.d.	
Caruso	23	aggressive	n.d.	n.d.	n.d.	n.d.	n.d.	No	n.d.	n.d.	n.d.	n.d.	n.d.	n.d.	
Lim	6	n.a.	Yes	No	No	n.d	n.d.	stage, E	Yes	No	No	Yes	No	No	IPI score
Komrokji	16	n.a.	No	No	n.d.	n.d	n.d.	stage	No	No	No	n.d.	n.d.	n.d.	IPI score
Borg	17	n.a.	n.d.	No	No	Yes	n.d.	stage	Yes	No	No	No	No	n.d.	IPI score
Yokoyama	19	n.a.	Yes	No	No	n.a.	n.d.	No	Yes	Yes	No	No	No	n.d.	IPI score
Goldschmidt	18	n.a.	No	n.d.	n.d.	n.a.	n.d.	n.d.	Yes	No	No	No	No	n.d.	
Byun	20	n.a.	Yes	Female	No	n.a.	n.d.	n.d.	n.d.	n.d.	Yes	No	No	n.d.	albumin <4
Lekovic	10	n.a.	No	No	n.d.	n.a	n.d.	n.d.	n.d.	n.d.	No	No	No	n.d.	fibrinogen
Borchmann	9	n.a.	n.d.	No	No	n.d	n.d.	Yes	n.d.	Yes	No	No	No	No	
Gebhart	21	n.a.	n.d.	n.d.	n.d.	n.d	n.d.	n.d.	n.d.	n.d.	n.d.	n.d.	n.d.	n.d.	LAC
Hultcrantz	29	n.a.	n.d.	n.d.	n.d.	n.d	n.d.	n.d.	n.d.	n.d.	n.d.	n.d.	n.d.	n.d.	
Gangaraju	26	n.d.	n.d.	n.d.	Yes	n.d	Yes	n.d.	n.d.	n.d.	n.d.	n.d	n.d.	n.d.	GVHD

Abbreviations: BMI, body mass index; VTE, venous thromboembolism; Cmb, Comorbidities; ECOG, performance status according to ECOG scale; LDH, lactate dehydrogenase; Hb, hemoglobin; WBC, white blood cell count; plt, platelet count; KS, Khorana score; DLBCL, diffuse large B cell lymphoma; E, extranodal disease; Med, mediastinal involvement; IPI, international prognostic index; LAC, lupus anticoagulant; GVHD, graft versus host disease; n.d, not done; n.a., not assessable. * indicates that WBC < 1000/mm^3 during chemotherapy was a risk factor instead of the WBC > 11,000/mm^3 at diagnosis in the other studies. The studies by Yamshon and Zhang were not included into Table 2, as they do not report on VTE risk factors, but focus on particular clinical situations (therapy with lenalidomide and CVC).

4.1. Individual Patient-Related Factors

4.1.1. Age

Older age has been reported as a risk factor for VTE in several studies on cancer-associated thrombosis. Six retrospective studies (four single-center, two multicenter) from Asia and Italy found an increased risk for VTE in patients with NHL older than 60 or 65 years [6,8,19,20,22,30]. The majority of the patients included in these studies had diffuse large B cell lymphoma. Restricting the analysis to DLBCL, Park et al. confirmed the contribution of age older than 60 years to the VTE risk [30]. The odds ratios for older age in the five studies vary between 1.6 and 3.3. One population-based study from California analyzing data of 16,755 patients with NHL identified an age of 45 years and above as risk factor for VTE (HR, 1.4, 95% CI, 1.1–1.7) [27]. Data from other studies did not point to an association between age and risk of VTE in lymphomas (Table 2).

4.1.2. Gender

Studies on the association between gender and risk of VTE in lymphomas point to the female gender as a potential risk factor. However, data are far from being conclusive. Evidence for an association between female gender and VTE comes from three studies [15,20,22]. An increased risk for VTE was observed in a multicenter study on 235 Asian patients with PCNSL (HR 2.3; 95%; CI 1.1–5.0) [20]. Female gender was a risk factor for VTE in multivariate analysis of 422 lymphoma patients treated at the MD Anderson Cancer Center (OR 3.51; 95%, 1.67–7.40) [15]. The pooled analysis of 12 clinical trials from Italy identified female gender as a risk factor for severe VTE grade 3 or more [22]. However, the female gender was not associated with risk for VTE in 14 other studies (Table 2).

4.1.3. Obesity

Obesity is well known as being a VTE risk factor in the general population and is a variable in the Khorana CAT assessment score [3]. Data on an association between body mass index (BMI) and VTE risk in patients with lymphoma are inconsistent. Increased BMI was identified as a VTE risk factor in three studies, while six studies did not find an association (Table 2). Antic et al. found a BMI > 30 kg/m^2, present in only 1.5% of patients, as a strong risk factor both in univariate and multivariate analysis of 1820 patients with lymphomas (OR 10.7; 95% CI, 3.3–34.6), including this parameter as a variable in the ThroLy score [7]. In the analysis of 2730 male NHL patients of the VA Cancer Registry in the US, BMI > 30 kg/m^2 was present in 25% of patients and a moderate VTE risk factor in a competing risk model for VTE in the first year of NHL diagnosis (adjusted HR 1.6; 95% CI 1.08–2.37) [25]. A BMI > 25 kg/m^2 was identified as a VTE risk factor in long-term survivors following allogeneic transplantation for NHL [26]. However, BMI was not included in the analysis of VTE risk in the majority of published studies on lymphoma patients (Table 2).

4.1.4. Performance Status/Immobility

Immobility due to poor performance status, hospitalization, or post-surgery is one of the most important risk factors for VTE for patients with lymphoma as for other cancers. Khorana reported VTE events in 4.1% during hospitalization of cancer patients, which is clearly higher than the 1.6% incidence in the study cohort of cancer outpatients used for the development of the Khorana score [3,34]. Only one out of ten studies that analyzed performance status as a VTE risk factor in patients with lymphoma did not find an association between reduced performance status and VTE risk (Table 2) [16]. Most studies defined a reduction of the daily activity of the patient with variation from partial to complete immobilization corresponding to ECOG scale grade 2 or more as poor performance. This threshold is not only a VTE risk factor, but also a poor prognostic parameter for lymphoma-specific and overall survival in nearly all types of lymphoma, as it is one of the variables in the International Prognostic Index (IPI) [35]. The prevalence of reduced performance status in the study cohorts varied widely depending on the clinical setting and lymphoma type. The frequency of patients with a reduced performance status was lowest in ambulatory cohorts [7,12] and highest in a patient cohort with PCNSL (50%) [20]. In a population-based database from Denmark, the proportion of patients with reduced performance status was 17% [28]. The OR of reduced performance status for VTE ranged between 1.5 to 5.1 [6–8,12,17,20,28,30], with one outlier of 39.9 [19].

A lower threshold to define poor performance status as a VTE risk factor was found in the analysis of the Danish lymphoma database of 10,375 patients, setting the cut-point at ECOG grade 1 [28]. This corresponds to symptoms that do not interfere with daily activity and do not lead to increased immobility. In our single-center study, poor performance status was associated with a higher VTE localization to the lower extremities [8].

4.1.5. Comorbidity

Comorbidities such as congestive heart failure, renal, liver, and pulmonary disease have been reported as VTE risk factors in hospitalized cancer patients [36]. The impact of comorbidities on the VTE risk has been only rarely addressed in patients with lymphoma. Mahajan et al. used the California Cancer Registry coupled with the California Patient Discharge database to determine the incidence of first-time VTE in 16,755 patients with lymphoma and found that a greater number of chronic comorbid comorbidities was a strong predictor for VTE [27]. Patients with one or two comorbidities in addition to lymphoma were 2-fold and patients with three or more comorbidities were 4-fold more likely to develop VTE. The types of comorbid conditions were not reported. In the study by Park et al. on 686 patients, hypertension was significantly associated with VTE ($p = 0.017$), but was not maintained as a significant parameter in the competing risk analysis [30]. The diagnosis of coronary artery disease was identified as a risk factor for late VTE in long-term survivors with lymphoma following autologous transplantation [26].

4.1.6. Prior Thrombosis/Thrombophilia

A previous thrombosis has been reported in some studies to be associated with an increased risk for VTE after diagnosis of lymphoma and during treatment [7,12,17,25]. Data are not conclusive, as many studies did not register prior VTE as a variable, or the study size was too small, and no prior VTE in the study cohort had been observed [10,18–20]. Prior VTE is a relatively rare event. In the cohort of 2730 NHL patients of the Veteran's Administration Central Cancer Registry, a previous VTE was recorded in 1.6% of patients [25]. Data interpretation is further complicated by differences in the type of thrombotic event counted as prior thrombosis, as well as the lack of information between the time between the prior VTE and lymphoma diagnosis/treatment. Antic et al. combined prior VTE, myocardial infarction (MI), and stroke as a single variable to develop the ThroLy score [7]. This variable that was present in 1% of patients had the highest OR (14.1; 5% CI, 4.4–45) in the multivariate analysis and was assigned 2 points in the 7-parameter, 10-point predictive model for VTE, the ThroLy score. In a validation study of the ThroLy score in a single-center cohort of 428 patients, Rupa-Matysek et al. confirmed the presence of previous VTE/MI/stroke as a significant predictive parameter [12]. Sanfilippo et al. counted only VTE as prior thrombosis and found an adjusted hazard ratio of 4.73 (95% CI, 2.47–9.04) for a history of VTE [25]. One cannot exclude that some of the prior VTE could be already heralding events of the lymphoma activity [37]. In the analysis of our cohort of 857 patients with lymphoma, we counted 54 VTE that were present at diagnosis or occurred in the 6 months prior to the diagnosis as heralding event [8].

A genetic component appears to play a role in cancer-associated thrombosis [38,39]. The contribution of hereditary or acquired thrombophilia as a VTE risk factor in patients with lymphoma is yet to be explored in comprehensive studies. In a study on 70 patients with splenic marginal zone lymphoma, Gebhart et al. observed a high prevalence of anti-phospholipid antibodies [21]. Lupus anticoagulans activity was present in 9/70 (13%) patients and was associated with a higher VTE risk, in particular following splenectomy. In a cohort of 142 Japanese patients with DLBCL, the investigators screened for the possibility of inherited thrombophilia by measuring antithrombin activity, protein C activity, and protein S antigen only in the 15 patients that developed VTE [19]. None of them had inherited thrombophilia. We currently address the contribution of hereditary and acquired thrombophilia in an ongoing prospective study on the risk of VTE in patients with lymphoma (VANILLA study).

4.2. Lymphoma-Related Factors

4.2.1. Histology

Lymphoma histologies can be roughly divided into indolent and aggressive lymphomas, with the latter category including intermediate and highly-aggressive lymphoma types. The literature consistently reports that aggressive histology in NHL associates with increased VTE risk [7,8,12–14,22,23,25,27,28,30]. Aggressive histology has been identified in single-center, multi-center, and population-based cohorts. In the group of B cell-NHL, DLBCL is the most frequent subtype and is clearly at a higher VTE risk with respect to follicular and other indolent lymphoma [8,12,14,22,27]. Mantle cell lymphoma is considered an aggressive B cell lymphoma. Peripheral T cell lymphomas generally have a poor prognosis and are included in the group of lymphoma types with a higher risk for VTE [8,28]. Ten studies presented in Table 1 focus on one lymphoma type, most DLBCL. The actuarial incidence rate in the first year after diagnosis for DLBCL is about 10–12%. The incidence of VTE for localization of subtypes of aggressive B cell lymphoma to particular sites, as CNS and mediastinum are discussed in the next paragraph. In indolent lymphomas, the incidence rate varies between 1.5 and 4% [25,28]. The risk for VTE in the first year after diagnosis has been reported to be 4-fold higher in 2190 patients with Waldenstroem's macroglobulinemia/lymphoplasmocytic lymphoma with respect to a control population, identified through Swedish registries [29]. The total incidence of VTE in patients with Hodgkin lymphoma treated in the GHSG is 3.3% [9].

4.2.2. Site of Disease

Lymphoma localization to the CNS has the highest VTE risk ever reported in patients with lymphoma. In a series of 42 patients with primary CNS lymphoma (PCNSL), Goldschmidt reported VTE in 24 patients (59.5%) [18]. In a multicenter study from Korea including 235 patients with PCNSL, 33 patients (14%) developed VTE during the 21 months follow-up period [20]. In our single-center study including 857 patients with lymphoma, we found that the 33 patients with PCNSL had a peak VTE incidence of 27.2% [8]. In a single-center study from Korea, brain involvement in 51 of 686 patients was associated with 19.6% incidence rate of VTE, translating into a 2.04-fold (95% CI, 1.03–6.30) increased risk [30]. In a Danish population-based study CNS involvement that was present in 287 of 10,375 patients was associated with a cumulative 2-year incidence of VTE of only 8.4% increasing the VTE risk by 2.52 fold (95% CI, 1.54–4.12) compared to patients without CNS involvement [28]. This study reported a lower VTE incidence among all lymphoma patients compared with prior studies.

Mediastinal localization as a bulky disease is another site of particular risk for VTE. In a series of 42 patients with primary mediastinal B cell lymphoma, 15 patients (35.7%) developed VTE [10]. In 10/15 patients the thrombosis was present at diagnosis. Antic et al. identified mediastinal and extranodal localization as VTE risk factors [7]. In particular, mediastinal involvement was associated with an 8-fold increased VTE risk, while extranodal localization increased the risk for VTE by the factor 2.3. In the ThroLy score Antic et al. assigned two points to mediastinal involvement and one point to extranodal localization [7]. Both factors were confirmed in the studies by Rupa-Matysek [12,13]. We found bulky disease defined as 10 cm independent of mediastinal localization as a risk factor both in univariate and multivariate analysis with an OR of 3.23 (95% CI, 1.85–5.63) [8].

4.2.3. Stage of the Disease

A higher tumor burden results in a higher risk for VTE, and VTE, in turn, is a marker of tumor aggressiveness and poor prognosis [27]. Parameters for tumor burden are the stage of disease according to the Ann Arbor staging system, with stage I/II considered localized disease, stage III with disease extension on both sides of the diaphragm, and stage IV with disease spreading to extranodal organs as the advanced stage. The advanced-stage disease has been associated with the VTE risk in large cohort studies on B-NHL (HR 1.49; 95% CI 1.0–2.00 [25]; and 1.5; 95% CI, 1.2–1.7 [27]) and in DLBCL case series (3.31, 95% CI, 1.55–7.09 [6]; and 2.8, 95% CI, 1.1–6.8 [17]). Six studies did not find a significant association between stage and VTE risk [14–16,19,22,23].

4.2.4. Laboratory Variables

Laboratory variables included in the Khorana risk assessment model for VTE in cancer are a pre-chemotherapy platelet count of 350×10^9/L or more, hemoglobin level less than 100 g/L, and pre-chemotherapy WBC count $> 11 \times 10^9$/L [3]. There is no study that indicates that the platelet count is a VTE risk factor in lymphomas (11 negative studies) (Table 2). A WBC count $> 11 \times 10^9$/L has been identified as VTE risk factor only in two studies on lymphomas [6,12], while nine other studies were negative [7–10,15,17,19,20,28]. In the same line, data on anemia are inconsistent; seven studies did not find an association of pre-chemotherapy hemoglobin levels with VTE risk [6,8,9,12,17,19,28], one study found an association only in univariate analysis [25], and the only study that identified Hb < 100 g/L as VTE risk factor also in multivariate analysis was the study by Antic et al. [7]

Alterations of other laboratory values have been occasionally been associated with an increased VTE risk in lymphoma. Elevated levels of LDH indicating a more aggressive disease were predictive of VTE in some studies [8,28,30,40], but not in others [6,15–17,20,25]. Low albumin levels that were associated to VTE risk in the study form our institute [8] and a study on PCNSL from Korea [20] might be indicators of inflammatory status, as albumin inversely correlates with IL-6 levels [41]. Higher IL-6, IL-10, RANTES, and IP-10 levels, but not TNF alpha, were associated with increased VTE risk in a cohort of 322 patients with DLBCL form Korea; however, no parameter retained statistical significance at the multivariable analysis [6]. Another emerging parameter is the mean platelet volume (MPV) [42,43]. A lower MPV has been associated with the risk of VTE in cohorts of patients with DLBCL and HL, however, with varying cut-points [44,45].

4.2.5. International Prognostic Index (IPI)

The International Prognostic Index (IPI) has been for more than 25 years the most widely-used prognostic score to predict prognosis in aggressive lymphomas [35]. As all of the factors that compose the IPI have been—albeit variably—associated with an increased VTE risk in lymphomas, such as age, stage, performance status, LDH levels and the number of extranodal sites, it appears consequential that the IPI score has also been found to be associated with VTE risk in several studies [6,13,16,17,19].

4.2.6. Time after Diagnosis

The VTE risk in lymphoma patients is the highest upfront during the first months after lymphoma diagnosis and thereafter decreases over time. This upfront risk may be related to the tumor burden and the start of chemotherapy as contributing factors. Zhou et al. reported that 64% (51/80) of the patients with venous thromboembolism experienced the event before or during the first three cycles of therapy [15]. The most frequently-reported median time to VTE was about 2 months [6,17,20,22,30]. For patients with DLBCL, Sanfilippo et al. reported a VTE incidence rate of 10% during the 6 months treatment period and a drop to 2% in the post-treatment period from 6 months to 2 years [25]. Caruso et al. concluded from a meta-analysis of 18 studies that 95% of VTE occurred during the treatment period and only 1.2% in the follow-up period [23].

The presence of a VTE prior to the start of chemotherapy is particularly frequent in patients with local venous compression. Lekovic et al. found a high incidence rate in PBMCL with mediastinal masses (35.7%), and 10/15 (66.7%) VTE were already present at diagnosis [10]. The proportion of VTE occurring before the start of therapy of all VTE that had been observed varied between 16/80 (20%) 10/27 (37%) and 54/95 (57%) in three retrospective single-center studies [8,14,16]. These figures are much lower in pooled analyses of study protocols and meta-analyses. Caruso et al. calculated a 3.8% proportion of VTE at disease presentation in the meta-analysis of 18 studies [23]. The analysis of three protocols of the German Hodgkin Study group revealed only a few events between diagnosis and the start of chemotherapy (5/175, 2.9%) [9]. In the pooled analysis of 12 study protocols, only VTE occurrences after study enrolment were registered [22]. Differences in cohort compositions and in reporting VTE events before the start of therapy may contribute to the heterogeneity of the results.

4.2.7. Type of Therapeutic Regimen

The contribution of single chemotherapeutic agents to the VTE risk is often difficult to isolate from other contributing risk factors, as therapeutic regimens may vary according to the aggressiveness of the disease. Patients with advanced stage Hodgkin lymphoma treated with BEACOPP instead of ABVD have a higher VTE risk [9]. The randomized comparison between BEACOPP schedules administered every 14 days instead of 21 days was associated with a higher VTE incidence rate [9]. Sanfilippo et al. found that the addition of doxorubicin to the CVP regimen increased the VTE risk in patients with B cell lymphomas (DLBCL and FL) [25]. This difference remained significant even when adjusting for histology, as DLBCL patients were much more likely to receive doxorubicin. Regimens that contain methotrexate and/or doxorubicin such as hyper-CVAD, CHOP, and ABVD been described to be associated with an increased VTE risk in a single-center study from the MD Anderson Cancer Center of 422 patients with a variety of lymphomas when compared to regimens not including these two drugs [15]. Lenalidomide is associated with an increased risk for VTE in myeloma. A recent meta-analysis showed that the rate of VTE in B-cell NHL patients treated with lenalidomide in clinical trials is similar to the rate in multiple myeloma [24]. The VTE rate appears to be lowest for lenalidomide combined with a biologic (0.49/100 patient-cycles) compared with single-agent lenalidomide (1.07) or its combination with chemotherapy (0.89) [24].

4.2.8. Indwelling Central Venous Catheters

Indwelling central venous catheters (CVC) are associated with increased risk of VTE also in patients with lymphoma. There are only a few studies systematically addressing the VTE risk of CVC [11,28,30]. Some studies report CVC-related VTE without formally analyzing CVC as a risk factor [14,19,28], and one study excluded CVC-related upper extremity DVT [27]. In a single-center study from China, the incidence of upper-extremity deep vein thrombosis related to the presence of a peripherally-inserted CVC (PICC) was 7.1% (40/565) in patients with lymphoma, without significant differences between lymphomas, but significantly higher than in patients with other cancers (209/7463, 2.80%) [11]. In a study from Korea on 686 patients with lymphoma, the incidence of VTE in patients with a CVC (42/460, 9.1%) was higher than in patients without a catheter (12/226, 5.3%, $p = 0.042$) [30]. However, only three of the 42 cases were catheter-related venous thrombosis, suggesting that in most patients, VTE was not directly associated with the presence of CVC, but was due to other contributing factors such as chemotherapy. In a study linking the Danish lymphoma database with the Danish patient registry, Lund found that in 1453 of 10,375 (14%) patients CVC were used, and the use of a CVC was associated with a 6.67-fold increase in the risk of VTE (95% CI: 1.18) [28]. However, coding in the registry did not allow for reliable identification of upper-extremity VTE in order to establish a link between CVC and CVC-related VTE.

4.2.9. Supportive Care Agents

Cytopenias and the administration of erythropoiesis stimulating agents (ESA) and myeloid growth factors, such as granulocyte colony stimulating factor (G-CSF), have been identified as risk factors for cancer-associated thromboses [3]. Supports with ESA were associated with an increased risk of VTE and mortality in patients with cancer [3]. This has not been specifically addressed in studies on VTE risk in lymphoma patients with lymphoma. Anemia and neutropenia during chemotherapy have been associated with the VTE risk in the study by Anti et al., and could be indicators of the use of growth factors, but formal proof is missing in lymphoma patients [7].

5. Risk Assessment Models

International guidelines recommend risk factor assessment in patients with cancer [4,5]. The most widely-used model was developed by Khorana et al. for patients receiving chemotherapy in an outpatient setting [3]. Five studies assessed this model in a cohort of exclusively lymphoma patients [6,8,9,13,22]. Santi et al. found that a Khorana score of ≥3 was associated with the incidence of VTE in a pooled analysis of 12 lymphoma studies [22]. Four other studies failed to find evidence for an association [6,9,13]. In the same line, analyses of patient cohorts focusing on specific cancer sites, such as pancreatic cancer or lung cancer, showed poor performance of the Khorana score [46,47]. A recent meta-analysis revealed that the predictive power of the Khorana score was not homogenous across various types of cancer [48]. The pan-cancer Khorana score does not capture the disease-specific characteristics associated with VTE risk, and clinicians should be cautious when applying the Khorana score as a universal risk assessment tool.

Moreover, the sensitivity of the Khorana score is quite poor. Most VTE events in cancer patients occur outside the high-risk group [49]. In a meta-analysis on 27,849 patients, only 23.4% of VTE occurred in the 17.4% of patients with a high-risk (>3) Khorana score [49]. When decreasing the threshold to include also patients with a risk score of 2, the detection rate increased to 55.2% of VTE events in a patient cohort that included 47% of the cancer population [49].

Variations of the Khorana risk score have been developed to improve risk assessment that include additional parameters, such as metastatic disease, vascular compression, and previous VTE, such as in the ONKOTEV score [50] or combining clinical and genetic risk factors in the TiC Onco score [51]. Pabinger et al. identified the tumor-site risk category as the only parameter of the Khorana score to predict VTE in the Cancer and Thrombosis Study (CATS) cohort of 1423 patients [52]. Combining tumor-site category and D-dimer values, the authors developed a simple and VTE risk model validated in an independent patient cohort. The CATS cohort included 249 patients with lymphoma (17%), while the validation cohort of 832 patients did not contain lymphoma patients. This VTE risk score merits further exploration in lymphoma patients.

Recently, Antic et al. developed a lymphoma-specific, 7-parameter 10-point score they termed ThroLy score [7] that was validated so far in one single-center study [12]. Similar to the Khorana score, the performance of the ThroLy score is limited by a high frequency of VTE occurring in the low-risk group. In a validation study by Rupa-Matysek, 48% of VTE occurred in the low-risk group of the ThroLy score that comprised 75% of patients [12].

We developed a simple score based on only 3 parameters, CNS involvement, bulky disease and performance status, with CNS involvement defining the highest risk group, and patients with ether bulky disease and/or reduced performance status as high-risk patients, and all other patients as standard-risk patients [8]. The predictive performance of our score is quite good when compared to the Khorana and ThroLy scores. Our VTE score identified 82% of VTE in the high-risk group that consisted of 48% of patients [8]. If the performance will be confirmed in validation studies, this score would provide a simple tool for VTE risk stratification and could be useful in designing studies on primary prophylaxis for higher-risk patients.

Further studies are clearly needed to develop robust lymphoma-specific VTE scores. As VTE risk may change during therapy due to periods of immobilization, positioning of CVC, or changes in therapeutic regimens, the development of dynamic risk models might be more helpful to guide VTE prophylaxis.

6. Treatment and Prophylaxis of VTE in Lymphomas

There are no lymphoma-specific guidelines for treatment or prophylaxis of VTE. VTE should be treated in accordance with international guidelines for patients with cancer, such as those endorsed by the International Society on Thrombosis and Haemostasis [4] or the American Society of Oncology [5]. In brief, these guidelines recommend low-molecular-weight heparin (LMWH) for the initial treatment of established VTE in patients with cancer when creatinine clearance is ≥30 mL per min. [4]. After 6 months, termination or continuation of anticoagulation should be based on an individual evaluation of the benefit–risk ratio, tolerability, drug availability, patient preference, and cancer activity. For the treatment of symptomatic catheter-related thrombosis, the international guidelines recommend anticoagulant treatment for a minimum of 3 months, and as long as the CVC is in place [4].

Thrombocytopenia can develop during chemotherapy and treatment of VTE. An expert panel endorsed by the Gruppo Italiano Malattie Ematologiche dell'Adulto Working Party on Thrombosis and Haemostasis produced a formal consensus about platelet cut-offs for safe treatment with LMWH in patients with hematological neoplasms and thrombocytopenia [53]. Dose modifications of LMWH for platelet counts < 50 × 10^9/L are recommended. In clinical practice, risk factors for bleeding and VTE have to be considered to balance the risk in the individual patient, as localization to particular sites could potentially increase the bleeding risk (e.g., localization of the lymphoma in the gastrointestinal or the central nervous system).

The use of direct oral anticoagulants (DOAC) is emerging as a safe and effective alternative to subcutaneous LMWH for the treatment of cancer-associated VTE. Four randomized clinical trials showed that DOAC were non-inferior to LMWH for the treatment of cancer-associated VTE without an increased risk of major bleeding [54–57]. Only a few patients with hematological malignancies were enrolled, and the proportion of lymphoma patients was lower than 5%.

In the Hokusai VTE cancer study, 40 of 1050 (3.8%) patients had lymphoma [54]. The primary outcome was the composite of recurrent VTE or major bleeding. The DOAC edoxaban was not inferior to LWMH. In a recent subgroup analysis, data for 111 patients with hematological malignancies including the 40 patients with lymphoma were presented, and no difference in the primary outcome during the 12-month observation period between edoxaban and dalteparin was observed (8.9% and 10.9%) [58].

The SELECT D trial randomized 406 patients with active cancer and VTE to either rivaroxaban or dalteparin [55]. No differences were observed between them in the primary outcome, which was recurrent VTE. Only 10 (2.5%) patients had hematological cancers.

In the ADAM VTE trial, the safety of the DOAC apixaban was compared to LMWH in 300 cancer-associated VTE [56]. The primary outcome was major bleeding, and secondary outcomes included VTE recurrence and a composite of major plus clinically-relevant non-major bleeding (CRNMB). No major bleedings were observed in the apixaban arm, and VTE recurrence was lower in the apixaban arm. Only 16/300 (5.3%) patients had lymphoma.

In the Caravaggio trial, apixaban was compared to dalteparin for the treatment of cancer-associated VTE [57]. Dalteaparin was noninferior to dalteparin without an increased risk of major bleeding. Of the 1155 enrolled patients, 85 (7.3%) had hematological malignancies, and a sub-analysis of the small number of hematological malignancies did not reveal a difference between the two arms.

International guidelines do not recommend routine primary VTE prophylaxis with LMWH in ambulatory patients receiving systemic anti-cancer therapy [4]. Guidelines recommend prophylaxis with LMWH or fondaparinux when creatinine clearance is ≥30 mL/min, or with unfractionated heparin in hospitalized patients with cancer and reduced mobility [4]. Reduced mobility expressed by the ECOG performance status is a risk factor in 9/10 studies addressing this parameter in patients with lymphoma (Table 2). Therefore, hospitalization associated with conditions limiting the patient's mobility should be a reason for thromboprophylaxis.

The guidelines do recommend primary prophylaxis in ambulatory patients who are receiving systemic anti-cancer therapy at intermediate-to-high risk of VTE, identified by cancer type (i.e., pancreatic) or by a validated risk assessment model (i.e., a Khorana score ≥ 2), and not actively bleeding or not at a high risk of bleeding [4]. As there is no widely-accepted and validated VTE risk assessment model for lymphomas, no general recommendations for primary prophylaxis in ambulatory patients with lymphoma receiving systemic anti-cancer therapy can be given. Data on the use of LMWH in the studies presented in this review are insufficient to draw any conclusion on the role of primary prophylaxis. The decision to start primary prophylaxis in ambulatory patients with lymphoma should be based on individual evaluation of the benefit–risk ratio, taking into consideration the VTE risk factors described in this review, tolerability, patient preference, and risk of bleeding. We consider localization to the CNS, venous compression by a locally-advanced mass, and reduced performance status as the major VTE risk factors, and consider primary prophylaxis in these patients when they are at low risk for bleeding. The role of primary prophylaxis in ambulatory patients with lymphoma has to be addressed in prospective clinical trials.

Recently, DOACs have also been compared to the use of placebo as primary prophylaxis to prevent cancer-associated VTE in high-risk patients, identified by the Khorana score (>2). In the AVERT trial, 574 patients were randomized, and the occurrence of VTE was lower in the apixaban group (4.2% vs.10.2%), while major bleeding was increased (3.5% vs.1.8%) [59]. A total of 145 (25.2%) patients with lymphoma were included. Outcomes according to disease groups were not reported. In the CASSINI trial randomizing 841 patients, rivaroxaban reduced the occurrence of VTE during the treatment period when compared to placebo (2.6% vs. 6.4%) without increasing the risk of major bleeding [60]. However, there was no difference in the VTE incidence when the analysis was extended to the full observation period of 180 days. Separate outcome for the 59 (7.0%) patients with lymphoma were not reported.

Primary VTE prophylaxis with DOACs is an interesting perspective that has to be further explored in randomized studies specifically designed for patients with lymphoma. Potential interactions with chemotherapeutic drugs involving metabolism via cytochrome P450 system is of concern. A prerequisite for the design of a randomized study is the validation of the recently-published VTE risk models for lymphomas, as the performance of the Khorana score is low in this category of patients.

7. Conclusions

Lymphomas are among the neoplasias at high risk for VTE. Aggressive lymphomas have about a 10–15% incidence rate of VTE in the first year. This risk is even higher when the disease is localized in the CNS or causes a mediastinal mass. The risk is the highest upfront, from diagnosis to the first cycles of antineoplastic treatment. Extensive disease activity, immobility, the positioning of CVC, and administration of chemotherapy with anthracyclines all contribute to the VTE risk upfront. Previous VTE is a risk factor, but well-conducted studies exploring genetic background as a contributing factor are missing. Assessment scores for VTE that were developed for patients with solid tumors, such as the Khorana score, do not predict the VTE risk in lymphoma patients. In the absence of a validated risk score, no evidence-based recommendation for VTE prophylaxis in ambulatory patients undergoing anti-neoplastic treatment can be given. Individual evaluation of the risk-benefit ratio considering the risk factors described in this review is the current strategy. Prospective studies on primary prophylaxis specifically designed for patients with lymphoma are warranted. Moreover, studies to gain more insight into pathogenetic factors that induce VTE in lymphomas are needed.

Author Contributions: Conceptualization, S.H. and V.D.S.; original draft preparation, S.H.; selection and review of the papers, writing review and editing, S.H., F.B., A.C., E.M., E.A., F.D., S.B., E.R. and V.D.S.; supervision, V.D.S. All authors have read and agreed to the published version of the manuscript.

Funding: This research received no external funding.

Conflicts of Interest: The authors declare no conflict of interest.

References

1. Khorana, A.A.; Francis, C.W.; Culakova, E.; Kuderer, N.M.; Lyman, G.H. Thromboembolism is a leading cause of death in cancer patients receiving outpatient chemotherapy. *J. Thromb. Haemost.* **2007**, *5*, 632–634. [CrossRef] [PubMed]

2. Lyman, G.H.; Culakova, E.; Poniewierski, M.S.; Kuderer, N.M. Morbidity, mortality and costs associated with venous thromboembolism in hospitalized patients with cancer. *Thromb. Res.* **2018**, *164*, S112–S118. [CrossRef] [PubMed]
3. Khorana, A.A.; Kuderer, N.M.; Culakova, E.; Lyman, G.H.; Francis, C.W. Development and validation of a predictive model for chemotherapy-associated thrombosis. *Blood* **2008**, *111*, 4902–4907. [CrossRef] [PubMed]
4. Farge, D.; Frere, C.; Connors, J.M.; Ay, C.; Khorana, A.A.; Munoz, A.; Brenner, B.; Kakkar, A.; Rafii, H.; Solymoss, S.; et al. 2019 international clinical practice guidelines for the treatment and prophylaxis of venous thromboembolism in patients with cancer. *Lancet Oncol.* **2019**, *20*, e566–e581. [CrossRef]
5. Key, N.S.; Khorana, A.A.; Kuderer, N.M.; Bohlke, K.; Lee, A.Y.Y.; Arcelus, J.I.; Wong, S.L.; Balaban, E.P.; Flowers, C.R.; Francis, C.W.; et al. Venous Thromboembolism Prophylaxis and Treatment in Patients with Cancer: ASCO Clinical Practice Guideline Update. *J. Clin. Oncol.* **2020**, *38*, 496–520. [CrossRef]
6. Lim, S.H.; Woo, S.-Y.; Kim, S.; Ko, Y.H.; Kim, W.S.; Kim, S.J. Cross-sectional Study of Patients with Diffuse Large B-Cell Lymphoma: Assessing the Effect of Host Status, Tumor Burden, and Inflammatory Activity on Venous Thromboembolism. *Cancer Res. Treat.* **2016**, *48*, 312–321. [CrossRef]
7. Antic, D.; Milic, N.; Nikolovski, S.; Todorovic, M.; Bila, J.; Djurdjevic, P.; Andjelic, B.; Djurasinovic, V.; Sretenovic, A.; Vukovic, V.; et al. Development and validation of multivariable predictive model for thromboembolic events in lymphoma patients. *Am. J. Hematol.* **2016**, *91*, 1014–1019. [CrossRef]
8. Hohaus, S.; Tisi, M.C.; Bartolomei, F.; Cuccaro, A.; Maiolo, E.; Alma, E.; D'Alo, F.; Bellesi, S.; Rossi, E.; De Stefano, V. Risk factors for venous thromboembolism in patients with lymphoma requiring hospitalization. *Blood Cancer J.* **2018**, *8*, 54. [CrossRef]
9. Borchmann, S.; Muller, H.; Hude, I.; Fuchs, M.; Borchmann, P.; Engert, A. Thrombosis as a treatment complication in Hodgkin lymphoma patients: A comprehensive analysis of three prospective randomized German Hodgkin Study Group (GHSG) trials. *Ann. Oncol. Off. J. Eur. Soc. Med. Oncol.* **2019**, *30*, 1329–1334. [CrossRef]
10. Lekovic, D.; Miljic, P.; Mihaljevic, B. Increased risk of venous thromboembolism in patients with primary mediastinal large B-cell lymphoma. *Thromb. Res.* **2010**, *126*, 477–480. [CrossRef]
11. Zhang, X.; Huang, J.-J.; Xia, Y.; Li, C.-F.; Wang, Y.; Liu, P.-P.; Bi, X.-W.; Sun, P.; Lin, T.-Y.; Jiang, W.-Q.; et al. High risk of deep vein thrombosis associated with peripherally inserted central catheters in lymphoma. *Oncotarget* **2016**, *7*, 35404–35411. [CrossRef] [PubMed]
12. Rupa-Matysek, J.; Brzezniakiewicz-Janus, K.; Gil, L.; Krasinski, Z.; Komarnicki, M. Evaluation of the ThroLy score for the prediction of venous thromboembolism in newly diagnosed patients treated for lymphoid malignancies in clinical practice. *Cancer Med.* **2018**, *35*, 5. [CrossRef] [PubMed]
13. Rupa-Matysek, J.; Gil, L.; Kazmierczak, M.; Baranska, M.; Komarnicki, M. Prediction of venous thromboembolism in newly diagnosed patients treated for lymphoid malignancies: Validation of the Khorana Risk Score. *Med. Oncol.* **2017**, *35*, 5. [CrossRef] [PubMed]
14. Mohren, M.; Markmann, I.; Jentsch-Ullrich, K.; Koenigsmann, M.; Lutze, G.; Franke, A. Increased risk of venous thromboembolism in patients with acute leukaemia. *Br. J. Cancer* **2006**, *94*, 200–202. [CrossRef] [PubMed]
15. Zhou, X.; Teegala, S.; Huen, A.; Ji, Y.; Fayad, L.; Hagemeister, F.B.; Gladish, G.; Vadhan-Raj, S. Incidence and risk factors of venous thromboembolic events in lymphoma. *Am. J. Med.* **2010**, *123*, 935–941. [CrossRef] [PubMed]
16. Komrokji, R.S.; Uppal, N.P.; Khorana, A.A.; Lyman, G.H.; Kaplan, K.L.; Fisher, R.I.; Francis, C.W. Venous thromboembolism in patients with diffuse large B-cell lymphoma. *Leuk. Lymphoma* **2006**, *47*, 1029–1033. [CrossRef]
17. Borg, I.H.; Bendtsen, M.D.; Bogsted, M.; Madsen, J.; Severinsen, M.T. Incidence of venous thromboembolism in patients with diffuse large B-cell lymphoma. *Leuk. Lymphoma* **2016**, *57*, 2771–2776. [CrossRef]
18. Goldschmidt, N.; Linetsky, E.; Shalom, E.; Varon, D.; Siegal, T. High incidence of thromboembolism in patients with central nervous system lymphoma. *Cancer* **2003**, *98*, 1239–1242. [CrossRef]
19. Yokoyama, K.; Murata, M.; Ikeda, Y.; Okamoto, S. Incidence and risk factors for developing venous thromboembolism in Japanese with diffuse large b-cell lymphoma. *Thromb. Res.* **2012**, *130*, 7–11. [CrossRef]
20. Byun, J.M.; Hong, J.; Yoon, S.-S.; Koh, Y.; Ock, C.-Y.; Kim, T.M.; Lee, J.H.; Kim, S.-H.; Lee, J.-O.; Bang, S.-M.; et al. Incidence and characteristics of venous thromboembolism in Asian patients with primary central nervous system lymphoma undergoing chemotherapy. *Thromb. Res.* **2019**, *183*, 131–135. [CrossRef]

21. Gebhart, J.; Lechner, K.; Skrabs, C.; Sliwa, T.; Muldur, E.; Ludwig, H.; Nosslinger, T.; Vanura, K.; Stamatopoulos, K.; Simonitsch-Klupp, I.; et al. Lupus anticoagulant and thrombosis in splenic marginal zone lymphoma. *Thromb. Res.* **2014**, *134*, 980–984. [CrossRef] [PubMed]

22. Santi, R.M.; Ceccarelli, M.; Bernocco, E.; Monagheddu, C.; Evangelista, A.; Valeri, F.; Monaco, F.; Vitolo, U.; Cortelazzo, S.; Cabras, M.G.; et al. Khorana score and histotype predicts incidence of early venous thromboembolism in non-Hodgkin lymphomas. A pooled-data analysis of 12 clinical trials of Fondazione Italiana Linfomi (FIL). *Thromb. Haemost.* **2017**, *117*, 1615–1621. [CrossRef]

23. Caruso, V.; Di Castelnuovo, A.; Meschengieser, S.; Lazzari, M.A.; de Gaetano, G.; Storti, S.; Iacoviello, L.; Donati, M.B. Thrombotic complications in adult patients with lymphoma: A meta-analysis of 29 independent cohorts including 18,018 patients and 1149 events. *Blood* **2010**, *115*, 5322–5328. [CrossRef] [PubMed]

24. Yamshon, S.; Christos, P.J.; Demetres, M.; Hammad, H.; Leonard, J.P.; Ruan, J. Venous thromboembolism in patients with B-cell non-Hodgkin lymphoma treated with lenalidomide: A systematic review and meta-analysis. *Blood Adv.* **2018**, *2*, 1429–1438. [CrossRef]

25. Sanfilippo, K.M.; Wang, T.F.; Gage, B.F.; Luo, S.; Riedell, P.; Carson, K.R. Incidence of venous thromboembolism in patients with non-Hodgkin lymphoma. *Thromb. Res.* **2016**, *143*, 86–90. [CrossRef]

26. Gangaraju, R.; Chen, Y.; Hageman, L.; Wu, J.; Francisco, L.; Kung, M.; Ness, E.; Parman, M.; Weisdorf, D.J.; Forman, S.J.; et al. Risk of venous thromboembolism in patients with non-Hodgkin lymphoma surviving blood or marrow transplantation. *Cancer* **2019**, *125*, 4498–4508. [CrossRef]

27. Mahajan, A.; Wun, T.; Chew, H.; White, R.H. Lymphoma and venous thromboembolism: Influence on mortality. *Thromb. Res.* **2014**, *133*, S23–S28. [CrossRef]

28. Lund, J.L.; Ostgard, L.S.; Prandoni, P.; Sorensen, H.T.; de Nully Brown, P. Incidence, determinants and the transient impact of cancer treatments on venous thromboembolism risk among lymphoma patients in Denmark. *Thromb. Res.* **2015**, *136*, 917–923. [CrossRef]

29. Hultcrantz, M.; Pfeiffer, R.M.; Bjorkholm, M.; Goldin, L.R.; Turesson, I.; Schulman, S.; Landgren, O.; Kristinsson, S.Y. Elevated risk of venous but not arterial thrombosis in Waldenstrom macroglobulinemia/lymphoplasmacytic lymphoma. *J. Thromb. Haemost.* **2014**, *12*, 1816–1821. [CrossRef]

30. Park, L.C.; Woo, S.; Kim, S.; Jeon, H.; Ko, Y.H.; Kim, S.J.; Kim, W.S. Incidence, risk factors and clinical features of venous thromboembolism in newly diagnosed lymphoma patients: Results from a prospective cohort study with Asian population. *Thromb. Res.* **2012**, *130*, e6–e12. [CrossRef]

31. Abdol Razak, N.B.; Jones, G.; Bhandari, M.; Berndt, M.C.; Metharom, P. Cancer-Associated Thrombosis: An Overview of Mechanisms, Risk Factors, and Treatment. *Cancers* **2018**, *10*, 380. [CrossRef] [PubMed]

32. Falanga, A.; Russo, L.; Verzeroli, C. Mechanisms of thrombosis in cancer. *Thromb. Res.* **2013**, *131* (Suppl. 1), S59–S62. [CrossRef]

33. Falanga, A.; Russo, L.; Milesi, V.; Vignoli, A. Mechanisms and risk factors of thrombosis in cancer. *Crit. Rev. Oncol. Hematol.* **2017**, *118*, 79–83. [CrossRef] [PubMed]

34. Khorana, A.A.; Francis, C.W.; Culakova, E.; Kuderer, N.M.; Lyman, G.H. Frequency, risk factors, and trends for venous thromboembolism among hospitalized cancer patients. *Cancer* **2007**, *110*, 2339–2346. [CrossRef] [PubMed]

35. A predictive model for aggressive non-Hodgkin's lymphoma. *New Engl. J. Med.* **1993**, *329*, 987–994. [CrossRef] [PubMed]

36. Khorana, A.A.; Francis, C.W.; Culakova, E.; Fisher, R.I.; Kuderer, N.M.; Lyman, G.H. Thromboembolism in hospitalized neutropenic cancer patients. *J. Clin. Oncol.* **2006**, *24*, 484–490. [CrossRef]

37. White, R.H.; Chew, H.K.; Zhou, H.; Parikh-Patel, A.; Harris, D.; Harvey, D.; Wun, T. Incidence of venous thromboembolism in the year before the diagnosis of cancer in 528,693 adults. *Arch. Intern. Med.* **2005**, *165*, 1782–1787. [CrossRef]

38. Blom, J.W.; Doggen, C.J.M.; Osanto, S.; Rosendaal, F.R. Malignancies, prothrombotic mutations, and the risk of venous thrombosis. *JAMA* **2005**, *293*, 715–722. [CrossRef]

39. Pabinger, I.; Ay, C.; Dunkler, D.; Thaler, J.; Reitter, E.-M.; Marosi, C.; Zielinski, C.; Mannhalter, C. Factor V Leiden mutation increases the risk for venous thromboembolism in cancer patients—Results from the Vienna Cancer and Thrombosis Study (CATS). *J. Thromb. Haemost.* **2015**, *13*, 17–22. [CrossRef]

40. Yokoyama, K. Thrombosis in Lymphoma Patients and in Myeloma Patients. *Keio J. Med.* **2015**, *64*, 37–43. [CrossRef]

41. Hohaus, S.; Massini, G.; Giachelia, M.; Vannata, B.; Bozzoli, V.; Cuccaro, A.; D'Alo', F.; Larocca, L.M.; Raymakers, R.A.P.; Swinkels, D.W.; et al. Anemia in Hodgkin's lymphoma: The role of interleukin-6 and hepcidin. *J. Clin. Oncol.* **2010**, *28*, 2538–2543. [CrossRef]
42. Riedl, J.; Kaider, A.; Reitter, E.-M.; Marosi, C.; Jager, U.; Schwarzinger, I.; Zielinski, C.; Pabinger, I.; Ay, C. Association of mean platelet volume with risk of venous thromboembolism and mortality in patients with cancer. Results from the Vienna Cancer and Thrombosis Study (CATS). *Thromb. Haemost.* **2014**, *111*, 670–678. [PubMed]
43. Ferroni, P.; Guadagni, F.; Riondino, S.; Portarena, I.; Mariotti, S.; La Farina, F.; Davi, G.; Roselli, M. Evaluation of mean platelet volume as a predictive marker for cancer-associated venous thromboembolism during chemotherapy. *Haematologica* **2014**, *99*, 1638–1644. [CrossRef] [PubMed]
44. Rupa-Matysek, J.; Gil, L.; Baranska, M.; Dytfeld, D.; Komarnicki, M. Mean platelet volume as a predictive marker for venous thromboembolism in patients treated for Hodgkin lymphoma. *Oncotarget* **2018**, *9*, 21190–21200. [CrossRef] [PubMed]
45. Rupa-Matysek, J.; Gil, L.; Kroll-Balcerzak, R.; Baranska, M.; Komarnicki, M. Mean platelet volume as a predictive marker for venous thromboembolism and mortality in patients treated for diffuse large B-cell lymphoma. *Hematol. Oncol.* **2017**, *35*, 456–464. [CrossRef] [PubMed]
46. van Es, N.; Franke, V.F.; Middeldorp, S.; Wilmink, J.W.; Buller, H.R. The Khorana score for the prediction of venous thromboembolism in patients with pancreatic cancer. *Thromb. Res.* **2017**, *150*, 30–32. [CrossRef]
47. Mansfield, A.S.; Tafur, A.J.; Wang, C.E.; Kourelis, T.V.; Wysokinska, E.M.; Yang, P. Predictors of active cancer thromboembolic outcomes: Validation of the Khorana score among patients with lung cancer. *J. Thromb. Haemost.* **2016**, *14*, 1773–1778. [CrossRef]
48. van Es, N.; Ventresca, M.; Di Nisio, M.; Zhou, Q.; Noble, S.; Crowther, M.; Briel, M.; Garcia, D.; Lyman, G.H.; Macbeth, F.; et al. The Khorana score for prediction of venous thromboembolism in cancer patients: An individual patient data meta-analysis. *J. Thromb. Haemost.* **2020**. [CrossRef]
49. Mulder, F.I.; Candeloro, M.; Kamphuisen, P.W.; Di Nisio, M.; Bossuyt, P.M.; Guman, N.; Smit, K.; Buller, H.R.; van Es, N. The Khorana score for prediction of venous thromboembolism in cancer patients: A systematic review and meta-analysis. *Haematologica* **2019**, *104*, 1277–1287. [CrossRef]
50. Cella, C.A.; Di Minno, G.; Carlomagno, C.; Arcopinto, M.; Cerbone, A.M.; Matano, E.; Tufano, A.; Lordick, F.; De Simone, B.; Muehlberg, K.S.; et al. Preventing Venous Thromboembolism in Ambulatory Cancer Patients: The ONKOTEV Study. *Oncologist* **2017**, *22*, 601–608. [CrossRef]
51. Munoz Martin, A.J.; Ortega, I.; Font, C.; Pachon, V.; Castellon, V.; Martinez-Marin, V.; Salgado, M.; Martinez, E.; Calzas, J.; Ruperez, A.; et al. Multivariable clinical-genetic risk model for predicting venous thromboembolic events in patients with cancer. *Br. J. Cancer* **2018**, *118*, 1056–1061. [CrossRef] [PubMed]
52. Pabinger, I.; van Es, N.; Heinze, G.; Posch, F.; Riedl, J.; Reitter, E.-M.; Di Nisio, M.; Cesarman-Maus, G.; Kraaijpoel, N.; Zielinski, C.C.; et al. A clinical prediction model for cancer-associated venous thromboembolism: A development and validation study in two independent prospective cohorts. *Lancet Haematol.* **2018**, *5*, e289–e298. [CrossRef]
53. Napolitano, M.; Saccullo, G.; Marietta, M.; Carpenedo, M.; Castaman, G.; Cerchiara, E.; Chistolini, A.; Contino, L.; De Stefano, V.; Falanga, A.; et al. Platelet cut-off for anticoagulant therapy in thrombocytopenic patients with blood cancer and venous thromboembolism: An expert consensus. *Blood Transfus.* **2019**, *17*, 171–180. [PubMed]
54. Raskob, G.E.; van Es, N.; Verhamme, P.; Carrier, M.; Di Nisio, M.; Garcia, D.; Grosso, M.A.; Kakkar, A.K.; Kovacs, M.J.; Mercuri, M.F.; et al. Edoxaban for the Treatment of Cancer-Associated Venous Thromboembolism. *New Engl. J. Med.* **2018**, *378*, 615–624. [CrossRef] [PubMed]
55. Young, A.M.; Marshall, A.; Thirlwall, J.; Chapman, O.; Lokare, A.; Hill, C.; Hale, D.; Dunn, J.A.; Lyman, G.H.; Hutchinson, C.; et al. Comparison of an Oral Factor Xa Inhibitor With Low Molecular Weight Heparin in Patients With Cancer With Venous Thromboembolism: Results of a Randomized Trial (SELECT-D). *J. Clin. Oncol.* **2018**, *36*, 2017–2023. [CrossRef] [PubMed]
56. McBane, R.D., 2nd; Wysokinski, W.E.; Le-Rademacher, J.G.; Zemla, T.; Ashrani, A.; Tafur, A.; Perepu, U.; Anderson, D.; Gundabolu, K.; Kuzma, C.; et al. Apixaban and dalteparin in active malignancy-associated venous thromboembolism: The ADAM VTE trial. *J. Thromb. Haemost.* **2020**, *18*, 411–421. [CrossRef]

57. Agnelli, G.; Becattini, C.; Meyer, G.; Munoz, A.; Huisman, M.V.; Connors, J.M.; Cohen, A.; Bauersachs, R.; Brenner, B.; Torbicki, A.; et al. Apixaban for the Treatment of Venous Thromboembolism Associated with Cancer. *New Engl. J. Med.* **2020**, *382*, 1599–1607. [CrossRef]
58. Mulder, F.I.; van Es, N.; Kraaijpoel, N.; Di Nisio, M.; Carrier, M.; Duggal, A.; Gaddh, M.; Garcia, D.; Grosso, M.A.; Kakkar, A.K.; et al. Edoxaban for treatment of venous thromboembolism in patient groups with different types of cancer: Results from the Hokusai VTE Cancer study. *Thromb. Res.* **2020**, *185*, 13–19. [CrossRef]
59. Carrier, M.; Abou-Nassar, K.; Mallick, R.; Tagalakis, V.; Shivakumar, S.; Schattner, A.; Kuruvilla, P.; Hill, D.; Spadafora, S.; Marquis, K.; et al. Apixaban to Prevent Venous Thromboembolism in Patients with Cancer. *New Engl. J. Med.* **2019**, *380*, 711–719. [CrossRef]
60. Khorana, A.A.; Soff, G.A.; Kakkar, A.K.; Vadhan-Raj, S.; Riess, H.; Wun, T.; Streiff, M.B.; Garcia, D.A.; Liebman, H.A.; Belani, C.P.; et al. Rivaroxaban for Thromboprophylaxis in High-Risk Ambulatory Patients with Cancer. *New Engl. J. Med.* **2019**, *380*, 720–728. [CrossRef]

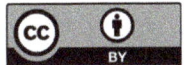 © 2020 by the authors. Licensee MDPI, Basel, Switzerland. This article is an open access article distributed under the terms and conditions of the Creative Commons Attribution (CC BY) license (http://creativecommons.org/licenses/by/4.0/).

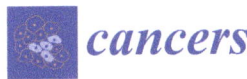

Review

Venous Thromboembolism in Cancer Patients on Simultaneous and Palliative Care

Silvia Riondino [1,2], Patrizia Ferroni [2], Girolamo Del Monte [3], Vincenzo Formica [1], Fiorella Guadagni [2] and Mario Roselli [1,*]

[1] Department of Systems Medicine, Medical Oncology, University of Rome, Tor Vergata, 00133 Rome, Italy; silviariondino2@gmail.com (S.R.); vincenzo.formica@ptvonline.it (V.F.)
[2] Department of Human Sciences and Quality of Life Promotion, San Raffaele Roma Open University, 00166 Rome, Italy; patrizia.ferroni@sanraffaele.it (P.F.); fiorella.guadagni@sanraffaele.it (F.G.)
[3] Department of Palliative Care, San Raffaele Cassino, Clinical Center, 03043 Cassino, Italy; girolamo.delmonte@sanraffaele.it
* Correspondence: mario.roselli@uniroma2.it; Tel.: +39-06-20903372; Fax: +39-06-20903806

Received: 9 March 2020; Accepted: 2 May 2020; Published: 6 May 2020

Abstract: Simultaneous care represents the ideal integration between early supportive and palliative care in cancer patients under active antineoplastic treatment. Cancer patients require a composite clinical, social and psychological management that can be effective only if care continuity from hospital to home is guaranteed and if such a care takes place early in the course of the disease, combining standard oncology care and palliative care. In these settings, venous thromboembolism (VTE) represents a difficult medical challenge, for the requirement of acute treatments and for the strong impact on anticancer therapies that might be delayed or, even, totally discontinued. Moreover, cancer patients not only display high rates of VTE occurrence/recurrence but are also more prone to bleeding and this forces clinicians to optimize treatment strategies, balancing between hemorrhages and thrombus formation. VTE prevention is, therefore, regarded as a double-edged sword. Indeed, while on one hand the appropriate use of antithrombotic agents can reduce VTE occurrence, on the other it significantly increases the bleeding risk, especially in the frail patients who present with multiple co-morbidities and poly-therapy that can interact with anticoagulant drugs. For these reasons, thromboprophylaxis should start while active cancer treatment is ongoing, according to a simultaneous care model in a patient-centered perspective.

Keywords: simultaneous care; integrated care; venous thromboembolism; thromboprophylaxis

1. Integrated Palliative Care and Simultaneous Care

In the new era of personalized medicine, one of the recognized priorities regards the role of integration of early supportive and palliative care with cancer-directed treatments, the so-called "simultaneous care" [1]. It has been widely acknowledged that such an integrated model of care may have a positive effect on patients' quality of life (QoL) as well as on other patient outcomes [2].

The very notion of "simultaneous care" has stem from the necessity of an earlier integration between oncology and palliative care and from the observation that earlier interventions resulted in reduced depression and symptom burden, decreased hospital care, improved QoL and prolonged survival [3–5]. This concept has been implemented by the World Health Organization (WHO), stating that palliative care is already applicable early in the course of illness, in conjunction with other therapies that are intended to prolong life [6].

The concept of palliative care has thus substantially developed from its initial meaning of care for the dying, towards a more complete, yet complex, integrated approach focused on patient centered care. Indeed, the WHO describes "palliative care" as an approach that improves the quality of life of patients and their families facing the problems associated with life-threatening illness, through the prevention and relief of suffering by means of early identification and impeccable assessment and treatment of pain and other distresses, at physical, psychosocial and spiritual level [6].

Although historically supportive care has been developed to counter and mitigate the side effects of cancer treatment, such as chemotherapy-induced nausea and vomiting (CINV) or neutropenia, while palliative care is intended when the patient is "out of therapy," when active cancer treatments are no longer available, symptom management is the shared goal of both care settings. The European Society of Medical Oncology (ESMO) also encourages the role of supportive care at all stages of the disease and considers palliative care focused on treatments that take place when active anticancer therapies are no more indicated [7]. The transition between simultaneous and palliative care should be taken following the evaluation of some "guiding" indexes, including disease progression, worsening of performance and/or nutritional status, weight loss and symptom burden [8,9]. The integration of oncology treatment and palliative care is steered by a patient's centered approach and, by virtue of this integration, treatment outcome must be continuously evaluated and redefined during the progression of the disease and must always be aimed at controlling symptoms and at maintaining the longest possible well-being [8], in order to ensure compliance to a congruent treatment.

In this light, to the National Comprehensive Cancer Network (NCCN) guidelines, patients should be screened at every visit, starting from the very beginning and during follow-ups and checked for the following items—1) uncontrolled symptoms; 2) moderate to severe distress related to cancer diagnosis and therapy; 3) serious comorbid physical, psychiatric and psychosocial conditions; 4) life expectancy of 6 months or less; 5) patient or family concerns about the disease course and decision-making; and/or 6) a specific request for palliative care by the patient or family [10].

Accordingly, three different scenarios can be delineated, in which cancer patients can fluidly move during the course of their disease—primary, secondary and tertiary palliative care [11]. Although all settings require professional skills aimed at performing basic assessments and management of physical symptoms, including the evaluation of the drug-induced ones, socio-psychological problems and caregiver support, primary palliative care can occur both as outpatient setting for ambulatory patients and in the home setting, secondary palliative cares are provided in specialized cancer centers at inpatient- and outpatient- levels and tertiary palliative care requires the presence of palliative care specialists [11]. In the perspective of changes, the simultaneous care also overcomes the drawback relative to life expectancy of 6 months or less [10] which, unlike what has been implied so far in the concept of palliative care, is no longer considered in a temporal viewpoint but in a symptomatic one.

The changes introduced in the new conception of oncology care have thus led to include not only active anticancer under this model but also strategies aimed at primary prevention, early diagnosis, cure, survival-prolongation, supportive treatment and tertiary prevention, including rehabilitation that, together with continuous care and palliative care, extends during the whole course of the disease and even beyond. Indeed, in cancer survivals, physical symptoms and psychological distress altering and affecting their QoL, continuous care should be provided, being capable to improve the perceptions of their lives [12]. Current guidelines recommend the early integration of PC for patients with cancer [3,13], due to the demonstrated positive relationship between early integration of PC and improvements in QoL of both patients and caregivers, associated with a reduced access to pointless interventions and incongruent emergency department accesses [14–17].

Despite these considerations and recommendations, cancer patients are often referred to PC late in their disease course. Towards the final phases of the disease, home-based care is particularly important, because it can prevent inadequate hospital admissions and allows patients to live in their own environment where, however, they must be dynamically evaluated in order to identify their needs that change over time in response to treatment or disease progression. Patients' needs must be always used in the decision making process and discussed with the patients themselves, in a patient-centered approach [11]. Patient "centeredness" has been defined as "care that is respectful of and responsive to, individual patient preferences, needs and values and ensuring that patient values guide all clinical decisions" [18]. In this light, the aim of patient-centeredness is to personalize treatment and care to the specific needs of each patient and to modulate the care accordingly.

2. Incidence of VTE in Palliative Cancer Patients—A Road Map Approaching Simultaneous Care

Starting from 1995, the National Council for Hospice and Specialist Palliative Care Services has set a systematic data collection of minimum standard (The Minimum Data Set (MDS)) to inform and analyze the activity of Palliative Care Services. MDS methods have been adopted worldwide by most of Palliative Care Organizations and have allowed consistent data comparison, including venous thromboembolism (VTE) in specialist palliative care units (SPCUs) [19].

VTE in its two tightly related clinical entities, deep vein thrombosis (DVT) and pulmonary embolism (PE) [20], is commonly considered as one of the preventable sequelae that can afflict hospitalized patients. In cancer patients VTE occurs in approximately 20% cases [21] and PE is associated with a mortality rate up to 30% [22,23]. Although representing the extreme expression of a manifest disease, asymptomatic manifestations, including disseminated intravascular coagulation, occur rather frequently and are often detected at time of restaging.

VTE incidence increases with age, represents a frequent complication of the more advanced stages and is significantly worsened by anticancer treatments such as platinum-, fluoropyrimidine- and gemcitabine-containing chemotherapy regimens, immune-modulatory drugs such as thalidomide, lenalidomide and pomalidomide, estrogen receptor inhibitor tamoxifen, antiangiogenic drugs, administered both alone and in combination and by concomitant supportive therapies (i.e., granulocyte-colony stimulating factors, erythropoiesis stimulating agents and glucocorticoids) [24–28]. The highest association with VTE is observed for multiple clinical factors, including increased medical co-morbidities and treatment associated with multiple drugs. The association between VTE and cancer appears to be time-dependent, with most VTE events occurring within the first 6 months after cancer diagnosis and the first 3 months of chemotherapy [25,29,30]. If on one hand surgery and medical treatment, catheters, chemo-radiotherapy and co-morbidities contribute to increase thrombosis risk [31], on the other some co-morbidities and/or chemotherapy-related side effects, such as renal or hepatic insufficiency and thrombocytopenia, can affect the efficacy and safety of anticoagulation [32].

These factors associated with age and ECOG (Eastern Cooperative Oncology Group) performance status, indicative of the patient's level of function and mobility [33,34] are parameters that drive all decision making processes in cancer patients at risk for VTE and which should indicate not only those who might benefit from thromboprophylaxis but also those who are fit for receiving it. Indeed, the increased risk of VTE occurrence and/or recurrence requires a tight balance with the anticoagulation-associated major bleeding complications [35–37]. The interplay between VTE and cancer has been further confirmed by considering that ~20% of patients with an episode of unprovoked VTE will be diagnosed with cancer within one year from VTE occurrence [38] and that patients with malignancies are more prone than others to develop recurrent VTE despite appropriate anticoagulant therapy [29,35,37].

In centers adhering to MDS standards, admission to Nursing Homes with a diagnosis of symptomatic VTE is reported to be overall (independently of cancer diagnosis) ~4% [39], while ~1% of new symptomatic VTE are recorded during residency [40]. These figures significantly increase for SPCUs dealing with advanced cancer patients, with a recorded ~10% prevalence [41].

In a study by Soto-Cárdenas et al., 712 patients attending the SPCU in a three-year period of observation presented a symptomatic VTE in 9.98% of cases (n = 71) [42]. Lung and colorectal cancer were most prevalent primary tumors (14% and 13%, respectively) and for the vast majority of patients (88.7%) symptomatic VTE occurred in the outpatient setting and was itself the cause of admission to SPCU.

Two studies have also investigated the incidence of asymptomatic VTE in these sceneries. Johnson et al. have analyzed the presence of cloths in deep veins (DVT) of 258 hospice cancer inpatients by means of light reflection rheography. The prevalence of DVT was 52% (n = 135) and being bedridden and hypoalbuminemia were independent risk factors at multivariate analysis [43].

In a prospective longitudinal trial, the HIDDen trial, 273 SPCU cancer patients from the UK, with a life expectancy >5 days, were screened for asymptomatic DVT by using bilateral femoral vein ultrasonography within 48 h of admission [44]. Stringent follow-up was also carried out with weekly repeated ultrasonography up to 3 weeks after admission. As expected, study population was relatively elderly (mean age 68 years) and with a poor Karnofsky performance status (mean score: 49).

Consistent results with Johnson's study were demonstrated, with an incidence of DVT of 34% and being bedbound in the 12 weeks preceding study recruitment as a significant risk factor [44].

Albuminemia was not confirmed to be associated with DVT diagnosis (p = 0.43). Interestingly, only four additional patients were diagnosed with DVT during the three weeks of follow-up.

Overall, these data confirmed that the prevalence of VTE among palliative care unit (PCU) patients is impressive (35–50%), however how much it might truly affect QoL in this cancer setting is still highly debated, although in terms of increasing anxiety, patients consider VTE a physically and emotionally distressing phenomenon that overlaps the underlying malignancy and strongly decreases their QoL. The PELICAN study [45], performed by interviewing a small population of cancer patients in order to assess their perception of the newly diagnosis of cancer-associated thrombosis (CAT), has identified three stages that were described as "life before CAT," "initial diagnosis and treatment of CAT" and "living with CAT," each one associated with specific patient needs. The study showed that only an exhaustive information by the clinical staff with respect to clinical intervention and process was capable to guarantee compliance to anticoagulant treatment and distress reduction [45].

2.1. VTE Current Guidelines

2.1.1. VTE Prophylaxis

In the light of all the above, it is evident that VTE prevention in cancer patients is of great importance due to the difficult management of thromboembolic events that increase morbidity, interfere with the anticancer treatments causing drug administration delay or discontinuation, affect patient's QoL and influence disease outcome [46].

As regard primary thromboprophylaxis, there is an unanimous consent from all major international guidelines to recommend thromboprophylaxis only in patients hospitalized for acute medical illness and in patients undergoing major surgery, while no thromboprophylaxis is recommended in ambulatory patients receiving chemotherapy due to the limited documented benefits counterbalanced by an increased risk of bleeding [35,47–53]. Therefore, clinicians are left with the decision to start an anticoagulant prophylaxis in selected high risk categories of patients after careful assessment of the risk of mortality and morbidity associated with possible bleeding events. Although most cancer patients are not recommended to receive prophylactic anticoagulation from VTE, NCCN guidelines suggest prophylactic anticoagulation or aspirin use in patients with multiple myeloma receiving thalidomide, lenalidomide or pomalidomide treatment [47]. The recently updated ASCO guidelines introduced the use of direct oral anticoagulants (DOACs) in VTE prophylaxis and treatment by stating that the use of primary prophylaxis "should" be offered to cancer patients hospitalized for an acute illness or reduced mobility and it "may" be offered to hospitalized solid cancer patients without additional risk factors, provided the risk of bleeding is absent [54]. In a context of critically ill patients such as those in the Intensive Care Units (ICU), anticoagulants should be administered until mobility is restored [55]. All patients with malignant disease undergoing major surgery should be offered thromboprophylaxis with either unfractionated heparin (UFH) or low-molecular weight heparins (LMWHs) unless contraindicated because of active bleeding or high bleeding risk or other contraindications and should be commenced preoperatively [54]. From the above, it is clear the urge to identify those subjects to be treated with antithrombotic prophylaxis. To the purpose of evaluating VTE risk in cancer patients, the Khorana Score (KS), a user-friendly VTE risk predictor based on the evaluation of pre-chemotherapy routinely available variables, has been developed and, despite the acknowledged limitations, has been adopted in the decision making processes (Table 1) [56]. According to KS, patients with a score ≥3 are classified as high-risk, those with a score 1–2 are classified as intermediate-risk and patients with a score = 0 as low-risk ones [56].

Table 1. The Khorana risk assessment model for cancer patients prior to chemotherapy start [56].

Patient's Characteristics	Score
Site of cancer Very high risk (stomach, pancreas, brain)	2
High risk (lung, lymphoma, gynecologic, bladder, myeloma, testicular or kidney)	1
Platelet count ≥350 × 10^9/L	1
Hemoglobin level <6.2 mmol/L or use of red cell growth factors	1
Leukocyte count >11 × 10^9/L	1
Body mass index ≥35 kg/m^2	1

The total score represents three risk groups of patients: 0 = low risk, 1–2 = intermediate risk, 3 = high risk.

Although routine thromboprophylaxis is still not recommended for all cancer outpatients receiving chemotherapy, current guidelines encourage to evaluate patients at higher risk of VTE by means of KS and recommend thromboprophylaxis with LMWH or DOACs, either apixaban or rivaroxaban, to those patients which have been assigned a risk score ≥2 and not actively bleeding or not at high risk of bleeding [54,57,58]. These considerations find the highest application in patients under a simultaneous care therapeutic program.

Two large randomized controlled studies using DOACs for VTE primary prevention and incorporating KS to target intermediate to high-risk patients, evaluated the efficacy and safety of apixaban 2.5 mg twice daily (AVERT) [59] or rivaroxaban 10 mg daily (CASSINI) [57] in ambulatory cancer patients. Both DOACs significantly reduced the risk of VTE in the primary analysis (5.2% on DOACs and 9.3% on placebo; 95% CI, 0.34–0.90; $p = 0.02$) although at the expense of an increased risk of major bleeding (2.0% on DOACs and 1.0% on placebo; 95% CI, 0.80–4.82; $p = 0.14$) and clinically relevant non-major bleeding (4.6% on DOACs and 3.4% on placebo; 95% CI, 0.80–2.27; $p = 0.26$). However, the net benefit of DOACs considering VTE prevention vs. major bleeding, was in favor of an overall risk reduction of 2.8% with DOACs [60].

Other Standard Committees recommend the Khorana risk score as a tool to identify patients with very high risk of VTE [61,62], although acknowledging that the score has insufficient precision in certain settings, such as lung and pancreas cancers [63–65].

Other authors have tried to improve the Khorana score performance and proposed modifications by adding biomarkers, types of chemotherapy or performance status [52,66,67]. A recently published review aimed at the optimization of thromboprophylaxis in cancer patients has been considering all these aspects and suggested that prediction scores might be developed for specific cancer sites [68]. Pabinger et al. [69] developed and validated a nomogram that included only tumor site risk category and D-dimer to assess the risk of VTE in chemotherapy-treated cancer patients [69]. Pabinger's nomogram was validated in an external cohort by Ferroni and co-workers for cumulative 6-month VTE risk prediction. [70].

All these models, designed to punctually evaluate ambulatory cancer patients before the starting of a new chemotherapy regimen, do not consider, nor apply, to those admitted to palliative care or hospices. However, they well fit to cancer patients under simultaneous care, thus still under active anticancer treatment. Indeed, among the patients for whom anticoagulation is of uncertain benefit there are listed patient receiving end-of-life/hospice care [54]. Hence, primary thromboprophylaxis for VTE is differently considered in the two setting, palliative and simultaneous (Table 2). The latter might be assimilated to that of the ambulatory cancer patients and evaluated accordingly.

Table 2. Recommendation guidelines for thromboprophylaxis in cancer patients. Differences between palliative care and ambulatory (in which patients on simultaneous care can be reconsidered) settings.

Guideline	Recommendation	
	Palliative Care	Ambulatory Setting
National Institute for Health and Clinical Excellence (NICE) [71]	TP should be considered for hospitalised palliative care patients, taking into account temporary increases in thrombotic risk factors, risk of bleeding, likely life expectancy and the views of patient and caregivers. Exceptions are patients in the last days of life.	Not specifically addressed. TPX is not indicated in patients receiving cancer-modifying treatments such as RT, CHT or immunotherapy, unless they are also at increased risk of VTE for other reasons than cancer. Consider for people receiving CHT for pancreatic cancer or myeloma (in association with thalidomide, pomalidomide or lenalidomide and steroids).
American College of Chest Physicians (ACCP) [51]	No guidelines in palliative care. Recommended in immobilized outpatients with solid tumors but opposed in immobilized patients at nursing homes.	TPX is not recommended routinely but it is suggested in those patients with additional risk factors for VTE and who are at low risk of bleeding
British Committee for standards in Haematology (BCSH) [62]	Antithrombotic use aimed solely at increasing life expectancy in patients with cancer but without a history of VTE, is not recommended	Outpatients with active cancer should be assessed for thrombosis risk; TPX should be considered for high risk patients and offered to patients with myeloma receiving thalidomide or lenalidomide, unless contraindicated
National Comprehensive Cancer Network (NCCN) [47]	No guidelines in palliative care. Routine TPX use should be limited to clinical trials only	Patients with a KS score ≥3 could be considered for VTE prophylaxis on an individual basis, after discussions with patients/caregivers regarding the potential risks and benefits. Prophylactic anticoagulation or aspirin use in patients with multiple myeloma receiving thalidomide, lenalidomide or pomalidomide treatment, is suggested
American Society of Clinical Oncology (ASCO) [54]	No guidelines in palliative care. TPX should not be the life-prolonging procedure. Can be considered in selected high-risk cancer outpatients	Routine TPX should not be offered. In high-risk outpatients (KS≥ 2) it may be offered provided there are no significant risk factors for bleeding nor drug interactions. Patients with multiple myeloma receiving thalidomide- or lenalidomide-based regimens with chemotherapy and/or dexamethasone should be offered pharmacologic thromboprophylaxis with either aspirin or LMWH for lower-risk pts and LMWH for higher-risk pts
European Society for Medical Oncology (ESMO) [52]	No guidelines in palliative care setting	Routine TPX is not recommended apart from select populations of cancer patients with solid tumours or in categories of patients with myeloma.
International Society on Thrombosis and Haemostasis (ISTH) [60]	No guidelines in palliative care setting	Primary TPX is suggested in cancer patients starting chemotherapy with a KS ≥2, no drug-drug interactions and not at high risk for bleeding
International Initiative on Thrombosis and Cancer (ITAC) [61]	No guidelines in palliative care setting. TPX is suggested in hospitalised patients with reduced mobility	Primary prophylaxis is not recommended routinely but indicated in patients with locally advanced or metastatic pancreatic cancer treated with systemic anticancer therapy and who have a low risk of bleeding
Italian Association of Medical Oncology AIOM [72]	No guidelines in palliative care setting	TPX is not routinely recommended in patients at low risk but it can be considered only in high risk patients receiving chemo- or hormone-therapy.
Canadian Consensus Recommendations [32]	No guidelines in palliative care setting. Hospitalized patients with active malignancy and acute illness or decreased mobility should receive TPX in the absence of contraindications.	TPX is not routinely recommended. May be considered for very selected high-risk patients receiving chemotherapy.

CHT: chemotherapy; KS: Khorana Score; RT: Radiotherapy; TPX: Thromboprophylaxis; VTE: Venous thromboembolism.

In the dynamic evaluation of patients in simultaneous care, VTE risk assessment might benefit from the inclusion of all these indexes and scores that might combine for the optimization of a unique, inclusive score. As recently outlined by our research group, artificial intelligence (AI) can be used to analyze a huge amount of clinical variables thus representing a solid instrument to build a predictive tool for VTE risk assessment in chemotherapy-treated cancer outpatients [73,74]. This tool has proven extremely useful in selecting VTE risk predictors [73], resulting in a significant improvement of VTE risk prediction performance over the KS [56] and also over the nomogram proposed by Pabinger et al. [69] and can be easily applied to different situations/populations, thus in patients that move from one intensity of care to another, even in the palliative setting.

2.1.2. VTE Treatment and Prevention of Recurrence

Active cancer is a strong risk factor also for VTE recurrence and VTE patients with active cancer should be treated with prolonged anticoagulation therapy as long as the disease is considered active. This, however, poses serious challenging problems due to the increased risk of hemorrhages in this setting of patients, thus a careful evaluation should be performed on a case-by-case basis, since both the differences in the rate of VTE recurrence incidence and major bleeding events are dependent on the cancer type and stage and on associated co-morbidities. Indeed, according to the RIETE study results, cancer patients with VTE recurrence, particularly if the event is a PE, are at a 3-fold increased risk of death [75]. Thus, in cancer patients with established VTE, according to the American Society on clinical Oncology (ASCO) guidelines, initial anticoagulation may involve LMWH, UFH, fondaparinux or rivaroxaban. For long-term anticoagulation, LMWH, edoxaban or rivaroxaban should be used for at least 6 months and preferred to Vitamin K antagonists, which may be used if LMWH or DOACs are not accessible. Further prolongation of anticoagulation for patients with active cancer, should be reserved only to selected patients with metastatic cancer or those receiving chemotherapy [54]. The guidelines released by the Scientific and Standardization Committee (SSC) of the International Society on Thrombosis and Hemostasis (ISTH) [58] suggested the use of LMWHs for cancer patients with an acute diagnosis of VTE and a high risk of bleeding, indicating edoxaban and rivaroxaban as an acceptable alternative if there are no drug–drug interactions with the current systemic therapy. With regard to rivaroxaban, results from the SELECT-D study, showed that it was indeed efficacious in reducing the rate of recurrent VTE compared with LMWH but at the cost of more bleeding, both major and clinically relevant nonmajor bleeding (CRNMB) [76]. A very recent trial (the Caravaggio trial) assessing the efficacy and safety of apixaban during the initial 6-month treatment of venous thromboembolism in patients enrolled without limitation of cancer type and anticancer treatment in order to be consistent with the cancer distribution in the general population, demonstrated a noninferiority of this DOAC (10 mg twice daily for the first 7 days, followed by 5 mg twice daily) as compared to subcutaneous dalteparin, in terms of recurrent VTE (5.6% vs. 7.9%, respectively) and major bleeding (3.8% vs. 4.0%, respectively), including gastrointestinal ones [77].

After 6 months' treatment, the need for extending anticoagulation requires reassessment in a risk vs. benefit manner, taking into account patient's preferences [47,71]. The Hokusai VTE Cancer trial, designed to compare, for 6 to 12 months, edoxaban with dalteparin for VTE treatment in patients with predominantly advanced cancer and acute symptomatic or incidental venous thromboembolism, demonstrated a noninferiority of edoxaban with respect to dalteparin in the composite outcome of recurrent venous thromboembolism or major bleeding [78]. Indeed, a post-hoc analysis of the Hokusai-VTE Cancer study patients, demonstrated that an extended treatment (beyond 6 months) with oral edoxaban was as effective and safe as subcutaneous dalteparin [79]. Results from a phase III, multicenter, randomized, double-blind, trial (EVE Trial) assessing apixaban 2.5 mg vs. 5 mg twice daily for 12 months for the secondary VTE prevention in cancer patients who have completed 6 months (but no more than 12 months) of anticoagulation (NCT03080883) are awaited [80].

NCCN guideline recommend lifelong anticoagulation for non-catheter-related cancer DVT or PE while cancer is active, under treatment or if risk factors for recurrence persist [47].

The final treatment strategy should thus be designed by the physician after shared decision-making with the patients, incorporating their preferences and values [58]. In this light, a particular cluster of patients for whom the risk of recurrent VTE and the advantages of oral therapy need to be carefully balanced, is represented by those with gastrointestinal cancer, given their increased risk of bleeding [81].

Patients who have recurrent VTE while on VKA therapy (in the therapeutic range) or on DOACs (dabigatran, rivaroxaban, apixaban or edoxaban) should switch to treatment with LMWH at least temporarily, while in those with VTE recurrence during LMWH, the dose of LMWH should be increased [82].

One important aspect that should be considered and discussed with patients in order to ensure compliance to anticoagulant treatment is the patient's preference regarding the modality of drug administration. In fact, some patients find tablets more convenient, thus welcoming DOACs, while others accept low-molecular-weight heparin injections as part of their treatment, despite some drawbacks [83].

In spite of the above, the vast majority of the studies performed to assess the best choice/duration of anticoagulant treatment were not directed to the frailest cancer patients, those with poor performance status or a life expectancy lower than 3 months, in which bleeding and recurrent thromboses are increased [84] and that represent a cluster of hospitalized patients that must be considered separately.

2.2. Role of Anticoagulants in Simultaneous and Palliative Care

More than 60 years ago, the first randomized trial on thromboprophylaxis demonstrated that adequate oral anticoagulants were able to significantly reduce new symptomatic VTE occurrence and death while containing excessive hemorrhagic side effects in patients undergoing hip fracture surgery [85]. Since then, a number of randomized controlled trials (RCTs), have confirmed that prevention of VTE is feasible and can possibly be considered as the commonest pharmacologically avoidable acute hospital death [86]. RCTs on prevention or treatment of VTE in cancer patients are mainly focused on settings of active oncological therapies and an estimated life expectancy inferior to three months, such as that attributed to subjects on palliative care, was invariable an exclusion criteria for RCTs [87].

The use of anticoagulants and in particular of LMWHs in hospices and SPCUs is controversial. The real effectiveness of full dose anticoagulants in SPCUs is perceived as minimal, since their benefit in terms of VTE-related symptom relief may be outweighed by excessive risk of bleeding in frail cancer patients [88].

Many patients are admitted with a history of VTE and are on stable LMWH at entry. However, subcutaneous administration, often twice a day, is undoubtedly considered as an extraordinary distress for patients who are symptomatic and compromised. No clear data exist on the impact of LMWHs in delaying or relieving VTE-related symptoms, and, although not the primary objective for palliative care, still no data are available on survival prolongation.

In palliative care, anticoagulants are perceived as unnecessary and their use is generally limited. The highly prevalent VTE in cancer patients on palliation is considered more a negligible epiphenomenon of the deteriorated clinical conditions of the near-end-of-life period than a leading cause of premature death or significant contributor of symptom burden.

Results from the HIDDen trial showed that DVT was not associated with reduced survival ($p = 0.45$) and the use of anticoagulants did not reduce DVT incidence ($p = 0.17$). Moreover, DVT was not associated to symptom burden, except from a significant association with limb edema ($p = 0.009$) [44].

Cai et al. performed a Medline, Embase and the Cochrane Library systematic review searching for studies assessing thromboprophylaxis in palliative care. Among a total of 22 original reports, use of thromboprophylaxis ranged between 4% and 53% [89].

More recently, Noble et al. have reviewed patients attending a clinic for CAT and, by using death notification cross-references, selected those dying within 2 years from CAT clinic referral ($n = 214$). Half of them were found to continue LMWH until death and 11% up to 7 days prior death. Even though no VTE-related symptoms were recorded possibly due to the high therapy adherence, a substantial incidence of clinically relevant bleeding was notified (7%) [90].

In the above-mentioned study by Soto-Cárdenas et al. [42], after VTE diagnosis all patients received LMWH. Consistent hemorrhagic complications were reported (11.3%) and some patients died because of the bleeding (4%). However, in a relevant percentage of cases the death was considered to be VTE-related instead, despite the start of full dose LMWH. Authors concluded that the risk/benefit ratio in this specific cancer population need to be attentively evaluated.

Similar incidence of bleeding complication has been recorded in a French cohort of palliative care cancer patients ($n = 1091$). Overall, bleeding occurred in 10% of patients and in the majority of cases was associated with LMWH. Pharmacological thromboprophylaxis was associated with a nearly 50% increased risk of hemorrhagic event in this patient population (HR: 1.48, $p = 0.04$) [91].

For patients on active anti-cancer treatment, NCCN guidelines recommend indefinite anticoagulation when CAT is diagnosed [47]. However, the real clinical impact of such an approach seems to be of limited value in the palliation setting mainly because of the very short life expectancy. In the above-mentioned HIDDen trial, almost two third (61%) of screened patients did not meet the inclusion criteria because of a believed life expectancy <5 days [44].

These evidences, taken together with the substantial bleeding risk of anticoagulants, suggest that treatment should be started/continued in highly selected cases when a worsening in symptom burden is feared. Moreover, they highlight the need for robust clinical study in the palliative care population to assess the best strategy for VTE prevention and treatment and the most accurate measurable end points relevant to the advanced cancer population [92].

The necessity of VTE risk assessment tools and thromboprophylaxis for patients admitted to palliative care units in order to identify those at higher risk, led to the development of guidelines especially focused on patients admitted to either acute or palliative care settings—the Pan Birmingham Cancer Network (PBCN) palliative-modified Thromboembolic Risk Factors (THRIFT) Consensus Group criteria [93]. The PBCNP Guideline for VTE primary prophylaxis suggests that all patients, regardless of diagnosis, should be assessed through a three-step process involving—1) general assessment; 2) assessment of the benefits of prophylaxis; 3) palliative team decision. The last step, to be also discussed with the patient, considers the appropriateness of treatment weighing up not only the associated risks and benefits but also the burden of monitoring and allows designing a strategy of therapy choice, duration and monitoring.

2.3. The Integrated Model

An integrated system of multilevel networks is the optimal way to guarantee the patient access to palliative care and pain therapy. The "network," as such, is designed to promote patient care continuity, from hospital to home and coordinates the structures and professionals dedicated to providing the service in a context of simultaneous care. Simultaneous care represents the new paradigm of care for cancer patients and requires a cultural and organizational change necessary to share goals, values and programming at the level of operating units, multidisciplinary groups, oncology departments and territorial services. This modality of management and treatment of advanced disease is aimed at associating, in a systematic way, palliative care with anticancer therapies, obtaining not only a benefit on QoL parameters but in some cases, even an extension of survival.

It has become evident that the problems and needs of patients affected by advanced neoplasia and their family members start long before the end of life phase, so that simultaneous care can be considered as the set of global care interventions aimed at both the patients and to family members and, more generally, to caregivers. This concept was implemented in 2012 by ASCO that recommended considering the combination of standard cancer care and palliative care early in the course of the disease, for all patients with metastatic cancer and/or with symptomatic disease [13]. Indeed, an increasing number of patients are admitted to palliative care units or residential hospices for brief periods necessary for symptom assessment and management and are then subsequently discharged home to continue active anticancer treatments, with discharge rates of about 60% [94–96].

The integrated management model should be considered the most suitable approach to improve care for people with oncological pathologies, whose effective treatments are necessarily modulated on the different levels of severity. Due to the complexity of the neoplastic pathology, a close collaboration between the many specialists is required in the form of multidisciplinary meetings between specialists from different disciplines. It is, therefore, necessary to identify integrated care and organizational pathways and to use validated multi-dimensional tests for patients in the metastatic phase, to detect and respond to all symptoms and care needs.

According to our own experience, in order to guarantee users a coordinated information flow and a single access to home services, it is essential that the palliative care network, with regard to its home activities, be coordinated and closely connected with a reference Operating Center for the Services of home care. We have, thus, stipulated local operating protocols, agreed upon and predefined between the Central and the Dispensing Subjects constituting the network, which safeguard the patient's freedom of choice. These protocols will have to consider all the phases of the specific care process for the end of life (reporting, evaluation, acceptance and definition of the care plan, verification of the results), which must be carried out jointly by the general practitioner, the staff of the PCU and the Operating Center of the Home Care Service. Furthermore, for patients included in a home-based palliative care program we have considered appropriate to provide for the direct delivery of drugs (in particular analgesic drugs including opioids and anticoagulants). The cooperative process that ascertains the need, plans, implements, coordinates, controls and evaluates options and services in response to an individual's demand in order to achieve quality and economically efficient outcomes is defined as Case Management. The Case Management model in Oncology in general and in our Unit in particular, is configured as a highly innovative project having been applied for the first time to sections of the population classified as "fragile," that is, with great difficulty in accessing and autonomously following medical care and access to the hospital. The model is outlined as a new tool in the course of treating the disease; the person and his centrality have been placed at the base of the realization of the program—"there is no cure for the disease without personal care."

Patients with medium/low intensity of care (defined as "no-therapy" with hospice transfer/home assistance) are those with advanced cancer, for which health interventions are no longer capable to provide satisfactory results in terms of medium-long term regression-stabilization of neoplastic disease.

Indeed, when cancer patients reach a limited life expectancy, quality of life and symptom relief often represent more important endpoints than survival. These outcome measures are subjective and not always reported [97]. Considering that the vast majority of patients admitted to hospices are at moderate to high risk of developing a VTE during their stay [93], the possibility of an early integration of VTE preventive strategies, in a simultaneous care program, might help overcoming the problem of deciding in favor or against thromboprophylaxis in a context of palliation.

In 2006, the Food and Drug Administration (FDA) introduced the concept of patient-reported outcomes measures (PROMs) for those measures that best reflect the patients' perceptions, for an optimal monitoring of symptoms from the primary cancer diagnosis and during follow-up care [98]. Advances in information technologies permits to collect PROMs by means of electronic tools, namely electronic PRO (ePRO). The development of such tools allowing the integration of PROMs with patient-related data from hospital and laboratory sources warrants a follow-up at several levels, also at distance, with data that can be automatically transferred in real time to a computer server [99–102]. Moreover, all clinically relevant actions based on PRO scores can be added to the patient's electronic medical record, thus allowing the health-care providers to be always aware of patient conditions and to move smoothly from an active treatment to palliation.

Novel tools allowing routine assessment of PROs via smartphone and tablet applications have proven user friendly to patients, with a low loss of data and with the possibility to monitor patient compliance to pharmacotherapy [102,103].

3. Physicians' Perspectives

Specific guidelines for management of VTE in palliative care patients are lacking and administration of anticoagulants relies mainly on physicians' clinical judgement. Expertise and individual clinical judgment is pivotal in the decision-making process, however it might be more influenced by incidental factors and personal convictions than by objective evidence.

In general, palliative care physicians are less prone to prescribing anti-coagulants and the perceived imminent death for most of cancer patients on palliation is considered the main reason, thus impeding the appropriate prevention of VTE-related symptoms in some cases. On the other hand, in certain sets of cancer patients, such as pancreatic ones, an early VTE episode at the beginning of chemotherapy administered for palliation, represents a poor prognostic factor [104].

In a factorial survey conducted in Canada among 62 medical oncologists (MOs) and 73 palliative care physicians (PCPs), MOs were twice more likely to prescribe anti-coagulants in specific VTE risk conditions (OR: 2.09, $p < 0.001$) [105]. In the multivariable analysis, being a medical oncologist was an independent factor associated with anticoagulant prescription, together with medical conditions that indicate a possibly longer overall survival (such acute care hospital admission or reversible cause for admission) and low risk of bleeding.

PCPs have culturally and historically less attitude towards intensive interventions, however specific differences in the training programme between MOs and PCPs might contribute to different medical decisions in the same clinical scenarios and specific guidelines are eagerly needed to harmonize the standard treatment in this context.

Similar results were found in a smaller study surveying a diverse panel of 20 physicians constituted of experts in palliative care, oncology, blood coagulation and intensive care. Again, PCPs were less likely to indicate thromboprophylaxis.

This possibly nihilistic approach among PCPs (VTE perhaps conceived as one of the possible terminal causes of an imminent death) is in contrast with the increasing percentage of patients being discharged from the palliative care settings because admitted and treated for reversible causes for brief periods [106]. Conversely, larger consensus might come from the inclusion of patients in the simultaneous care setting under the category of ambulatory cancer patients, for which a constant evaluation of pros and cons should indicate the appropriate timing and risks of anticoagulation. Simultaneous cares are indeed increasingly involved in the earlier phases of the cancer journey when active anticancer treatments are still delivered and intensive interventions are required [95]. Specific decision-making tools are necessary to avoid under-treatment also in the field of CAT and since the continuum of care paradigm is in constant change, a major effort should be made in this area to achieve a broad consensus on how to manage VTE. Figure 1 depicts a proposed algorithm for the management of the best anticancer strategy to cancer patients under a simultaneous care program that includes palliative care interventions with active antineoplastic treatment and cannot ignore an initial VTE risk evaluation.

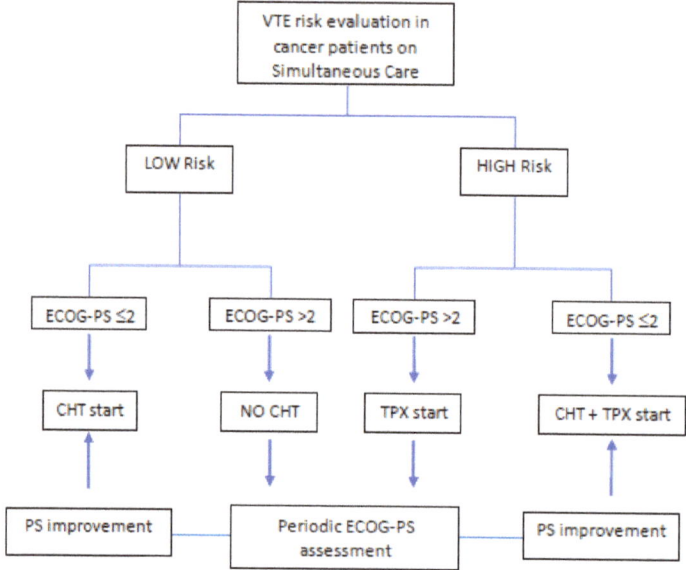

Figure 1. Proposed algorithm for a therapeutic strategy based on the evaluation of venous thromboembolism (VTE) risk in patients with advanced cancer on a simultaneous care program. The classical category of the Intermediate-risk patients defined by the Khorana score is no longer included, since the integration of detailed programs and evaluations allows a more specific discrimination among patients [68–70,73]. CHT: Chemotherapy; ECOG-PS: ECOG-Performance Status; TPX: Thromboprophylaxis.

4. Conclusions

People are living longer thus the aging population associated with increased multimorbidity, chronic diseases and disability is growing and is living longer with metastatic disease for which it is receiving more and more chemotherapy and palliative therapies.

In palliative clinical practice, oncologists are frequently faced with the task of determining the appropriate, if any, anticoagulation strategy in their patients. The first crossroads is represented by the necessity to establish whether risk of VTE occurrence overcomes the risk of fatal bleeding. Secondly, the possibility to switch the patient to active anticancer treatment during his/her staying should be determined. Indeed, anticoagulant therapy may have important side effects that could cause cancer treatment discontinuation and could even result in patient's death. Finally, when patients are diagnosed with VTE, the period in which VTE occurred, either before or during admission, could guide the decisions to start anticoagulation. Information regarding prognostic VTE-related factors and predictors would assist oncologists in predicting the occurrence of VTE and in determining active cancer treatment as well as anticoagulant therapy in clinical practice. On the other hand routine risk assessment for VTE in all patients admitted to a hospice is not usual and hospices are managing patients who are not imminently dying. Thus, it is important a careful evaluation of the effects of VTE and its related events on QoL and, conversely, those of anticoagulant treatment. In this light, the possibility to realize algorithms that include patient's age, co-morbidities and polypharmacy, might enhance the sensitivity of existing available biomarkers and might allow the discovery of new, more specific, ones along with the development of appropriate testing for this particular cluster of patients. This will represent a fundamental step to avoid delays of VTE thromboprophylaxis and to allow an early start during the course of the active cancer treatment, according to a simultaneous care model.

Funding: This work has been partially supported by the European Social Fund, under the Italian Ministry of Economic Development—NET4HEALTH ("HORIZON 2020" PON I&C 2014-2020—F/050383/01-03/X32).

Conflicts of Interest: The Authors declare no conflict of interest.

References

1. Zagonel, V.; Torta, R.; Franciosi, V.; Brunello, A.; Biasco, G.; Cattaneo, D.; Cavanna, L.; Corsi, D.; Farina, G.; Fioretto, L.; et al. Early Integration of Palliative Care in Oncology Practice: Results of the Italian Association of Medical Oncology (AIOM) Survey. *J. Cancer* **2016**, *7*, 1968–1978. [CrossRef] [PubMed]
2. Jordan, K.; Aapro, M.; Kaasa, S.; Ripamonti, C.; Scotté, F.; Strasser, F.; Young, A.; Bruera, E.; Herrstedt, J.; Keefe, D.; et al. European Society for Medical Oncology (ESMO) position paper on supportive and palliative care. *Ann. Oncol.* **2018**, *29*, 36–43. [CrossRef] [PubMed]
3. Temel, J.S.; Greer, J.A.; Muzikansky, A.; Gallagher, E.R.; Admane, S.; Jackson, V.A.; Dahlin, C.M.; Blinderman, C.D.; Jacobsen, J.; Pirl, W.F.; et al. Early palliative care for patients with metastatic non-small-cell lung cancer. *New Engl. J. Med.* **2010**, *363*, 733–742. [CrossRef] [PubMed]
4. Bakitas, M.; Lyons, K.D.; Hegel, M.T.; Balan, S.; Brokaw, F.C.; Seville, J.; Hull, J.G.; Li, Z.; Tosteson, T.D.; Byock, I.R.; et al. Effects of a palliative care intervention on clinical outcomes in patients with advanced cancer: The project ENABLE II randomized controlled trial. *JAMA* **2009**, *302*, 741–749. [CrossRef] [PubMed]
5. Gaertner, J.; Siemens, W.; Meerpohl, J.J.; Antes, G.; Meffert, C.; Xander, C.; Stock, S.; Mueller, D.; Schwarzer, G.; Becker, G. Effect of specialist palliative care services on quality of life in adults with advanced incurable illness in hospital, hospice or community settings: Systematic review and meta-analysis. *BMJ* **2017**, *357*, j2925. [CrossRef]
6. WHO. Definition of Palliative Care. Available online: https://www.who.int/cancer/palliative/definition/en/ (accessed on 3 May 2020).
7. Cherny, N.I.; Catane, R.; Kosmidis, P. ESMO Taskforce on Supportive and Palliative Care. ESMO takes a stand on supportive and palliative care. *Ann. Oncol.* **2003**, *14*, 1335–1337. [CrossRef]
8. Rochigneux, P.; Raoul, J.L.; Beaussant, Y.; Aubry, R.; Goldwasser, F.; Tourignand, C.; Morin, L. Use of chemotherapy near the end of life: What factors matter? *Ann. Oncol.* **2017**, *28*, 809–817. [CrossRef]
9. Peppercorn, J.M.; Smith, T.J.; Helft, P.R.; Debono, D.J.; Berry, S.R.; Wollins, D.S.; Hayes, D.M.; Von Roenn, J.H.; Schnipper, L.E. American Society of Clinical Oncology. American Society of Clinical Oncology statement: Toward individualized care for patients with advanced cancer. *J. Clin. Oncol.* **2011**, *29*, 755–760. [CrossRef]
10. Levy, M.H.; Adolph, M.D.; Back, A.; Block, S.; Codada, S.N.; Dalal, S.; Deshields, T.L.; Dexter, E.; Dy, S.M.; Knight, S.J.; et al. NCCN (National Comprehensive Cancer Network). Palliative care. *J. Natl. Compr. Canc. Netw.* **2012**, *10*, 1284–1309. [CrossRef]
11. Kaasa, S.; Loge, J.H.; Aapro, M.; Albreht, T.; Anderson, R.; Bruera, E.; Brunelli, C.; Caraceni, A.; Cervantes, A.; Currow, D.C.; et al. Integration of oncology and palliative care: A Lancet Oncology Commission. *Lancet Oncol.* **2018**, *19*, e588–e653. [CrossRef]
12. Mayer, D.K.; Nasso, S.F.; Earp, J.A. Defining cancer survivors, their needs and perspectives on survivorship health care in the USA. *Lancet Oncol.* **2017**, *18*, e11–e18. [CrossRef]
13. Smith, T.J.; Temin, S.; Alesi, E.R.; Abernethy, A.P.; Balboni, T.A.; Basch, E.M.; Ferrell, B.R.; Loscalzo, M.; Meier, D.E.; Paice, J.A.; et al. American Society of Clinical Oncology provisional clinical opinion: The integration of palliative care into standard oncology care. *J. Clin. Oncol.* **2012**, *30*, 880–887. [CrossRef] [PubMed]
14. Formica, V.; Fossile, E.; Pellegrino, R.; Fatale, M.; Mari, M.; Rabuffetti, M.; Benedetto, F.R.; Visconti, G.; Bollero, E.; Roselli, M. The Medical Care Continuity (MCC) project. A pilot study of video-assisted home care within the eTEN European Community program. The Italian experience. *Support. Care Cancer* **2009**, *17*, 471–478. [CrossRef] [PubMed]
15. Mazanec, P.; Daly, B.J.; Pitorak, E.; Kane, D.; Wile, S.; Wolen, J. A new model of palliative care for oncology patients with advanced disease. *J. Hosp. Palliat. Nurs.* **2009**, *11*, 324–331. [CrossRef]
16. Ferris, F.D.; Bruera, E.; Cherny, N.; Cummings, C.; Currow, D.; Dudgeon, D.; Janjan, N.; Strasser, F.; von Gunten, C.F.; Von Roenn, J.H. Palliative cancer care a decade later: Accomplishments, the need, next steps—From the American Society of Clinical Oncology. *J. Clin. Oncol.* **2009**, *27*, 3052–3058. [CrossRef]

17. Barton, M.K. Early outpatient referral to palliative care services improves end-of-life care. *J. Clin.* **2014**, *64*, 223–224. [CrossRef]
18. Institute of Medicine (US) Committee on Quality of Health Care in America. *Crossing the Quality Chasm: A New Health System for the 21st Century*; National Academies Press (US): Washington, DC, USA, 2001.
19. Jack, B.A.; Littlewood, C.; Eve, A.; Murphy, D.; Khatri, A.; Ellershaw, J.E. Reflecting the scope and work of palliative care teams today: An action research project to modernise a national minimum data set. *Palliat. Med.* **2009**, *23*, 80–86. [CrossRef]
20. Battinelli, E.M.; Murphy, D.L.; Connors, J.M. Venous thromboembolism overview. *Hematol. Oncol. Clin. N. Am.* **2012**, *26*, 345–367. [CrossRef]
21. Lyman, G.H.; Khorana, A.A.; Kuderer, N.M.; Lee, A.Y.; Arcelus, J.I.; Balaban, E.P.; Clarke, J.M.; Flowers, C.R.; Francis, C.W.; Gates, L.E.; et al. Venous thromboembolism prophylaxis and treatment in patients with cancer: American Society of Clinical Oncology Clinical Practice Guideline Update. *J. Clin. Oncol.* **2013**, *31*, 2189–2204. [CrossRef]
22. Gao, S.; Escalante, C. Venous thromboembolism and malignancy. *Expert Rev. Anticancer Ther.* **2004**, *4*, 303–320. [CrossRef]
23. Paskauskas, S.; Pundzius, J.; Barauskas, G. Venous thromboembolism and prophylaxis in cancer patients. *Medicina* **2008**, *44*, 175–181. [CrossRef] [PubMed]
24. Prandoni, P.; Piccioli, A.; Girolami, A. Cancer and venous thromboembolism: An overview. *Haematologica* **1999**, *84*, 437–445. [PubMed]
25. Roselli, M.; Ferroni, P.; Riondino, S.; Mariotti, S.; Laudisi, A.; Vergati, M.; Cavaliere, F.; Palmirotta, R.; Guadagni, F. Impact of chemotherapy on activated protein C-dependent thrombin generation—Association with VTE occurrence. *Int. J. Cancer* **2013**, *133*, 1253–1258. [CrossRef] [PubMed]
26. Bohlius, J.; Wilson, J.; Seidenfeld, J.; Piper, M.; Schwarzer, G.; Sandercock, J.; Trelle, S.; Weingart, O.; Bayliss, S.; Brunskill, S. Erythropoietin or darbepoetin for patients with cancer. *Cochrane Database Syst. Rev.* **2006**, *3*, CD003407.
27. Ferroni, P.; Formica, V.; Roselli, M.; Guadagni, F. Thromboembolic events in patients treated with anti-angiogenic drugs. *Curr. Vasc. Pharmacol.* **2010**, *8*, 102–113. [CrossRef]
28. Johannesdottir, S.A.; Horváth-Puhó, E.; Dekkers, O.M.; Cannegieter, S.C.; Jørgensen, J.O.; Ehrenstein, V.; Vandenbroucke, J.P.; Pedersen, L.; Sørensen, H.T. Use of glucocorticoids and risk of venous thromboembolism: A nationwide population-based case-control study. *JAMA Intern. Med.* **2013**, *173*, 743–752. [CrossRef]
29. Douketis, J.D.; Foster, G.A.; Crowther, M.A.; Prins, M.H.; Ginsberg, J.S. Clinical risk factors and timing of recurrent venous thromboembolism during the initial 3 months of anticoagulant therapy. *Arch. Intern. Med.* **2000**, *160*, 3431–3436. [CrossRef]
30. Di Nisio, M.; Ferrante, N.; De Tursi, M.; Iacobelli, S.; Cuccurullo, F.; Büller, H.R.; Feragalli, B.; Porreca, E. Incidental venous thromboembolism in ambulatory cancer patients receiving chemotherapy. *Thromb. Haemost.* **2010**, *104*, 1049–1054.
31. Dickmann, B.; Ahlbrecht, J.; Ay, C.; Dunkler, D.; Thaler, J.; Scheithauer, W.; Quehenberger, P.; Zielinski, C.; Pabinger, I. Regional lymph node metastases are a strong risk factor for venous thromboembolism: Results from the Vienna Cancer and Thrombosis Study. *Haematologica* **2013**, *98*, 1309–1314. [CrossRef]
32. Easaw, J.C.; Shea-Budgell, M.A.; Wu, C.M.; Czaykowski, P.M.; Kassis, J.; Kuehl, B.; Lim, H.J.; MacNeil, M.; Martinusen, D.; McFarlane, P.A.; et al. Canadian consensus recommendations on the management of venous thromboembolism in patients with cancer. Part 1: Prophylaxis. *Curr. Oncol.* **2015**, *22*, 133–143. [CrossRef]
33. Dutia, M.; White, R.H.; Wun, T. Risk assessment models for cancer-associated venous thromboembolism. *Cancer* **2012**, *118*, 3468–3476. [CrossRef] [PubMed]
34. Kroger, K.; Weiland, D.; Ose, C.; Neumann, N.; Weiss, S.; Hirsch, C.; Urbanski, K.; Seeber, S.; Scheulen, M.E. Risk factors for venous thromboembolic events in cancer patients. *Ann. Oncol.* **2006**, *17*, 297–303. [CrossRef] [PubMed]
35. Prandoni, P.; Lensing, A.W.; Piccioli, A.; Bernardi, E.; Simioni, P.; Girolami, B.; Marchiori, A.; Sabbion, P.; Prins, M.H.; Noventa, F.; et al. Recurrent venous thromboembolism and bleeding complications during anticoagulant treatment in patients with cancer and venous thrombosis. *Blood* **2002**, *100*, 3484–3488. [CrossRef] [PubMed]
36. Riondino, S.; Guadagni, F.; Formica, V.; Ferroni, P.; Roselli, M. Gender differences in cancer-associated venous thromboembolism. *Curr. Med. Chem.* **2017**, *24*, 2589–2601. [CrossRef] [PubMed]

37. Al-Samkari, H.; Connors, J.M. Managing the competing risks of thrombosis, bleeding and anticoagulation in patients with malignancy. *Blood. Adv.* **2019**, *3*, 3770–3779. [CrossRef] [PubMed]
38. Heit, J.A.; Spencer, F.A.; White, R.H. The epidemiology of venous thromboembolism. *J. Thromb. Thrombolysis* **2016**, *41*, 3–14. [CrossRef]
39. Reardon, G.; Pandya, N.; Nutescu, E.A.; Lamori, J.; Damaraju, C.V.; Schein, J.; Bookhart, B. Incidence of venous thromboembolism in nursing home residents. *J. Am. Med. Dir. Assoc.* **2013**, *14*, 578–584. [CrossRef]
40. Gomes, J.P.; Shaheen, W.H.; Truong, S.V.; Brown, E.F.; Beasley, B.W.; Gajewski, B.J. Incidence of venous thromboembolic events among nursing home residents. *J. Gen. Intern. Med.* **2003**, *18*, 934–936. [CrossRef]
41. Merminod, T.; Zulian, G.B. Diagnosis of venous thromboembolism in cancer patients receiving palliative care. *J. Pain Symptom Manag.* **2000**, *19*, 238–239. [CrossRef]
42. Soto-Cárdenas, M.J. Venous thromboembolism in patients with advanced cancer under palliative care: Additional risk factors, primary/secondary prophylaxis and complications observed under normal clinical practice. *Palliat. Med.* **2008**, *22*, 965–968. [CrossRef]
43. Johnson, M.J.; Sproule, M.W.; Paul, J. The prevalence and associated variables of deep venous thrombosis in patients with advanced cancer. *Clin. Oncol. (R Coll Radiol).* **1999**, *11*, 105–110. [CrossRef] [PubMed]
44. White, C.; Noble, S.I.R.; Watson, M.; Swan, F.; Allgar, V.L.; Napier, E.; Nelson, A.; McAuley, J.; Doherty, J.; Lee, B.; et al. Prevalence, symptom burden and natural history of deep vein thrombosis in people with advanced cancer in specialist palliative care units (HIDDen): A prospective longitudinal observational study. *Lancet Haematol.* **2019**, *6*, e79–e88. [CrossRef]
45. Noble, S.; Prout, H.; Nelson, A. Patients' Experiences of LIving with CANcer-associated thrombosis: The PELICAN study. *Patient Prefer. Adherence* **2015**, *24*, 337–345. [CrossRef] [PubMed]
46. Vergati, M.; Della-Morte, D.; Ferroni, P.; Cereda, V.; Tosetto, L.; La Farina, F.; Guadagni, F.; Roselli, M. Increased risk of chemotherapy-associated venous thromboembolism in elderly patients with cancer. *Rejuvenation Res.* **2013**, *16*, 224–231. [CrossRef]
47. Streiff, M.B.; Holmstrom, B.; Angelini, D.; Ashrani, A.; Bockenstedt, P.L.; Chesney, C.; Fanikos, J.; Fenninger, R.B.; Fogerty, A.E.; Gao, S.; et al. NCCN Guidelines Insights: Cancer-Associated Venous Thromboembolic Disease, Version 2.2018. *J. Natl. Compr. Canc. Netw.* **2018**, *16*, 1289–1303. [CrossRef]
48. Alikhan, R.; Cohen, A.T.; Combe, S.; Samama, M.M.; Desjardins, L.; Eldor, A.; Janbon, C.; Leizorovicz, A.; Olsson, C.G.; Turpie, A.G.; et al. Risk factors for venous thromboembolism in hospitalized patients with acute medical illness: Analysis of the MEDENOX Study. *Arch. Intern. Med.* **2004**, *164*, 963–968. [CrossRef]
49. Gross, C.P.; Galusha, D.H.; Krumholz, H.M. The impact of venous thromboembolism on risk of death or hemorrhage in older cancer patients. *J. Gen. Intern. Med.* **2007**, *22*, 321–326. [CrossRef]
50. Ruíz-Giménez, N.; Suárez, C.; González, R.; Nieto, J.A.; Todolí, J.A.; Samperiz, A.L.; Monreal, M.; RIETE Investigators. Predictive variables for major bleeding events in patients presenting with documented acute venous thromboembolism. Findings from the RIETE Registry. *Thromb. Haemost.* **2008**, *100*, 26–31.
51. Kahn, S.R.; Lim, W.; Dunn, A.S.; Cushman, M.; Dentali, F.; Akl, E.A.; Cook, D.J.; Balekian, A.A.; Klein, R.C.; Le, H.; et al. Prevention of VTE in nonsurgical patients: Antithrombotic therapy and prevention of thrombosis, 9th ed: American College of Chest Physicians evidence-based clinical practice guidelines. *Chest* **2012**, *141*, e195S–e226S. [CrossRef]
52. Ay, C.; Kamphuisen, P.W.; Agnelli, G. Antithrombotic therapy for prophylaxis and treatment of venous thromboembolism in patients with cancer: Review of the literature on current practice and emerging options. *ESMO Open* **2017**, *2*, e000188. [CrossRef]
53. Becattini, C.; Verso, M.; Muñoz, A.; Agnelli, G. Updated meta-analysis on prevention of venous thromboembolism in ambulatory cancer patients. *Haematologica* **2019**, *105*, 838–848. [CrossRef] [PubMed]
54. Key, N.S.; Khorana, A.A.; Kuderer, N.M.; Bohlke, K.; Lee, A.Y.Y.; Arcelus, J.I.; Wong, S.L.; Balaban, E.P.; Flowers, C.R.; Francis, C.W.; et al. Venous Thromboembolism Prophylaxis and Treatment in Patients With Cancer: ASCO Clinical Practice Guideline Update. *J. Clin. Oncol.* **2020**, *38*, 496–520. [CrossRef] [PubMed]
55. Minet, C.; Potton, L.; Bonadona, A.; Hamidfar-Roy, R.; Somohano, C.A.; Lugosi, M.; Cartier, J.C.; Ferretti, G.; Schwebel, C.; Timsit, J.F. Venous thromboembolism in the ICU: Main characteristics, diagnosis and thromboprophylaxis. *Crit. Care* **2015**, *19*, 287. [CrossRef] [PubMed]
56. Khorana, A.A.; Kuderer, N.M.; Culakova, E.; Lyman, G.H.; Francis, C.W. Development and validation of a predictive model for chemotherapy-associated thrombosis. *Blood* **2008**, *111*, 4902–4907. [CrossRef] [PubMed]

57. Khorana, A.A.; Soff, G.A.; Kakkar, A.K.; Vadhan-Raj, S.; Riess, H.; Wun, T.; Streiff, M.B.; Garcia, D.A.; Liebman, H.A.; Belani, C.P.; et al. Rivaroxaban for thromboprophylaxis in high-risk ambulatory patients with cancer. *New Engl. J. Med.* **2019**, *380*, 720–728. [CrossRef]
58. Khorana, A.A.; Noble, S.; Lee, A.Y.Y.; Soff, G.; Meyer, G.; O'Connell, C.; Carrier, M. Role of direct oral anticoagulants in the treatment of cancer-associated venous thromboembolism: Guidance from the SSC of the ISTH. *J. Thromb. Haemost.* **2018**, *16*, 1891–1894. [CrossRef]
59. Carrier, M.; Abou-Nassar, K.; Mallick, R.; Tagalakis, V.; Shivakumar, S.; Schattner, A.; Kuruvilla, P.; Hill, D.; Spadafora, S.; Marquis, K.; et al. AVERT Investigators. Apixaban to prevent venous thromboembolism in patients with cancer. *New. Engl. J. Med.* **2019**, *380*, 711–719. [CrossRef]
60. Wang, T.F.; Zwicker, J.I.; Ay, C.; Pabinger, I.; Falanga, A.; Antic, D.; Noble, S.; Khorana, A.A.; Carrier, M.; Meyer, G. The use of direct oral anticoagulants for primary thromboprophylaxis in ambulatory cancer patients: Guidance from the SSC of the ISTH. *J. Thromb. Haemost.* **2019**, *17*, 1772–1778. [CrossRef]
61. Farge, D.; Frere, C.; Connors, J.M.; Ay, C.; Khorana, A.A.; Munoz, A.; Brenner, B.; Kakkar, A.; Rafii, H.; Solymoss, S.; et al. for the International Initiative on Thrombosis and Cancer (ITAC) advisory panel. 2019 international clinical practice guidelines for the treatment and prophylaxis of venous thromboembolism in patients with cancer. *Lancet Oncol.* **2019**, *20*, e566–e581. [CrossRef]
62. Watson, H.G.; Keeling, D.M.; Laffan, M.; Tait, R.C.; Makris, M. British Committee for Standards in H. guideline on aspects of cancer-related venous thrombosis. *Br. J. Haematol.* **2015**, *70*, 640–648. [CrossRef]
63. Noble, S.; Alikhan, R.; Robbins, A.; Macbeth, F.; Hood, K. Predictors of active cancer thromboembolic outcomes: Validation of the Khorana score among patients with lung cancer: Comment. *J. Thromb. Haemost.* **2017**, *15*, 590–591. [CrossRef] [PubMed]
64. Kruger, S.; Haas, M.; Burkl, C.; Goehring, P.; Kleespies, A.; Roeder, F.; Gallmeier, E.; Ormanns, S.; Westphalen, C.B.; Heinemann, V.; et al. Incidence, outcome and risk stratification tools for venous thromboembolism in advanced pancreatic cancer—A retrospective cohort study. *Thromb. Res.* **2017**, *157*, 9–15. [CrossRef] [PubMed]
65. Van Es, N.; Franke, V.F.; Middeldorp, S.; Wilmink, J.W.; Büller, H.R. The Khorana score for the prediction of venous thromboembolism in patients with pancreatic cancer. *Thromb. Res.* **2017**, *150*, 30–32. [CrossRef] [PubMed]
66. Pelzer, U.; Sinn, M.; Stieler, J.; Riess, H. Primary pharmacological prevention of thromboembolic events in ambulatory patients with advanced pancreatic cancer treated with chemotherapy? *Dtsch. Med. Wochenschr.* **2013**, *138*, 2084–2088. [PubMed]
67. Verso, M.; Di Nisio, M. Management of venous thromboembolism in cancer patients: Considerations about the clinical practice guideline update of the American society of clinical oncology. *Eur. J. Intern. Med.* **2020**, *71*, 4–7. [CrossRef]
68. Mulder, F.I.; Bosch, F.T.M.; van Es, N. Primary Thromboprophylaxis in Ambulatory Cancer Patients: Where Do We Stand? *Cancers* **2020**, *12*, 367. [CrossRef]
69. Pabinger, I.; van Es, N.; Heinze, G.; Posch, F.; Riedl, J.; Reitter, E.M.; Di Nisio, M.; Cesarman-Maus, G.; Kraaijpoel, N.; Zielinski, C.C.; et al. A clinical prediction model for cancer-associated venous thromboembolism: A development and validation study in two independent prospective cohorts. *Lancet Haematol.* **2018**, *5*, e289–e298. [CrossRef]
70. Ferroni, P.; Roselli, M.; Zanzotto, F.M.; Guadagni, F. Artificial intelligence for cancer-associated thrombosis risk assessment. *Lancet Haematol.* **2018**, *5*, e391. [CrossRef]
71. National Institute for Health and Care Excellence. Venous Thromboembolism in over 16s: Reducing the Risk of Hospital-Acquired Deep Vein Thrombosis or Pulmonary Embolism. Last updated: August 2019. 2018. Available online: https://www.nice.org.uk/guidance/ng89 (accessed on 3 May 2020).
72. AIOM: Linee guida "Tromboembolismo venoso nei pazienti con tumori solidi". 2018. Available online: https://www.aiom.it/linee-guida-aiom-tromboembolismo-venoso-nei-pazienti-con-tumori-solidi-2019/ (accessed on 3 May 2020).
73. Ferroni, P.; Zanzotto, F.M.; Scarpato, N.; Riondino, S.; Nanni, U.; Roselli, M.; Guadagni, F. Risk Assessment for venous thromboembolism in chemotherapy-treated ambulatory cancer patients: A machine learning approach. *Med. Decis. Mak.* **2017**, *37*, 234–242. [CrossRef]
74. Riondino, S.; Ferroni, P.; Zanzotto, F.M.; Roselli, M.; Guadagni, F. Predicting VTE in Cancer Patients: Candidate Biomarkers and Risk Assessment Models. *Cancers* **2019**, *11*, 95. [CrossRef]

75. Trujillo-Santos, J.; Ruiz-Gamietea, A.; Luque, J.M.; Samperiz, A.L.; Garcia-Bragado, F.; Todoli, J.A.; Monreal, M. RIETE Investigators. Predicting recurrences or major bleeding in women with cancer and venous thromboembolism. Findings from the RIETE Registry. *Thromb. Res.* **2009**, *123*, S10–S15. [CrossRef]
76. Young, A.M.; Marshall, A.; Thirlwall, J.; Chapman, O.; Lokare, A.; Hill, C.; Hale, D.; Dunn, J.A.; Lyman, G.H.; Hutchinson, C.; et al. Comparison of an Oral Factor Xa Inhibitor With Low Molecular Weight Heparin in Patients With Cancer With Venous Thromboembolism: Results of a Randomized Trial (SELECT-D). *J. Clin. Oncol.* **2018**, *36*, 2017–2023. [CrossRef] [PubMed]
77. Agnelli, G.; Becattini, C.; Meyer, G.; Muñoz, A.; Huisman, M.V.; Connors, J.M.; Cohen, A.; Bauersachs, R.; Brenner, B.; Torbicki, A.; et al. Apixaban for the Treatment of Venous Thromboembolism Associated with Cancer. *New Engl. J. Med.* **2020**, *382*, 1599–1607. [CrossRef] [PubMed]
78. Raskob, G.E.; van Es, N.; Verhamme, P.; Carrier, M.; Di Nisio, M.; Garcia, D.; Grosso, M.A.; Kakkar, A.K.; Kovacs, M.J.; Mercuri, M.F.; et al. Edoxaban for the treatment of cancer-associated venous thromboembolism. *New Engl. J. Med.* **2017**, *378*, 615–624. [CrossRef] [PubMed]
79. Di Nisio, M.; van Es, N.; Carrier, M.; Wang, T.F.; Garcia, D.; Segers, A.; Weitz, J.; Buller, H.; Raskob, G. Extended treatment with edoxaban in cancer patients with venous thromboembolism: A post-hoc analysis of the Hokusai-VTE Cancer study. *J. Thromb. Haemost.* **2019**, *17*, 1866–1874. [CrossRef] [PubMed]
80. McBane, R.D., 2nd; Loprinzi, C.L.; Ashrani, A.; Lenz, C.J.; Houghton, D.; Zemla, T.; Le-Rademacher, J.G.; Wysokinski, W.E. Extending venous thromboembolism secondary prevention with apixaban in cancer patients: The EVE trial. *Eur. J. Haematol.* **2020**, *104*, 88–96. [CrossRef] [PubMed]
81. Mulder, F.I.; van Es, N.; Kraaijpoel, N.; Di Nisio, M.; Carrier, M.; Duggal, A.; Gaddh, M.; Garcia, D.; Grosso, M.A.; Kakkar, A.K.; et al. Edoxaban for treatment of venous thromboembolism in patient groups with different types of cancer: Results from the Hokusai VTE Cancer study. *Thromb. Res.* **2020**, *185*, 13–19. [CrossRef]
82. Kearon, C.; Akl, E.A.; Ornelas, J.; Blaivas, A.; Jimenez, D.; Bounameaux, H.; Huisman, M.; Kingm, C.S.; Morris, T.A.; Sood, N.; et al. Antithrombotic Therapy for VTE Disease: CHEST Guideline and Expert Panel Report. *Chest* **2016**, *149*, 315–352. [CrossRef]
83. Hutchinson, A.; Rees, S.; Young, A.; Maraveyas, A.; Date, K.; Johnson, M.J. Oral anticoagulation is preferable to injected but only if it is safe and effective: An interview study of patient and carer experience of oral and injected anticoagulant therapy for cancer-associated thrombosis in the select-d trial. *Palliat. Med.* **2019**, *33*, 510–517. [CrossRef]
84. Noble, S.; Sui, J. The treatment of cancer associated thrombosis: Does one size fit all? Who should get LMWH/warfarin/DOACs? *Thromb. Res.* **2016**, *140*, S154–S159. [CrossRef]
85. Sevitt, S.; Gallagher, N.G. Prevention of venous thrombosis and pulmonary embolism in injured patients. A trial of anticoagulant prophylaxis with phenindione in middle-aged and elderly patients with fractured necks of the femur. *Lancet* **1959**, *2*, 981–989. [CrossRef]
86. Geerts, W. Prevention of venous thromboembolism: A key patient safety priority. *J. Thromb. Haemost.* **2009**, *7*, 1–8. [CrossRef] [PubMed]
87. Rocque, G.B.; Barnett, A.E.; Illig, L.C.; Eickhoff, J.C.; Bailey, H.H.; Campbell, T.C.; Stewart, J.A.; Cleary, J.F. Inpatient hospitalization of oncology patients: Are we missing an opportunity for end-of-life care? *J. Oncol. Pract.* **2013**, *9*, 51–54. [CrossRef] [PubMed]
88. Chin-Yee, N.; Tanuseputro, P.; Carriera, M.; Noble, S. Thromboembolic disease in palliative and end-of-life care: A narrative review. *Thromb. Res.* **2019**, *175*, 84–89. [CrossRef]
89. Cai, R.; Zimmermann, C.; Krzyzanowska, M.; Granton, J.; Hannon, B. Thromboprophylaxis for inpatients with advanced cancer in palliative care settings: A systematic review and narrative synthesis. *Palliat. Med.* **2019**, *33*, 486–499. [CrossRef]
90. Noble, S.; Banerjee, S.; Pease, N.J. Management of venous thromboembolism in far-advanced cancer: Current practice. *BMJ Support. Palliat. Care* **2019**. [CrossRef]
91. Tardy, B.; Picard, S.; Guirimand, F.; Chapelle, C.; Danel Delerue, M.; Celarier, T.; Ciais, J.F.; Vassal, P.; Salas, S.; Filbet, M.; et al. Bleeding risk of terminally ill patients hospitalized in palliative care units: The RHESO study. *J. Thromb. Haemost.* **2017**, *15*, 420–428. [CrossRef]
92. Noble, S. The challenges of managing cancer related venous thromboembolism in the palliative care setting. *Postgrad. Med. J.* **2007**, *83*, 671–674. [CrossRef]

93. Johnson, M.J.; McMillan, B.; Fairhurst, C.; Gabe, R.; Ward, J.; Wiseman, J.; Pollington, B.; Noble, S.I. Primary thromboprophylaxis in hospices: The association between risk of venous thromboembolism and development of symptoms. *J. Pain Symptom Manag.* **2014**, *48*, 56–64. [CrossRef]
94. Bryson, J.; Coe, G.; Swami, N.; Murphy-Kane, P.; Seccareccia, D.; Le, L.W.; Rodin, G.; Zimmermann, C. Administrative outcomes five years after opening an acute palliative care unit at a comprehensive cancer center. *J. Palliat. Med.* **2010**, *13*, 559–565. [CrossRef]
95. Hui, D.; Elsayem, A.; Palla, S.; De La Cruz, M.; Li, Z.; Yennurajalingam, S.; Bruera, E. Discharge outcomes and survival of patients with advanced cancer admitted to an acute palliative care unit at a comprehensive cancer center. *J. Palliat. Med.* **2010**, *13*, 49–57. [CrossRef] [PubMed]
96. Gartner, V.; Kierner, K.A.; Namjesky, A.; Kum-Taucher, B.; Hammerl-Ferrari, B.; Watzke, H.H.; Stabel, C.; AUPACS group. Thromboprophylaxis in patients receiving inpatient palliative care: A survey of present practice in Austria. *Support. Care Cancer.* **2012**, *20*, 2183–2187. [CrossRef] [PubMed]
97. Centeno, C.; Lynch, T.; Garralda, E.; Carrasco, J.M.; Guillen-Grima, F.; Clark, D. Coverage and development of specialist palliative care services across the World Health Organization European Region (2005-2012): Results from a European Association for Palliative Care Task Force survey of 53 Countries. *Palliat. Med.* **2016**, *30*, 351–362. [CrossRef] [PubMed]
98. US Food and Drug Administration. Patient-Reported Outcome Measures: Use in Medical Product Development to Support Labeling Iclaims. Guidance for industry. Available online: https://www.fda.gov/regulatory-information/search-fda-guidance-documents/patient-reported-outcome-measures-use-medical-product-development-support-labeling-claims (accessed on 10 February 2020).
99. Bennett, A.V.; Jensen, R.E.; Basch, E. Electronic patient-reported outcome systems in oncology clinical practice. *CA Cancer J. Clin.* **2012**, *62*, 337–347. [CrossRef]
100. Johansen, M.A.; Henriksen, E.; Horsch, A.; Schuster, T.; Berntsen, G.K. Electronic symptom reporting between patient and provider for improved health care service quality: A systematic review of randomized controlled trials. part 1: State of the art. *J. Med. Internet Res.* **2012**, *14*, e118. [CrossRef]
101. Rose, M.; Bezjak, A. Logistics of collecting patient-reported outcomes (PROs) in clinical practice: An overview and practical examples. *Qual. Life Res.* **2009**, *18*, 125–136. [CrossRef]
102. Hoppe, C.; Obermeier, P.; Muehlhans, S.; Alchikh, M.; Seeber, L.; Tief, F.; Karsch, K.; Chen, X.; Boettcher, S.; Diedrich, S.; et al. Innovative Digital Tools and Surveillance Systems for the Timely Detection of Adverse Events at the Point of Care: A Proof of Concept Study. *Drug Saf.* **2016**, *39*, 977–988. [CrossRef]
103. Benze, G.; Nauck, F.; Alt-Epping, B.; Gianni, G.; Bauknecht, T.; Ettl, J.; Munte, A.; Kretzschmar, L.; Gaertner, J. PROutine: A feasibility study assessing surveillance of electronic patient reported outcomes and adherence via smartphone app in advanced cancer. *Ann. Palliat. Med.* **2019**, *8*, 104–111. [CrossRef]
104. Kim, J.S.; Kang, E.J.; Kim, D.S.; Choi, Y.J.; Lee, S.Y.; Kim, H.J.; Seo, H.Y.; Kim, J.S. Early venous thromboembolism at the beginning of palliative chemotherapy is a poor prognostic factor in patients with metastatic pancreatic cancer: A retrospective study. *BMC Cancer* **2018**, *18*, 1260. [CrossRef]
105. Hannon, B.; Taback, N.; Zimmermann, C.; Granton, J.; Krzyzanowska, M. Medical oncologists' and palliative care physicians' opinions towards thromboprophylaxis for inpatients with advanced cancer: A cross-sectional study. *BMJ Support. Palliat. Care* **2019**. [CrossRef]
106. Noble, S.I.R.; Nelson, A.; Finlay, I.G. Factors influencing hospice thromboprophylaxis policy: A qualitative study. *Palliat. Med.* **2008**, *22*, 808–813. [CrossRef] [PubMed]

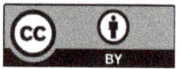

© 2020 by the authors. Licensee MDPI, Basel, Switzerland. This article is an open access article distributed under the terms and conditions of the Creative Commons Attribution (CC BY) license (http://creativecommons.org/licenses/by/4.0/).

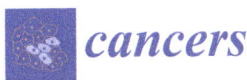

Review

Thromboprophylaxis in the End-of-Life Cancer Care: The Update

Ewa Zabrocka [1] and Ewa Sierko [2,3,*]

1. Department of Radiation Oncology, Stony Brook University, Stony Brook, New York, NY 11794, USA; ewa.zabrocka1@gmail.com
2. Department of Oncology, Medical University of Bialystok, 12 Ogrodowa St., 15-027 Bialystok, Poland
3. Comprehensive Cancer Center in Bialystok, 15-027 Bialystok, Poland
* Correspondence: ewa.sierko@iq.pl

Received: 30 January 2020; Accepted: 2 March 2020; Published: 5 March 2020

Abstract: Cancer patients are at increased risk for venous thromboembolism (VTE), which further increases with advanced stages of malignancy, prolonged immobilization, or prior history of thrombosis. To reduce VTE-related mortality, many official guidelines encourage the use of thromboprophylaxis (TPX) in cancer patients in certain situations, e.g., during chemotherapy or in the perioperative period. TPX in the end-of-life care, however, remains controversial. Most recommendations on VTE prophylaxis in cancer patients are based on the outcomes of clinical trials that excluded patients under palliative or hospice care. This translates to the paucity of official guidelines on TPX dedicated to this group of patients. The problem should not be underestimated as VTE is known to be associated with symptoms adversely impacting the quality of life (QoL), i.e., limb or chest pain, dyspnea, hemoptysis. In end-of-life care, where the assurance of the best possible QoL should be the highest priority, VTE prophylaxis may eliminate the symptom burden related to thrombosis. However, large randomized studies determining the benefits and risks profiles of TPX in patients nearing the end of life are lacking. This review summarized available data on TPX in this population, analyzed potential tools for VTE risk prediction in the view of this group of patients, and summarized the most current recommendations on TPX pertaining to terminal care.

Keywords: thromboprophylaxis; venous thromboembolism; cancer; hospice; palliative care units; low molecular weight heparin; deep vein thrombosis; pulmonary embolism

1. Introduction

Cancer is among well-recognized risk factors for venous thromboembolism (VTE) [1]. The relative risk of VTE in cancer patients compared to patients without cancer ranges between 4 and 7 [2]. The main forms of the thromboembolic disease include pulmonary embolism (PE) and deep vein thrombosis (DVT). Advanced cancer patients are at particularly increased risk for VTE, taking into account their diagnosis and usually poor performance status, resulting in a decreased level of activity or even immobilization [3]. The exact VTE incidence and prevalence in the population of cancer patients under hospice or palliative care have not been well investigated, and available reports are scant. Palliative care physicians have been found to underestimate the prevalence of VTE in hospice inpatients, and, in one study, they estimated the prevalence to be only 1–5% [4]. This is, however, a physician recall estimate, suggesting that VTE in hospice is not perceived as a common clinical problem. In a retrospective study, approximately 10% of 712 patients hospitalized in palliative care units (PCU) were found to have DVT on Doppler echography or PE on either computed tomography or ventilation/perfusion scintigraphy [5], although this likely did not reflect true prevalence since only the patients with clinical suspicion for VTE were tested. In fact, VTE prevalence in this population is most likely higher. Using a diagnostic bilateral femoral vein ultrasonography, White et al. [6] found that DVT involving femoral vein was present in about a third of advanced cancer patients admitted to PCU. In a prospective study by Johnson et al., DVT was found in as many as 52% of hospice inpatients [7]. However, the actual prevalence may be lower since light reflection rheography used to detect DVT in this study cannot distinguish between the external compression of the vein or obstruction of flow by thrombosis.

In cancer VTE studies, the primary outcome is often survival, whereas, in the palliative and hospice care population, the quality of life (QoL) is the most relevant outcome in clinical practice. The symptom burden associated with VTE, including dyspnea, chest or limb pain, and limb swelling, can adversely affect the QoL, but the reports on the actual symptom profile and severity in hospice and palliative care patient population are conflicting. Although half of the hospice patients in the study by Johnson et al. had radiographic suspicion of DVT, only 9% had VTE symptoms at the time of diagnosis [7]. On the other hand, the study of Soto-Cardenas et al. [5] revealed that half of PCU patients with DVT were suffering from localized pain, and 80% of those with PE reported dyspnea. The results of a recent observational study by White et al. [6] do not support these findings. Among the signs and symptoms of VTE, including limb pain, chest pain, breathlessness, hemoptysis, and lower extremity edema, only the latter is significantly more often found in PCU patients with DVT, indicating that symptom burden attributed to VTE may be, in fact, overestimated in this patient population. Aside from the physical aspect, VTE can also be a source of significant psychological distress, which by some cancer patients has been described as even worse than their cancer experiences [8]. Symptom control remains the mainstay of palliative care; therefore, symptom burden caused by VTE warrants the discussion on primary and secondary thromboprophylaxis in patients approaching the end of life.

Thromboprophylaxis is recommended for hospitalized cancer patients who do not have contraindications to such therapy [9]. However, it has not been commonly used in palliative and hospice care patients, which may result from the lack of official recommendations in that matter. Clinical trials investigating VTE prophylaxis in the population of cancer patients usually exclude palliative or hospice care patients [10]. Ethical factors likely play a major role in this approach since thromboprophylaxis (TPX) may be perceived as one of the ways of postponing the natural death, which would not be in line with the philosophy and foundations of palliative care. Nevertheless, it still remains questionable whether TPX can affect life expectancy in this group of patients. One prospective randomized study showed no statistically significant survival benefit of prophylactic nadroparin in hospitalized palliative care patients with an estimated life expectancy of ≤6 months [11]; however, only 20 patients were enrolled in the study. Another challenging aspect is also the degree of symptom relief by TPX, which is difficult to estimate due to the lack of standardized tools for QoL assessment. All these uncertainties seem to have a substantial impact on health care providers' decisions on prescribing anticoagulation for palliative care and hospice patients. The usefulness of TPX is also challenged by a recent observational study by White et al. [6], who investigated the prevalence and symptom burden of DVT as well as its association with TPX in 273 PCU patients. The average Karnofsky score was 49, indicating poor performance status. The study found no association between the presence or absence of DVT and TPX use [6], questioning the role of TPX in this population. There was no difference in survival between those with or without DVT.

The problem, however, should not be underestimated, particularly, nowadays when the perspective on hospice care has been changing. In 2010, almost one-fifth of hospice patients were discharged home in the United States [12], whereas discharge rate to home from PCUs was shown to be as high as 39% [13], pointing to the increasing role of these institutions is not only providing terminal care but also in improving patients' condition. This should be considered in the decision-making processes in these settings.

This paper reviewed the data on TPX in palliative care and hospice patients and summarized the updated recommendations on the TPX in this population.

2. Prevalence of Thromboprophylaxis in Hospices and Palliative Care Units

Thromboprophylaxis can be either primary—aimed at reducing the risk of VTE occurrence, or secondary—when the goal is to minimize the chances of recurrent VTE in patients with a known history of thrombosis. The prevalence of anticoagulation therapy at the end of life setting, both primary and secondary, varies across the institutions and countries. A study by Holmes et al. [14] showed that 9% (1557 out of 16,896) of lung cancer patients who were receiving home hospice care were prescribed TPX, although the type of TPX (primary vs. secondary) was not specified. Similar data were reported by Johnson et al. [15] in a retrospective study, demonstrating that primary TPX was being received by 6% of patients admitted to hospice in the UK. The use of TPX in hospice patients in another UK study was even lower, at 3.7% [16]. A retrospective cohort study by Kowalewska et al. [17] revealed that 6.7% of all (77 out of 1141) patients and 4.6% of cancer patients discharged from hospital to hospice care were prescribed antithrombotic therapy. It was shown that cancer patients, which constituted 60% of the study group, were significantly less likely to receive a prescription for anticoagulation, and the rationale for the de-escalation of TPX was increased bleeding risk, inconsistency with goals of care, or patient or family preference.

With regards to PCU, a retrospective analysis at Genevan PCU showed that TPX was used in 43% of cancer patients [18]. Likewise, the TPX prevalence was high (44%) in a French study, which enrolled 1199 PCU patients, 91% of whom were cancer patients [19]. A cross-sectional study on the prevalence of TPX among 134 PCU patients in Austria revealed that primary and secondary TPX was used in 49% of cancer patients, similarly to non-cancer patients (42%) [20], although there was a tendency to discontinuation of TPX upon admission to PCU. A similar trend was also reported by Legault et al. [21] in a retrospective analysis, revealing TPX prevalence of 44% on admission to PCU, followed by 87.7% TPX discontinuation rate within 72 hours of admission.

Although the data are limited, these results suggest that PCU patients are more likely to receive TPX compared to patients receiving hospice care (Table 1). It should be noted, however, that in some countries, e.g., United Kingdom, the terms "hospice" and "PCU" are synonymous; therefore, in those countries, active anti-cancer treatment and hospice care are not mutually exclusive. In contrast, in the United States, hospice patients usually no longer receive cancer-targeted therapies, and the vast majority hospice care is provided at home with the remainder of patients receiving hospice care in nursing homes or in-patient hospices, which are separated from acute care hospitals. These differences should be taken into account when comparing the data between the countries.

Table 1. Thromboprophylaxis (TPX) prevalence in hospice and palliative care units (PCU).

Authors	Thromboprophylaxis (TPX) Prevalence % (Number of Patients Receiving TPX/all Patients)	Type of TPX (Primary/Secondary)	% of Cancer Patients in the Study Group	Setting
Holmes et al. [14]	9 (1557/16,896)	No data	100	Hospice
Johnson et al. [15]	6 (68/1164)	Primary	82	Hospice
Gillon et al. [16]	3.7 (13/350)	Primary	77	Hospice
Kowalewska et al. [17]	4.6 (31/674)	Primary and secondary	100	Hospice
Pautex et al. [18]	43 (103/240)	No data	100	PCU
Tardy et al. [19]	44 (527/1199)	Primary	91	PCU
Gartner et al. [20]	49 (56/115)	Primary and secondary	100	PCU
Legault et al. [21]	44 (56/127)	Primary	92	PCU

The relatively low prevalence of TPX and the trend to its discontinuation after transitioning to hospice might also result from palliative care providers' belief that TPX should not be considered a priority in this setting, as shown in a qualitative study by Noble et al. [22]. The same study showed that, should TPX be proven effective in terms of symptom control, the providers were amenable to change of practice. A survey study among senior doctors in hospice inpatient units showed that although in 2000, 62% of physicians would stop TPX in patients with a high thrombotic risk who were intended for discharge home, in 2005, it was only 18% of respondents [23], suggesting an evolution of the approach to the TPX in this population.

3. Who Needs TPX?

Aside from its ethical aspect, clinical decision-making regarding TPX for hospice and palliative care cancer patients is challenging, also due to the heterogeneity of this population. Frequently, the patients may have contraindications to TPX, e.g., bleeding or thrombocytopenia [16], or the risks and benefits profile may be vague. A study by White et al. [6] revealed that previous VTE, being bedbound in the past 12 weeks, and lower limb edema were independent risk factors for VTE in PCU and hospice patients.

The clinical status of the patient also plays an important role in making decisions on TPX. A survey study among experts in palliative care, oncology, intensive care, and anticoagulation on whether they would use TPX on a virtual palliative care patient showed that all physicians opted to withdraw TPX in patients with Karnofsky index less than 10 [24]. Tools designed to select hospice or palliative care patients, who would benefit from TPX the most, would significantly aid in the decision-making process.

So far, the only available palliative-modified risk assessment tool is the pan Birmingham cancer network (PBCN) palliative-modified thromboembolic risk factors (THRIFT) score [15]. It includes a number of clinical risk factors to stratify patients to a high, intermediate, or low risk of VTE. The tool is not specific to cancer patients and was designed for use in a broadly defined palliative care population. A retrospective analysis of 1164 hospice inpatients in the U.K. revealed that a high/moderate THRIFT score had a high sensitivity (98.4%) but very low specificity (5.8%) in VTE risk prediction, suggesting the need of continued research in that matter.

Several models to predict the risk of VTE in cancer patients have been developed. Khorana score aims to identify ambulatory cancer patients at increased risk of VTE during chemotherapy [25]. It is a user-friendly tool based on routinely available predictive variables. Since this model has been tested in cancer patients receiving chemotherapy, it is questionable whether it should be applied to hospice or palliative care patients, the majority of whom do not continue active anti-neoplastic treatment. Moreover, 91.6% of patients in the study establishing Khorana score have shown eastern cooperative oncology group (ECOG) performance status of 0 to 1, whereas, in patients approaching the end of life, it is usually higher. Since the external validation of Khorana score has revealed a high proportion of patients falling into the intermediate-risk category (>50%) [26], several modifications of the Khorana score have been suggested, e.g., by addition of D-dimer and soluble P-selectin (Vienna score) [27]. However, a test for P-selectin is usually not available in routine clinical practice, making the use of this test infeasible. Another scoring system based on factors, such as Khorana score >2, previous VTE, metastatic disease, and vascular or lymphatic macroscopic compression, has been investigated in the ONKOTEV study [28] and has shown to have higher predictive power compared to Khorana score alone. Again, since the vast majority of patients in this trial were undergoing active anti-cancer treatment, the usefulness of the ONCOTEV score in PCU or hospice population not receiving cancer-targeted treatments is uncertain.

Recently, another prediction model for cancer-associated VTE, incorporating only one clinical factor (tumor-site category) and one biomarker (D-dimer), has been proposed [29]. Due to its simplicity, it may have the potential to become a useful tool for the screening of hospice/palliative care patients at increased risk for VTE, which could aid with decision-making regarding TPX in this setting. So far, this score has been validated only on a cohort of cancer patients of whom the majority were undergoing chemotherapy; therefore, further studies are required to investigate its utility in terminally ill cancer patients who can no longer benefit from active treatment.

Ferroni et al. [30] introduced an interesting VTE risk assessment model, which uses a combination of machine learning and artificial intelligence to design a set of VTE predictors, exploiting certain patterns in demographic, clinical, and biochemical data for VTE risk stratification. This method, similarly to the above, has been validated only in a cohort of cancer patients undergoing chemotherapy; however, due to its low cost, non-invasiveness, and user-friendly approach, it may be also a promising tool for VTE risk assessment in hospice or palliative care patients not receiving active anticancer treatment.

4. Thromboprophylaxis Agent Selection

There are various TPX methods used in clinical practice. However, due to the complexity and uniqueness of palliative care and hospice patient population, TPX agent selection may be challenging.

Vitamin K antagonists (VKAs), e.g., warfarin and acenocoumarin, have been used for decades in the management of cancer-related VTE. Nowadays, however, their use in clinical practice has become limited due to multiple interactions with food and medications used in cancer treatment. Patients receiving VKA require frequent monitoring of the clotting time (international normalized ratio, INR), which are not only cumbersome for patients but may also decrease treatment compliance [31]. Additionally, INR has been shown to be more labile in patients under hospice or palliative care due to, e.g., a high prevalence of liver dysfunction and malnutrition; therefore, more frequent INR monitoring may be necessary for this population [32].

Low-molecular-weight heparin (LMWH) is recommended as the first-line treatment of VTE in cancer patients due to its superiority over warfarin in the prevention of recurrent VTE without an increase in major bleeding complications [33]. LMWH has fewer interactions with other drugs and generally does not require frequent blood monitoring. However, hospice patients often have low body weight and impaired renal function, in which cases blood monitoring may be necessary. The controversy around LMWH use in terminally ill patients arises due to the need for daily painful injections, which are not in line with the philosophy of palliative medicine. However, as reported by Noble et al. [34], LMWH was found to be an acceptable intervention by palliative care cancer patients, and the only negative experience was bruising. LMWH was shown to have little or no influence on the QoL, in contrast to anti-embolic stockings, which were found to negatively impact the QoL [34]. Additionally, the results of a recent qualitative study on the treatment of cancer-associated thrombosis demonstrated that although the patients found taking tablets easier, they preferred injected anticoagulants if found to be more effective than tablets [35].

Fondaparinux, an indirect inhibitor of factor Xa, is frequently recommended for patients having contraindications to LMWH [36]. However, due to its dependence on renal clearance, its use in patients with advanced malignancy may be limited. Similar to LMWH, it is administered by deep subcutaneous injections, which may be found bothersome by some patients.

Novel oral anticoagulants (NOACs), which are direct inhibitors of coagulation factor IIa (dabigatran) and Xa (e.g., rivaroxaban, edoxaban, apixaban), have gained significant attention in the last decade. Several trials have shown that NOACs are effective and safe for the treatment of VTE [37], and cancer patients-subgroup analysis of these trials has revealed that NOACs are non-inferior to VKA in cancer patients [38–40]. However, these studies have excluded patients with renal or hepatic function impairment, both of which are frequent conditions in palliative or hospice patients. The analysis of NOACs use for the treatment of VTE in patients with advanced cancer has found a 5.5% and 20% risk of major and non-major bleeding, respectively [41]. Poor performance status is an independent factor for increased risk of bleeding. Therefore, the use of NOACs for VTE treatment in patients in advanced stages of malignancy remains questionable. There may be, however, a role for these medications in the primary TPX. A meta-analysis of randomized controlled trials investigating the use of NOACs in a total of 13,338 cancer patients for primary TPX has revealed that NOACs are effective in VTE prevention and does not increase the risk of major bleeding compared to placebo [42], although a subgroup analysis of advanced cancer patients has not been performed. Although non-invasiveness and no need for monitoring would make NOACs convenient for use in palliative care and hospice, the actual use may be limited in this setting due to decreased oral intake.

5. Current Recommendations

Based on the most recent guidelines issued by National Institute for Health and Care Excellence (NICE) [36], VTE prophylaxis should be considered for patients receiving palliative care; however, factors, including temporary increases in thrombotic risk factors, risk of bleeding, estimated life expectancy, and the views of the patient and their family members or carers, should be taken into account. This is different from previous NICE guidelines in which TPX in palliative care is recommended only for patients who have potentially reversible acute pathology [43]. It is emphasized not to offer VTE prophylaxis to people in the last days of life. Additionally, VTE prophylaxis should be reviewed daily. NICE recommends LMWH as a first-line agent and fondaparinux in case of contraindications to LMWH [36].

The most updated 10th edition of antithrombotic guidelines issued by the American College of Chest Physicians (CHEST) does not refer to VTE prevention among palliative care patients [32], although in 8th edition, TPX is considered acceptable for carefully selected group of palliative care patients, i.e., in whom it could prevent worsening of the QoL [44].

Current National Comprehensive Cancer Network (NCCN) guidelines support lifelong secondary TPX for patients with active cancer and a history of VTE [9]. Although TPX in a palliative care setting is not directly referred to in the recommendations, factors to consider before implementing VTE prophylaxis include lack of palliative benefits or any unreasonable burden of TPX (e.g., painful injections or frequent monitoring with phlebotomy).

In the most recent guideline update, the American Society of Clinical Oncology (ASCO) does not comment on TPX in palliative care [45]. Of note, therapeutic anticoagulation (i.e., VTE treatment) is not recommended for patients for whom anticoagulation is of uncertain benefit, including patients receiving end-of-life/hospice care or those with very limited life expectancy with no palliative or symptom reduction benefit. Whether this approach can be extrapolated to TPX remains uncertain.

The European Society for Medical Oncology (ESMO) guidelines on VTE management and prophylaxis do not refer to hospice patients [46]. For cancer patients with a history of VTE who are treated with palliative chemotherapy in the metastatic setting, an indefinite secondary TPX should be discussed with patients.

There is also no reference to the palliative care population in 2019 international clinical practice guidelines for the treatment and prophylaxis of venous thromboembolism in patients with cancer [47]. Of note, TPX is recommended for hospitalized cancer patients with reduced mobility and should not be routinely used in ambulatory cancer patients, including those receiving systemic anticancer therapy.

The above recommendations are summarized in Table 2. To our knowledge, the NICE guidelines are the only ones specifically addressing TPX in hospices or palliative care units.

Due to the lack of large, randomized studies on TPX in this setting, providers have to rely on their own assessment and experience. It has also become a more common practice to implement internal institutional policies on TPX [23]. Terminally ill patients wish to and should be, whenever possible, involved in the decision-making process regarding TPX, particularly where the evidence-based guidelines are lacking [34].

Table 2. Summary of guidelines for thromboprophylaxis in the palliative care setting.

Recommendation	Author	References
Thromboprophylaxis (TPX) should be considered for patients receiving palliative care; however, factors, including temporary increases in thrombotic risk factors, bleeding risk, estimated life expectancy, and the views of the patient and their family/carers, should be taken into account. TPX should not be offered to patients in the last days of life. TPX should be reviewed daily.	National Institute for Health and Clinical Excellence (NICE)	[36]
No guidelines on TPX in palliative care.	American College of Chest Physicians (ACCP)	[32]
No guidelines on TPX in palliative care. Before implementing VTE prophylaxis in all patients, factors to consider include lack of palliative benefits or any unreasonable burden of TPX.	National Comprehensive Cancer Network (NCCN)	[9]
No guidelines on TPX in palliative care.	American Society of Clinical Oncology (ASCO)	[45]
No guidelines on TPX in the hospice setting. Secondary TPX should be discussed with patients receiving palliative chemotherapy.	European Society for Medical Oncology (ESMO)	[46]
No guidelines on TPX in palliative care.	International clinical practice guidelines	[47]

6. Risks and Challenges

When considering TPX for cancer patients, increased risk of bleeding in this population remains an important issue. In a large, prospective study enrolling almost 3000 cancer patients, the abnormal renal function, metastatic disease, recent major bleeding, and recent immobility for more than 4 days were shown to be associated with a higher risk for both fatal PE and fatal bleeding [48]. Additionally, bodyweight <60 kg was an independent factor for fatal bleeding. Considering that hospice and palliative care patients frequently have a combination of these factors, bleeding risk in this subpopulation may be even higher, which may influence providers' decisions on TPX.

In the only one randomized study investigating prophylactic LMWH vs. placebo in 20 PCU patients with a life expectancy of ≤6 months, one VTE and one major bleeding occurred in the group receiving nadroparin ($p = 1$), whereas two minor bleedings occurred in the control group ($p = 0.474$) [11]. More light on bleeding risk in terminally ill PCU patients has been shed by a multicenter observational RHESO study [19]. Among twelve hundred patients on the study group, the majority of whom were cancer patients (91%), 44% were receiving primary or secondary TPX using LMWH or fondaparinux. The rate of clinically relevant bleeding, defined as a composite of a major bleeding and clinically relevant non-major bleeding, was 9.8% at 3 months. Bleeding occurred in 11% of patients who received TPX, and in 8.4% of those who did not, whereas the incidence of fatal bleeding was 2.1% vs. 1.8%, respectively. Cancer, recent bleeding, antiplatelet treatment, and TPX were found to be independent risk factors for clinically relevant bleeding, increasing the risk of the event 5.7, 3.4, 1.7, and 1.5 times, respectively.

Discussions on the TPX in terminal care should also include cost analysis. It has been calculated that if all immobile cancer patients were to receive prophylactic LMWH, the expenses for medications of a hospice would increase by almost 30% [49]. Costs involved in the TPX and management of potential bleeding events may be difficult to overcome since a lot of hospices are reimbursed on a fixed per diem basis—particularly in the United States—or they are supported primarily by charities.

7. Conclusions

Introducing uniform guidelines on TPX at the end of life care is encouraged. Ideally, they should be based on the results of clinical trials, focusing on this group of patients. The patient population should be carefully described with regard to the stage of the disease, goals of treatment, and nearness to the very end of life. The development of tools to predict VTE in this patient population would aid with decision-making regarding TPX. Although the risk of anticoagulation cannot be underestimated, there may be a group of patients who would benefit from symptomatic relief of TPX. Finally, the results of White et al. study [6] significantly challenge the appropriateness of TPX in advanced cancer patients with poor performance status, who are nearing the end of life.

Funding: This research received no external funding.

Conflicts of Interest: The authors declare no conflict of interest.

References

1. Bick, R.L. Alterations of hemostasis associated with malignancy: Etiology, pathophysiology, diagnosis and management. *Semin. Thromb. Hemost.* **1978**, *5*, 1–26. [CrossRef] [PubMed]
2. Timp, J.F.; Braekkan, S.K.; Versteeg, H.H.; Cannegieter, S.C. Epidemiology of cancer-associated venous thrombosis. *Blood* **2013**, *122*, 1712–1723. [CrossRef] [PubMed]
3. Wun, T.; White, R.H. Epidemiology of cancer-related venous thromboembolism. *Best Pract. Res. Clin. Haematol.* **2009**, *22*, 9–23. [CrossRef] [PubMed]
4. Johnson, M.J.; Sherry, K. How do palliative physicians manage venous thromboembolism? *Palliat. Med.* **1997**, *11*, 462–468. [CrossRef]
5. Soto-Cárdenas, M.J.; Pelayo-García, G.; Rodríguez-Camacho, A.; Segura-Fernández, E.; Mogollo-Galván, A.; Giron-Gonzalez, J.A. Venous thromboembolism in patients with advanced cancer under palliative care: Additional risk factors, primary/secondary prophylaxis and complications observed under normal clinical practice. *Palliat. Med.* **2008**, *22*, 965–968. [CrossRef]
6. White, C.; Noble, S.I.R.; Watson, M.; Swan, F.; Allgar, V.L.; Napier, E.; Nelson, A.; McAuley, J.; Doherty, J.; Lee, B.; et al. Prevalence, symptom burden, and natural history of deep vein thrombosis in people with advanced cancer in specialist palliative care units (HIDDen): A prospective longitudinal observational study. *Lancet Haematol.* **2019**, *6*, e79–e88. [CrossRef]
7. Johnson, M.J.; Sproule, M.W.; Paul, J. The prevalence and associated variables of deep venous thrombosis in patients with advanced cancer. *Clin. Oncol.* **1999**, *11*, 105–110. [CrossRef]
8. Seaman, S.; Nelson, A.; Noble, S. Cancer-associated thrombosis, low-molecular-weight heparin, and the patient experience: A qualitative study. *Patient Prefer. Adherence* **2014**, *8*, 453–461.
9. Clinical Practice Guidelines in Oncology: Cancer-Associated Venous Thromboembolic Disease, v.1.2019. National Comprehensive Cancer Network Web Site. Available online: https://www.nccn.org/professionals/physician_gls/pdf/vte.pdf (accessed on 19 October 2019).
10. Cai, R.; Zimmermann, C.; Krzyzanowska, M.; Granton, J.; Hannon, B. Thromboprophylaxis for inpatients with advanced cancer in palliative care settings: A systematic review and narrative synthesis. *Palliat. Med.* **2019**, *33*, 486–499. [CrossRef]
11. Weber, C.; Merminod, T.; Herrmann, F.R.; Zulian, G.B. Prophylactic anti-coagulation in cancer palliative care: A prospective randomised study. *Support. Care Cancer* **2008**, *16*, 847–852. [CrossRef]
12. Teno, J.M.; Plotzke, M.; Gozalo, P.; Mor, V. A national study of live discharges from hospice. *J. Palliat. Med.* **2014**, *17*, 1121–1127. [CrossRef] [PubMed]
13. Bryson, J.; Coe, G.; Swami, N.; Murphy-Kane, P.; Seccareccia, D.; Le, L.W.; Rodin, G.; Zimmermann, C. Administrative outcomes five years after opening an acute palliative care unit at a comprehensive cancer center. *J. Palliat. Med.* **2010**, *13*, 559–565. [CrossRef] [PubMed]
14. Holmes, H.M.; Bain, K.T.; Zalpour, A.; Luo, R.; Bruera, E.; Goodwin, J.S. Predictors of anticoagulation in hospice patients with lung cancer. *Cancer* **2010**, *116*, 4817–4824. [CrossRef] [PubMed]
15. Johnson, M.J.; McMillan, B.; Fairhurst, C.; Gabe, R.; Ward, J.; Wiseman, J.; Pollington, B.; Noble, S. Primary thromboprophylaxis in hospices: The association between risk of venous thromboembolism and development of symptoms. *J. Pain Symptom Manag.* **2014**, *48*, 56–64. [CrossRef]
16. Gillon, S.; Noble, S.; Ward, J.; Lodge, K.M.; Nunn, A.; Koon, S.; Johnson, M.J. Primary thromboprophylaxis for hospice inpatients: Who needs it? *Palliat. Med.* **2011**, *25*, 701–705. [CrossRef]
17. Kowalewska, C.A.; Noble, B.N.; Fromme, E.K.; McPherson, M.L.; Grace, K.N.; Furuno, J.P. Prevalence and Clinical Intentions of Antithrombotic Therapy on Discharge to Hospice Care. *J. Palliat. Med.* **2017**, *20*, 1225–1230. [CrossRef]

18. Pautex, S.; Vayne-Bossert, P.; Jamme, S.; Herrmann, F.; Vilarino, R.; Weber, C.; Burkhardt, K. Anatomopathological causes of death in patients with advanced cancer: Association with the use of anticoagulation and antibiotics at the end of life. *J. Palliat. Med.* **2013**, *16*, 669–674. [CrossRef]
19. Tardy, B.; Picard, S.; Guirimand, F.; Chapelle, C.; Danel Delerue, M.; Celarier, T.; Ciais, J.F.; Vassal, P.; Salas, S.; Filbet, M.; et al. Bleeding risk of terminally ill patients hospitalized in palliative care units: The RHESO study. *J. Thromb. Haemost.* **2017**, *15*, 420–442. [CrossRef]
20. Gartner, V.; Kierner, K.A.; Namjesky, A.; Kum-Taucher, B.; Hammerl-Ferrari, B.; Watzke, H.H.; Stabel, C. Thromboprophylaxis in patients receiving inpatient palliative care: A survey of present practice in Austria. *Support Care Cancer* **2012**, *20*, 2183–2187. [CrossRef]
21. Legault, S.; Tierney, S.; Sénécal, I. Evaluation of a thromboprophylaxis quality improvement project in a palliative care unit. *J. Pain Symptom Manag.* **2011**, *41*, 503–510. [CrossRef]
22. Noble, S.I.; Nelson, A.; Finlay, I.G. Factors influencing hospice thromboprophylaxis policy: A qualitative study. *Palliat. Med.* **2008**, *22*, 808–813. [CrossRef]
23. Noble, S.I.; Finlay, I.G. Have palliative care teams' attitudes toward venous thromboembolism changed? A survey of thromboprophylaxis practice across British specialist palliative care units in the years 2000 and 2005. *J. Pain Symptom Manag.* **2006**, *32*, 38–43. [CrossRef] [PubMed]
24. Kierner, K.A.; Gartner, V.; Schwarz, M.; Watzke, H.H. Use of thromboprophylaxis in palliative care patients: A survey among experts in palliative care, oncology, intensive care, and anticoagulation. *Am. J. Hosp. Palliat. Med.* **2008**, *25*, 127–131. [CrossRef] [PubMed]
25. Khorana, A.A.; Kuderer, N.M.; Culakova, E.; Lyman, G.H.; Francis, C.W. Development and validation of a predictive model for chemotherapy-associated thrombosis. *Blood* **2008**, *111*, 4902–4907. [CrossRef] [PubMed]
26. Mansfield, A.S.; Tafur, A.J.; Wang, C.E.; Kourelis, T.V.; Wysokinska, E.M.; Yang, P. Predictors of active cancer thromboembolic outcomes: Validation of the Khorana score among patients with lung cancer. *J. Thromb. Haemost.* **2016**, *14*, 1773–1778. [CrossRef]
27. Ay, C.; Dunkler, D.; Marosi, C.; Chiriac, A.L.; Vormittag, R.; Simanek, R.; Quehenberger, P.; Zielinski, C.; Pabinger, I. Prediction of venous thromboembolism in cancer patients. *Blood* **2010**, *116*, 5377–5382. [CrossRef]
28. Cella, C.A.; Di Minno, G.; Carlomagno, C.; Arcopinto, M.; Cerbone, A.M.; Matano, E.; Tufano, A.; Lordick, F.; De Simone, B.; Muehlberg, K.S.; et al. Preventing venous thromboembolism in ambulatory cancer patients: The ONKOTEV Study. *Oncologist* **2017**, *22*, 601–608. [CrossRef]
29. Pabinger, I.; van Es, N.; Heinze, G.; Posch, F.; Riedl, J.; Reitter, E.M.; Di Nisio, M.; Cesarman-Maus, G.; Kraaijpoel, N.; Zielinski, C.C.; et al. A clinical prediction model for cancer-associated venous thromboembolism: A development and validation study in two independent prospective cohorts. *Lancet Haematol.* **2018**, *5*, e289–e298. [CrossRef]
30. Ferroni, P.; Zanzotto, F.M.; Scarpato, N.; Riondino, S.; Guadagni, F.; Roselli, M. Validation of a Machine Learning Approach for Venous Thromboembolism Risk Prediction in Oncology. *Dis. Markers* **2017**, *2017*. [CrossRef]
31. Gerotziafas, G.T.; Mahé, I.; Elalamy, I. New orally active anticoagulant agents for the prevention and treatment of venous thromboembolism in cancer patients. *Ther. Clin. Risk Manag.* **2014**, *10*, 423–436. [CrossRef]
32. Kearon, C.; Akl, E.A.; Ornelas, J.; Blaivas, A.; Jimenez, D.; Bounameaux, H.; Huisman, M.; King, C.S.; Morris, T.A.; Sood, N.; et al. Antithrombotic therapy for VTE disease: CHEST guideline and expert panel report. *Chest* **2016**, *149*, 315–352. [CrossRef] [PubMed]
33. Farge, D.; Debourdeau, P.; Beckers, M.; Baglin, C.; Bauersachs, R.M.; Brenner, B.; Brilhante, D.; Falanga, A.; Gerotzafias, G.T.; Haim, N.; et al. International clinical practice guidelines for the treatment and prophylaxis of venous thromboembolism in patients with cancer. *J. Thromb. Haemost.* **2013**, *11*, 56–70. [CrossRef] [PubMed]
34. Noble, S.I.; Nelson, A.; Turner, C.; Finlay, I.G. Acceptability of low molecular weight heparin thromboprophylaxis for inpatients receiving palliative care: Qualitative study. *BMJ* **2006**, *332*, 577–580. [CrossRef] [PubMed]
35. Hutchinson, A.; Rees, S.; Young, A.; Maraveyas, A.; Date, K.; Johnson, M.J. Oral anticoagulation is preferable to injected, but only if it is safe and effective: An interview study of patient and carer experience of oral and injected anticoagulant therapy for cancer-associated thrombosis in the select-d trial. *Palliat. Med.* **2019**, *33*, 510–517. [CrossRef] [PubMed]

36. NICE. *Venous Thromboembolism in over 16s: Reducing the Risk of Hospital-Acquired Deep Vein Thrombosis or Pulmonary Embolism*; National Institute for Health and Care Excellence (NICE): London, UK, 2018; Available online: https://www.nice.org.uk/guidance/ng89 (accessed on 29 December 2019).
37. Rojas-Hernandez, C.M. The role of direct oral anticoagulants in cancer-related venous thromboembolism: A perspective beyond the guidelines. *Support. Care Cancer* **2018**, *26*, 711–720. [CrossRef]
38. Agnelli, G.; Buller, H.R.; Cohen, A.; Gallus, A.S.; Lee, T.C.; Pak, R.; Raskob, G.E.; Weitz, J.I.; Yamabe, T. Oral apixaban for the treatment of venous thromboembolism in cancer patients: Results from the AMPLIFY trial. *J. Thromb. Haemost.* **2015**, *13*, 2187–2191. [CrossRef]
39. Prins, M.H.; Lensing, A.W.; Brighton, T.A.; Lyons, R.M.; Rehm, J.; Trajanovic, M.; Davidson, B.L.; Beyer-Westendorf, J.; Pap, A.F.; Berkowitz, S.D.; et al. Oral rivaroxaban versus enoxaparin with vitamin K antagonist for the treatment of symptomatic venous thromboembolism in patients with cancer (EINSTEIN-DVT and EINSTEIN-PE): A pooled subgroup analysis of two randomised controlled trials. *Lancet Haematol.* **2014**, *1*, e37–e46. [CrossRef]
40. Schulman, S.; Goldhaber, S.Z.; Kearon, C.; Kakkar, A.K.; Schellong, S.; Eriksson, H.; Hantel, S.; Feuring, M.; Kreuzer, J. Treatment with dabigatran or warfarin in patients with venous thromboembolism and cancer. *Thromb. Haemost.* **2015**, *114*, 150–157.
41. Oyakawa, T.; Muraoka, N.; Iida, K.; Kusuhara, M.; Mori, K. Use of direct oral anti-coagulants for the treatment of venous thromboembolism in patients with advanced cancer: A prospective observational study. *Int. J. Clin. Oncol.* **2019**, *24*, 876–881. [CrossRef]
42. Barbarawi, M.; Zayed, Y.; Kheiri, B.; Gakhal, I.; Barbarawi, O.; Bala, A.; Alabdouh, A.; Abdalla, A.; Rizk, F.; Bachuwa, G.; et al. The role of anticoagulation in venous thromboembolism primary prophylaxis in patients with malignancy: A systematic review and meta-analysis of randomized controlled trials. *Thromb. Res.* **2019**, *181*, 36–45. [CrossRef]
43. Zabrocka, E.; Wojtukiewicz, M.Z.; Sierko, E. Thromboprophylaxis in cancer patients in hospice. *Adv. Clin. Exp. Med.* **2018**, *27*, 283–289. [CrossRef] [PubMed]
44. Geerts, W.H.; Bergqvist, D.; Pineo, G.F.; Heit, J.A.; Samama, C.M.; Lassen, M.R.; Colwell, C.W. Prevention of venous thromboembolism: American College of Chest Physicians Evidence-Based Clinical Practice Guidelines (8th edition). *Chest* **2008**, *133*, 381S–453S. [CrossRef] [PubMed]
45. Key, N.S.; Khorana, A.A.; Kuderer, N.M.; Bohlke, K.; Lee, A.Y.Y.; Arcelus, J.I.; Wong, S.L.; Balaban, E.P.; Flowers, C.R.; Francis, C.W.; et al. Venous thromboembolism prophylaxis and treatment in patients with cancer: ASCO clinical practice guideline update. *J. Clin. Oncol.* **2020**, *38*, 496–520. [CrossRef] [PubMed]
46. Mandalà, M.; Falanga, A.; Roila, F. Management of venous thromboembolism (VTE) in cancer patients: ESMO Clinical Practice Guidelines. *Ann. Oncol.* **2011**, *22*, 85–92. [CrossRef]
47. Farge, D.; Frere, C.; Connors, J.M.; Ay, C.; Khorana, A.A.; Munoz, A.; Brenner, B.; Kakkar, A.; Rafii, H.; Solymoss, S.; et al. 2019 international clinical practice guidelines for the treatment and prophylaxis of venous thromboembolism in patients with cancer. *Lancet Oncol.* **2019**, *20*, e566–e581. [CrossRef]
48. Monreal, M.; Falga, C.; Valdes, M.; Suarez, C.; Gabriel, F.; Tolosa, C.; Montes, J. Fatal pulmonary embolism and fatal bleeding in cancer patients with venous thromboembolism: Findings from the RIETE registry. *J. Thromb. Haemost.* **2006**, *4*, 1950–1956. [CrossRef]
49. Chambers, J.C. Prophylactic heparin in palliative care: ...to a challenging idea. *BMJ* **2006**, *332*, 729. [CrossRef]

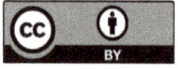

© 2020 by the authors. Licensee MDPI, Basel, Switzerland. This article is an open access article distributed under the terms and conditions of the Creative Commons Attribution (CC BY) license (http://creativecommons.org/licenses/by/4.0/).

MDPI
St. Alban-Anlage 66
4052 Basel
Switzerland
Tel. +41 61 683 77 34
Fax +41 61 302 89 18
www.mdpi.com

Cancers Editorial Office
E-mail: cancers@mdpi.com
www.mdpi.com/journal/cancers

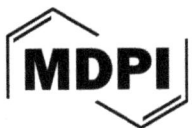

www.ingramcontent.com/pod-product-compliance
Lightning Source LLC
LaVergne TN
LVHW070726100526
838202LV00013B/1178